KEY TOPICS IN
OPHTHALMOLOGY
SECOND EDITION

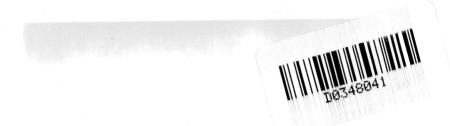

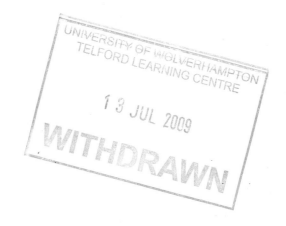

The KEY TOPICS Series

Advisors:

T.M. Craft *Department of Anaesthesia and Intensive Care, Royal United Hospital, Bath, UK*
C.S. Garrard *Intensive Therapy Unit, John Radcliffe Hospital, Oxford, UK*
P.M. Upton *Department of Anaesthesia, Royal Cornwall Hospital, Treliske, Truro, UK*

Anaesthesia, Third Edition, Clinical aspects
Obstetrics and Gynaecology, Second Edition
Accident and Emergency Medicine, Second Edition
Paediatrics, Second Edition
Orthopaedic Surgery
Otolaryngology, Second Edition
Ophthalmology, Second Edition
Psychiatry
General Surgery
Renal Medicine
Trauma
Chronic Pain
Oral and Maxillofacial Surgery
Oncology
Cardiovascular Medicine
Neurology
Neonatology
Gastroenterology
Thoracic Surgery
Respiratory Medicine
Orthopaedic Trauma Surgery
Critical Care
Evidence-Based Medicine

Forthcoming titles include:

Chronic Pain, Second Edition
Acute Poisoning
Urology
General Surgery, Second Edition
Clinical Research and Statistics
Cardiac Surgery

KEY TOPICS IN
OPHTHALMOLOGY

SECOND EDITION

Robert H. Taylor
FRCS, FRCOphth
Consultant Ophthalmologist,
York District Hospital, York, UK

Peter Shah
BSc (Hons), FRCOphth
Consultant Ophthalmologist,
Birmingham and Midland Eye Centre,
Birmingham, UK

Philip I. Murray
PhD, FRCS, FRCOphth
Professor of Ophthalmology,
The University of Birmingham and Birmingham and
Midland Eye Centre, Birmingham, UK

Michael A. Burdon
FRCOphth
Consultant Ophthalmologist, Selly Oak Hospital
and Birmingham and Midland Eye Centre, Birmingham, UK

Consultant Editor

Alex Levin
MD, MHSC, FRCSC
Department of Ophthalmology, Hospital for
Sick Children, Toronto, Canada

© BIOS Scientific Publishers Limited, 2001

First published 1995 (ISBN 1 87274 838 4)
Second Edition 2001 (ISBN 1 85996 178 9)

A CIP catalogue record for this book is available from the British Library.

ISBN 1 85996 178 9

BIOS Scientific Publishers Ltd
9 Newtec Place, Magdalen Road, Oxford OX4 1RE, UK
Tel. +44 (0)1865 726286. Fax +44 (0)1865 246823
World Wide Web home page: http://www.bios.co.uk/

Distributed exclusively in the United States, its dependent territories, Canada, Mexico, Central and South America, and the Caribbean by Springer-Verlag New York Inc, 175 Fifth Avenue, New York, USA, by arrangement with BIOS Scientific Publishers Ltd, 9 Newtec Place, Magdalen Road, Oxford OX4 1RE, UK.

Important Note from the Publisher
The information contained within this book was obtained by BIOS Scientific Publishers Ltd from sources believed by us to be reliable. However, while every effort has been made to ensure its accuracy, no responsibility for loss or injury whatsoever occasioned to any person acting or refraining from action as a result of information contained herein can be accepted by the authors or publishers.

The reader should remember that medicine is a constantly evolving science and while the authors and publishers have ensured that all dosages, applications and practices are based on current indications, there may be specific practices which differ between communities. You should always follow the guidelines laid down by the manufacturers of specific products and the relevant authorities in the country in which you are practising.

Production Editor: Andrea Bosher
Typeset by Jayvee Computer Services, Trivandrum, India
Printed by The Cromwell Press, Trowbridge, UK

CONTENTS

ABBREVIATIONS

AAION	arteritic anterior ischaemic optic neuropathy
AAU	acute anterior uveitis
AC/A	accommodative convergance / accommodation ratio
ACAID	anterior chamber-associated immune deviation
ACR	American College of Rheumatology
AION	anterior ischaemic optic neuropathy
AL	axial length
ANA	antinuclear antibody
ANCA	antineutrophil cytoplasmic antibodies
APCs	antigen-presenting cells
APCT	alternating prism cover test
APMPPE	acute posterior multifocal placoid pigment epitheliopathy
ARMD	age-related macular degeneration
ARN	acute retinal necrosis
AZOOR	acute zonal occult outer retinopathy
BHL	bilateral hilar lymphadenopathy
BRVO	branch retinal vein occlusion
CCDC	consultant in communicable disease control
CCF	carotico-cavernous fistula
CCTV	closed circuit television
CHAMPS	Controlled High Risk Subjects Avonex Multiple Sclerosis Prevention Study
CHD	coronary heart disease
CHS	Chediak–Higashi syndrome
CL	contact lens
CMO	cystoid macular oedema
CMV	cytomegalovirus
CMZ	carbimazole
CN	congenital-infantile nystagmus
CNS	central nervous system
CNV	choroidal neovascularization
CP	cicatricial pemphigoid
CRP	C-reactive protein
CRVO	central retinal vein occlusion
CSF	cerebrospinal fluid
CSNB	congenital stationary night blindness
CSR	central serous retinopathy
CXR	chest X-ray
dB	decibel
DCCT	Diabetic Control and Complications Study
DD	disc diameter
DGGE	denaturing gradient gel electrophoresis
DICC	drug-induced cicatrizing conjunctivitis
DIDMOAD	diabetes insipidus, diabetes mellitus, optic atrophy and deafness

DRS	Diabetic Retinopathy Study
DVD	dissociated vertical deviation
DUSN	diffuse unilateral subacute neuroretinitis
EBR	external beam radiation
EEC	ectrodactyly-electrodermal dysplasia-clefting
EOG	electro-oculogram
EPT	effective phako time
ERG	electroretinogram
ESR	erythrocyte sedimentation rate
ETDRS	Early Treatment Diabetic Retinopathy Study
ETOMS	Early Treatment of Multiple Sclerosis Study
EUA	examination under anaesthesia
EULAR	European League Against Rheumatism
EVS	Endophthalmitis Vitrectomy Study
FCPL	forced choice preferential looking
FDP	frequency-doubling perimetry
FFA	fundus fluorescein angiography
FHC	Fuchs' heterochromic cyclitis
5-HT	5-hydroxytryptamine
GCA	giant cell arteritis
HAART	highly active anti-retroviral therapy
HIV	human immunodeficiency
HPS	Hermansky–Pudlak syndrome
HRP	high-pass resolution perimetry
HRVO	hemicentral retinal vein occlusion
HSV	herpes simplex virus
ICA	internal carotid artery
ICE	iridocorneal endothelial syndrome
IgA	immunoglobulin A
IIH	idiopathic intracranial hypertension
ILAR	International League of Associations of Rheumatologists
INO	internuclear ophthalmoplegia
IOFB	intraocular foreign body
IOL	intraocular lenses
IOP	intraocular pressure
IPD	interpupillary distance
IRMA	intraretinal microvascular abnormalities
ISCEV	International Society for Clinical Electrophysiology of Vision
ISCR	intrastromal corneal rings
JCA	juvenile chronic arthritis
JIA	juvenile idiopathic arthritis
JRA	juvenile rheumatoid arthritis
LASIK	laser-assisted in-situ keratomileusis
LEA	Local Education Authority
LN	latent nystagmus
LPS	lumboperitoneal shunting

MDR	multiple drug resistance
MEWDS	multiple evanescent white dot syndrome
MHVI	multiple handicapped visually impaired
MRI	magnetic resonance imaging
MRV	magnetic resonance venography
MS	multiple sclerosis
NA	noradrenaline
NAION	non-arteritic anterior ischaemic optic neuropathy
NFL	nerve fibre layer
NIDDM	non-insulin-dependent diabetes mellitus
NNRTI	non-nucleoside reverse transcriptase inhibitors
NOAH	National Organization for Hypopigmentation and Albinism
NOT	nucleus of the optic tract
NPL	no perception of light
NTG	normal tension glaucoma
NVD	new vessels arising from the optic disc
NVE	new vessels arising from the retina and elsewhere
OA	ocular albinism
OCA	oculocutaneous albinism
ODEMS	optic disc oedema with macular star
OHT	ocular hypertension
ONSF	optic nerve sheath fenestration
ONTT	Optic Neuritis Treatment Trial
OSSN	ocular surface squamous neoplasia
PAN	periodic alternating nystagmus
PAS	peripheral anterior synechiae
PDE5	phosphodiesterase-5
PDR	proliferative diabetic retinopathy
PHPV	persistent hyperplastic primary vitreous
PI	protease inhibitors
PMMA	polymethylmethacrylate
POAG	primary open-angle glaucoma
POHS	presumed ocular histoplasmosis syndrome
PRP	pan-retinal photocoagulation
PTU	propylthiouracil
PVD	posterior vitreous detachment
PVR	proliferative vitreoretinopathy
PWS	port wine stain
RAI	radioactive iodine
RAPD	relative afferent pupil defect
RF	rheumatoid factor
RK	radial keratotomy
ROP	retinopathy of prematurity
RP	retinitis pigmentosa
RPE	retinal pigmented epithelial cells
RVO	retinal vein occlusion

SBS	shaken baby syndrome
SCG	superior cervical ganglion
SEN	Special Education Needs
SINS	surgically induced necrotizing scleritis
SITA	Swedish interactive threshold algorithm
SJS	Stevens–Johnson syndrome
SjS	Sjögren's syndrome
SLE	systemic lupus erythematosus
S-PRK	surface photorefractive keratectomy
SRNVM	sub-retinal neovascular membrane
SSCE	sequential sector conjunctival epitheliectomy
SSCP	single-strand conformation polymorphism
SWAP	short-wave automated perimetry
TAB	temporal artery biopsy
TEN	toxic epidermal necrolysis
TPF	tenacious proximal fusion
TRP1	tyrosinase-related protein 1
TSH	thyroid-stimulating hormone
UBM	ultrasound biomicroscopy
UKCCRG	UK Childhood Cancer Research Group
UKPDS	United Kingdom Prospective Diabetes Study
VEP	visual evoked potential
VI	visually impaired
VKH	Vogt–Koyanagi–Harada syndrome
VZV	varicella zoster virus
WESDR	Wisconsin Epidemiologic Study of Diabetic Retinopathy
WG	Wegener's granulomatosis
YAG	yttrium-aluminium-garnet

Names of Medical Substances

In accordance with directive 92/27/EEC, this book adheres to the following guidelines on naming of medicinal substances (rINN, Recommended International Non-proprietary Name; BAN, British Approved Name).

List 1 – Both names to appear

UK Name	rINN
[1]adrenaline	epinephrine
amethocaine	tetracaine
bendrofluazide	bendroflumethiazide
benzhexol	trihexyphenidyl
chlorpheniramine	chlorphenamine
dicyclomine	dicycloverine
dothiepin	dosulepin
eformoterol	formoterol
flurandrenolone	fludroxycortide
frusemide	furosemide
hydroxyurea	hydroxycarbamide
lignocaine	lidocaine
methotrimeprazine	levomepromazine
methylene blue	methylthioninium chloride
mitozantrone	mitoxantrone
mustine	chlormethine
nicoumalone	acenocoumarol
[1]noradrenaline	norepinephrine
oxypentifylline	pentoxyifylline
procaine penicillin	procaine benzylpenicillin
salcatonin	calcitonin (salmon)
thymoxamine	moxisylyte
thyroxine sodium	levothyroxine sodium
trimeprazine	alimemazine

List 2 – rINN to appear exclusively

Former BAN	rINN/new BAN
amoxycillin	amoxicillin
amphetamine	amfetamine
amylobarbitone	amobarbital
amylobarbitone sodium	amobarbital sodium
beclomethasone	beclometasone
benorylate	benorilate
busulphan	busulfan
butobarbitone	butobarbital
carticaine	articane
cephalexin	cefalexin
cephamandole nafate	cefamandole nafate
cephazolin	cefazolin
cephradine	cefradine
chloral betaine	cloral betaine
chlorbutol	chlorobutanol
chlormethiazole	clomethiazole
chlorathalidone	chlortalidone
cholecalciferol	colecalciferol
cholestyramine	colestyramine
clomiphene	clomifene
colistin sulphomethate sodium	colistimethate sodium
corticotrophin	corticotropin
cysteamine	mercaptamine
danthron	dantron
desoxymethasone	desoximetasone
dexamphetamine	dexamfetamine
dibromopropamidine	dibrompropamidine
dienoestrol	dienestrol
dimethicone(s)	dimeticone
dimethyl sulphoxide	dimethyl sulfoxide
doxycycline hydrochloride (hemihydrate hemiethanolate)	doxycycline hyclate
ethancrynic acid	etacrynic acid
ethamsylate	etamsylate
ethinyloestradiol	ethinylestradiol
ethynodiol	etynodiol
flumethasone	flumetasone
flupenthixol	flupentixol
gestronol	gestonorone
guaiphenesin	guaifenesin

[1] In common with the BP, precedence will continue to be given to the terms adrenaline and noradrenaline.

hexachlorophane   hexachlorophene   quinalbarbitone   secobarbital

hexamine hippurate   methenamine   riboflavine   riboflavin

    hippurate   sodium calciumedetate   sodium calcium

hydroxyprogesterone   hydroxyprogesterone   edetate

   hexanoate   caproate   sodium cromoglycate   sodium cromoglicate

indomethacin   indometacin   sodium ironedetate   sodium feredetate

lysuride   lisuride   sodium picosulphate   sodium picosulfate

methyl cysteine   mecysteine   sorbitan monostearate   sorbitan stearate

methylphenobarbitone   methylphenobarbital   stilboestrol   diethylstilbestrol

oestradiol   estradiol   sulphacetamide   sulfacetamide

oestriol   estriol   sulphadiazine   sulfadiazine

oestrone   estrone   sulphadimidine   sulfadimidine

oxethazaine   oxetacaine   sulphaguanadine   sulfaguanadine

pentaerythritol   pentaerithrityl   sulphamethoxazole   sulfamethoxazole

   tetranitrate   tetranitrate   sulphasalazine   sulfasalazine

phenobarbitone   phenobarbital   sulphathiazole   sulfathiazole

pipothiazine   pipotiazine   sulphinpyrazone   sulfinpyrazone

polyhexanide   polihexanide   tetracosactrin   tetracosactide

potassium cloazepate   dipotassium   thiabendazole   tiabendazole

    clorazepate   thioguanine   tioguanine

pramoxine   pramocaine   thiopentone   thiopental

prothionamide   protionamide   urofollitrophin   urofollitropin

PREFACE TO SECOND EDITION

It is with much delight that we find ourselves writing this second edition. We have received many compliments from trainee ophthalmologists as well as more senior colleagues regarding the contents of the first edition.

We have attempted to enhance the first text by adding new topics, re-writing most of the original, and deleting a few topics on the way.

This book is still aimed at ophthalmologists in training, particularly those who are studying for their final examinations. This book will not replace the many excellent comprehensive textbooks that already exist, but it is hoped it will compliment them.

Each topic is presented in a standard format, with the emphasis on identification and management of key problem areas. We have added in some tables but excluded photographs and diagrams. Each section ends with a set of key references.

The importance of assessing ophthalmic problems in the context of systemic disease and communication with other specialists in a multi-disciplinary approach to disease management remains a central theme.

We have taken care to try and exclude any factual errors and to include important recent advances in the subjects covered. We think it excels beyond the standard set in the first edition.

R.H. Taylor, P. Shah, P.I. Murray, M.A. Burdon, A. Levin

PREFACE TO FIRST EDITION

This book is aimed at ophthalmologists in training, particularly those who are studying for their final examinations. Many excellent comprehensive textbooks already exist and this text should be used as an adjunct to the larger reference books. Topics have been selected for a combination of reasons, including interest, importance of subject material, difficulty of concepts and examination orientation. Each topic is presented in a standard problem-orientated format, with the emphasis on identification and management of key problem areas. Each section ends with a set of key references which provide the reader with a direct entry into important recent literature.

Throughout the book we have attempted to achieve a constant style and emphasize certain principles. The importance of assessing ophthalmic problems in the context of systemic disease and communication with other specialists in a multi-disciplinary approach to disease management is a central theme.

During the period of preparing the text there have been many rapid developments within the field of ophthalmology. We have taken care to try and exclude any factual errors and to include important recent advances in the subjects covered. We hope that the reader finds the book interesting and useful, and can apply many of the principles in their clinical practice.

R.H. Taylor, P. Shah, P.I. Murray

CONTRIBUTORS

R.K. Aggarwal, Consultant Ophthalmologist, Southend General Hospital,
Westcliffe-on-Sea, UK

J.R. Ainsworth, Consultant Ophthalmologist, Birmingham Children's Hospital, Birmingham,

O. Backhouse, Specialist Registrar in Ophthalmology, Department of Ophthalmology,
York District Hospital, York, UK

A.P. Booth, Specialist Registrar in Ophthalmology, Eye Department,
York District Hospital, York, UK

S.E. Brodie, Associate Professor of Ophthalmology, Mount Sinai School of Medicine,
New York, NY 10029, USA

B. Burton, Moorfields Eye Hospital, London, UK

A. Butcher, Specialist Registrar in Medical Ophthalmology, Birmingham
Heartlands Hospital, Birmingham, UK

A.B. Callear, Consultant Ophthalmologist, Department of Ophthalmology,
Royal Shrewsbury Hospitals NHS Trust, Shrewsbury, UK

P. Chell, Consultant Ophthalmologist, Eye Department, Worcester Royal Infirmary,
Worcester, UK

J. Christmas, Head of Service: Visual Impairment, City of York Council, York, UK

C. Day, The University of Birmingham, Division of Medical Sciences, The Medical School,
Birmingham, UK

H. Devonport, Specialist Registrar in Ophthalmology, Eye Department,
York District Hospital, York, UK

P.M. Dodson, Consultant Physician, Birmingham Heartlands Hospital, UK

H.S. Dua, Professor of Ophthalmology, Department of Ophthalmology,
Queen's Medical Centre, Nottingham, UK

M. Fouladi, Consultant Ophthalmologist, William Harvey Hospital, Ashford, UK

J.M. Gibson, Consultant Ophthalmologist, Department of Ophthalmology,
Birmingham Heartlands Hospital, Birmingham, UK

K. Gregory-Evans, Senior Lecturer and Consultant Ophthalmologist, Imperial College
of Science, Technology and Medicine, The Western Eye Hospital, London, UK

J. Hamburger, Senior Lecturer in Oral Medicine, Birmingham Dental Hospital, UK

M. Hope-Ross, Consultant Ophthalmologist, Birmingham and Midland Eye Centre,
City Hospital Trust, Birmingham, UK

P. Jacobs, Consultant Ophthalmologist, York District Hospital, York, UK

T. Kipioti, Specialist Registrar in Ophthalmology, Eye Department,
York District Hospital, York, UK

D.E. Laws, Consultant Ophthalmologist, Ophthalmology Department,
Singleton Hospital, Wansea, UK

B. Leatherbarrow, Consultant Ophthalmic, Ocuplastic and Orbital Surgeon,
Manchester Royal Eye Hospital, Manchester, UK

G.A. Lee, International Research Fellow, City Hospital NHS Trust, Birmingham, UK

A.V. Levin, Associate Professor of Ophthalmology, Department of Ophthalmology,
Hospital for Sick Children, Toronto, Canada

R. Loh, Eye Department, St James's University Hospital, Leeds, UK

A. Morrell, Consultant Ophthalmologist, Eye Department, St. James University Hospital,
Leeds, UK

K.K. Nischal, Consultant Ophthalmologist, Eye Department,
Great Ormond Street Hospital, London, UK

A. O'Driscoll, Consultant Ophthalmologist, Warwick Hospital, Warwick, UK

C.M. Panton, Assistant Director of Electrophysiology, Department of Ophthalmology,
Hospital for Sick Children, Toronto, Canada

M. Papadopoulos, Moorfields Eye Hospital, London, UK

T. Potamitis, Consultant Ophthalmologist, Limassol, Cyprus

S. Ramanathan, Specialist Registrar in Ophthalmology,
Birmingham and Midland Eye Centre, City Hospital Trust, Birmingham, UK

S. Rauz, MRC Clinical Training Fellow, Birmingham and Midland Eye Centre,
Birmingham, UK

I. Rennie, Professor of Ophthalmology, Department of Ophthalmology and Orthoptics,
Royal Hallamshire Hospital, Sheffield, UK

C.O.S. Savage, The University of Birmingham, Division of Medical Sciences,
The Medical School, Birmingham, UK

H.C. Seward, Consultant Ophthalmologist, Croydon Eye Unit,
Mayday University Hospital, Thornton Heath, UK

F. Shah, Specialist Registrar in Dermatology, University Hospital Birmingham NHS Trust,
Birmingham, UK

P. Stavrou, Consultant Ophthalmologist, Birmingham and Midland Eye Centre,
City Hospital Trust, Birmingham, UK

S. Thakur, Specialist Registrar in Ophthalmology, Birmingham and Midland Eye Centre,
Birmingham, UK

M.D. Tsaloumas, Consultant Ophthalmologist, Birmingham and Midland Eye Centre, Birmingham, UK

G. Venables, Consultant Neurologist, Royal Hallamshire Hospital, Sheffield, UK

G. Walters, Specialist Registrar, Crofton, Wakefield, UK

S.-L. Watson, Specialist Registrar, Croydon Eye Unit, The Mayday University Hospital, Thornton Heath, UK

C.A. Westall, Director of Visual Electrophysiology, The Hospital for Sick Children, Toronto, Canada

A. Whallett, Consultant Rheumatologist, Dudley Heart Hospital, Dudley, UK

K. Whittaker, Specialist Registrar in Ophthalmology, Birmingham and Midland Eye Centre, City Hospital Trust, Birmingham, UK

H. Willshaw, Consultant Ophthalmologist, Birmingham Children's Hospital, Birmingham, UK

ACANTHAMOEBA

Tina Kipioti & Robert H. Taylor

Acanthamoeba keratitis was first recognized as a clinical entity in 1973 and it is now well established as a rare but potentially devastating corneal infection predominantly associated with contact lens wear. Five species have been reported to cause keratitis: *A. polyphaga*, *A. castellani*, *A. hatchetti*, *A. culbertsoni* and *A. rhysodes*, the first two being the ones most commonly encountered.

Problem

Despite the recent improvements in diagnosis and treatment, the frequent failure to recognize the condition at an early stage, the difficulty isolating the parasite from the cornea and the protracted clinical course make Acanthamoeba keratitis a difficult clinical problem which results in severe visual loss in over 15% of patients.

Background

The national Acanthamoeba keratitis study group conducted a multicentre survey in England between 1992 and 1996 and reported an annual incidence of 0.14 per 100 000 individuals in the UK. The incidence in the USA showed a dramatic increase in parallel with the growing popularity of soft contact lens (CL) wear. This was followed by a marked rise in the number of cases associated with the introduction of disposable soft CLs. However, all types of lenses have been incriminated, including PMMA, extended-wear soft and rigid gas-permeable. Well established risk factors are inappropriate disinfection regimens of CLs and CL cases, swimming with CLs in chlorinated water, lakes, rivers or in the sea and the use of non-sterile water (e.g. tap water or homemade saline) for rinsing CLs or their cases. Most non-CL-related cases are associated with trauma, usually minor, in rural, fishing or nautical environments or on building sites. A pattern of increased prevalence during the summer and early autumn months has been identified in several studies.

Acanthamoebae are free-living protozoa that can be isolated from soil, water, dust, sewage, hot tubs, air filters and cooling. The active trophozoite form can turn into a dormant cystic phase when environmental conditions become unfavourable. These cysts are very stable and resistant to desiccation, heat, cold, pH extremes and chemotherapy. Exposure to favourable conditions can trigger excystment within 3 days.

The pathogenesis is still largely unclear. Early clinical infection appears to involve the epithelium alone; the parasite adheres to mannose-containing glycoproteins of the corneal epithelium, which causes destruction of the epithelial cells, enabling entry into the stroma where secretion of collagenolytic enzymes that produce inflammation and necrosis occurs. Both trophozoites and cysts may exist simultaneously. Relapses after partially successful treatment are considered to be due to reactivation of the organism that has become encysted in the corneal stroma. Polymorphonuclear cells predominate in the host response but there may occasionally be mononuclear, epithelioid and foreign body giant cells suggestive of a granulomatous process.

Clinical features

The clinical presentation of Acanthamoeba keratitis is highly variable. It is usually unilateral but bilateral cases have been reported. The pain is characteristically described as severe and out of proportion to the clinical findings but this can be an unreliable clinical symptom. Other symptoms include photophobia, epiphora, redness and reduced vision.

Early infection is often confined to the epithelium, which demonstrates elevated epithelial lines or ridges. These can arborize to form pseudodendrites or true dendrites leading to a common misdiagnosis of herpes simplex virus (HSV) keratitis. The frequent finding of decreased corneal sensation in early infection and the occasional conjunctival follicle have also contributed to the misdiagnosis of HSV. Non-specific stromal infiltrates can develop. These can vary in appearance from barely discernible to necrotic, or circumscribed paracentral infiltrates that coalesce to form a ring. Infiltrates along corneal nerves are known as radial perineuritis and are diagnostic of Acanthamoeba. Satellite lesions may occur. Corneal neovascularization is uncommon. Eventually stromal thinning can lead to descemetocele formation and perforation.

Associated findings include occasional progression of the keratitis to limbitis and sectoral or nodular scleritis that contribute to the painful symptoms. The anterior chamber reaction can vary from trace cell and flare to hypopyon formation. However, treatment with topical steroids may often modify and mask the clinical signs and symptoms early on in the disease.

Diagnosis

Late diagnosis of the condition is often marked by resistance to medical and surgical therapy as well as poorer visual outcome, thus making early diagnosis of Acanthamoeba critical. The absence of a history of CL wear is associated with delayed diagnosis, increased need for surgery and more seriously impaired final vision. The higher clinical suspicion in CL patients seems to contribute to more prompt diagnosis of the condition.

Laboratory diagnosis is usually based on stains and culture of corneal scrapings. In cases of predominantly stromal involvement with little epithelial disease, corneal biopsy should be considered.

Smears are examined with the dye Calcofluor white under UV light which effectively demonstrates the walls of the cysts. Cultures should be plated on non-nutrient agar with an *E. coli* overlay. Plates should be incubated for 2 weeks at 25°C and 37°C before reported negative. Contact lenses, cases and CL solutions should be cultured as well.

Although not widely available, *in vivo* confocal microscopy is a non-invasive technique that enables direct visualization of cysts and trophozoites in the corneal stroma. Immunofluorescent assays, electron microscopy, Gram and Giemsa staining and polymerase chain reaction of epithelial samples or even tears can contribute to the diagnosis of Acanthamoeba in culture-negative cases.

Treatment

Although numerous effective antiamoebic antimicrobials have been made available, no optimum treatment has yet been established. There are four groups of chemotherapeutic agents acting against Acanthamoebae and they are usually used concurrently:

- Cationic antiseptics, which inhibit membrane function: polyhexamethylene biguanide (PHMB) and chlorhexidine.
- Aromatic diamidines, which inhibit DNA synthesis: propamidine isethionate (Brolene), pentamidine and hexamidine.
- Aminoglycosides, which inhibit protein synthesis: neomycin and paromomycin.
- Imidazoles, which destabilize cell walls: clotrimazole, fluconazole, ketoconazole.

Combinations of these agents produce additive (PHMB+ propamidine or neomycin) or synergistic effects (PHMB+ pentamidine). The most common initial approach is PHMB or chlorhexidine together with propamidine isethionate. If necessary, neomycin or an imidazole may be added. The drops are used initially hourly and then reduced according to clinical response. Treatment toxicity with PHMB, chlorhexidine and propamidine is rarely serious and usually consists only of stinging or punctuate keratopathy. Clinical relapses are quite common as therapy is tapered. Prudent use of topical steroid may reduce the length of antiamoebal treatment but does not seem to affect visual outcome. Steroids are usually reserved for patients with severe pain or associated iritis and should be discontinued before cessation of the anti-Acanthamoeba regimen. The mean duration of treatment is usually prolonged and between 20 and 40 weeks. Penetrating keratoplasty is only recommended for visual rehabilitation rather than for control of infection. It should be deferred until medical cure has been achieved. Pain control in patients with Acanthamoeba keratitis can be difficult and may require the use of narcotic analgesics. There may also be a role for therapeutic excimer laser ablation.

Prevention

The national Acanthamoeba keratitis study has demonstrated the highly preventable nature of this disease; the condition could have been avoided in 91% of the identified cases by refraining from inadvisable practices such as:

- non-sterile methods and solutions utilized for CLs;
- salt-tablet derived solutions;
- swimming with CLs.

No significant difference in effectiveness between peroxide-based and 'all in one' solutions has been demonstrated but peroxide seems to be superior in the absence of proper cleaning.

Further reading

Duguid IG, Dart JK, Morlet N, Allan BD, Matheson M, Ficker L, Tuft S. Outcome of Acanthamoeba keratitis treated with polyhexamethylene biguanide and propamidine. *Ophthalmology* 1997; **104**(10): 1587–92.

Hargrave SL, McCulley JP, Husseini Z. Results of a trial of combined propamidine isethionate and neomycin therapy for Acanthamoeba keratitis. Brolene Study Group. *Ophthalmology* 1999; **106**(5): 952–7.

Illingworth CD, Cook SD. Acanthamoeba keratitis (Review). *Survey of Ophthalmology* 1998; **42**(6): 493–508.

Illingworth CD, Cook SD, Karabatsas CH, Easty DL. Acanthamoeba keratitis: risk factors and outcome. *British Journal of Ophthalmology* 1995; **79**(12): 1078–82.

Lindquist TD. Treatment of Acanthamoeba keratitis. (Review). *Cornea* 1998; **17**(1): 11–6.

Mietz H, Font RL. Acanthamoeba keratitis with granulomatous reaction involving the stroma and the anterior chamber. *Archives of Ophthalmology* 1997; **115**(2): 259–63.

Niszl IA, Markus MB. Anti-Acanthamoeba activity of contact lens solutions. *British Journal of Ophthalmology* 1998; **82**(9): 1033–8.

Park DH, Palay DA, Daya SM, Stulting RD, Krachmer JH, Holland EJ. The role of topical corticosteroids in the management of Acanthamoeba keratitis. *Cornea* 1997; **16**(3): 277–83.

Radford CF, Lehmann OJ, Dart JK. Acanthamoeba keratitis: multicentre survey in England 1992–6. National Acanthamoeba keratitis study group. *British Journal of Ophthalmology* 1998; **82**(12): 1387–92.

Seal D, Hay J, Kirkness C, *et al.* Successful medical therapy of Acanthamoeba keratitis with topical chlorhexidine and propamidine. *Eye* 1996; **10**(4): 413–21.

Yang Z, Cao Z, Panjwani N. Pathogenesis of Acanthamoeba keratitis: carbohydrate-mediated host–parasite interactions. *Infection & Immunity* 1997; **65**(2): 439–45.

ACUTE RETINAL NECROSIS

Philip I. Murray

Acute retinal necrosis (ARN) is a necrotizing retinopathy with potentially devastating visual consequences. It usually occurs in the immunocompetent but has also been reported in immunocompromised patients with autoimmune disorders, cancer and organ transplants. It is infrequently seen in HIV infection. The main sight-threatening complication is retinal detachment, although an optic neuropathy can occur.

Problem

Confusion exists with regards to diagnosis, aetiology and management.

Background

The retinal necrosis is thought to result from the combined effect of intracellular viral replication with subsequent cell death and vascular occlusion secondary to acute vasculitis. The causes of ARN are the herpesviruses. Although most reported cases have been due to varicella zoster virus (VZV), others appear to be associated with herpes simplex virus (HSV), either types 1 or 2. Most cases are believed to be secondary to reactivation of a latent herpetic infection, and often patients have a prior history of dermatomal VZV (herpes zoster) or primary VZV (chickenpox) infection, or perioral blisters, presumably caused by HSV infection. Reactivation of the viral genome from the trigeminal ganglion may result in the development of ARN after transneural spread. Trauma-induced reactivation of latent congenital HSV-2 infection has been reported in a few cases of ARN. It is uncommon for healthy individuals to develop ARN simultaneously with cutaneous VZV or HSV infection. Despite being a clinical diagnosis, an aqueous (or vitreous) tap is usually performed to look for herpesviral DNA using the polymerase chain reaction. In a recent study on 28 patients (30 eyes), VZV DNA was detected in aqueous or vitreous samples of 13 patients (15 eyes), HSV-1 in 7 patients (7 eyes) and HSV-2 in 6 patients (6 eyes). All patients with ARN due to HSV-2 were younger than 25 years of age.

Clinical features

Prompt diagnosis and treatment are necessary to limit retinal damage and preserve vision. The diagnosis of ARN should be based solely on clinical appearance and course of infection. Standard diagnostic criteria have been developed by the American Uveitis Society. Clinical characteristics that must be seen include:

- One or more focus of retinal necrosis with discrete borders located in the peripheral retina, primarily involving the area adjacent to, or outside of, the major temporal vascular arcades. Macular lesions, although less common, do not preclude a diagnosis of ARN if they occur in the presence of peripheral lesions.
- Rapid progression of disease with advancement of lesion borders or development of new foci of necrosis if antiviral therapy has not been given.
- Circumferential spread of disease.

- Evidence of occlusive vasculopathy with arteriolar involvement. This is a very important clue to diagnosis.
- A prominent inflammatory reaction in the vitreous and anterior chamber.

Characteristics that support, but are not required for, a diagnosis of ARN include:

- Optic neuropathy/atrophy;
- Scleritis;
- Pain.

As the infection progresses, the leading edge of confluent retinal whitening advances toward the posterior pole. It may not progress posteriorly to the vascular arcades thus sparing the macula and central vision. In some patients, the retinal vasculitic component may be much more prominent than the retinal necrosis. Perivascular haemorrhages may be present but widespread areas of retinal haemorrhage are atypical. Optic disc swelling is a common feature of ARN.

Treatment

Without treatment, the inflammatory component of ARN typically burns out in 6 to 12 weeks, leaving behind a thin, atrophic retina with associated pigmentary changes. Classic retinal pigment epithelial alterations in a scalloped pattern clearly separate previously involved retina from spared retina. The mainstay of treatment is a course of intravenous aciclovir, usually 10 mg/kg tid for at least 14 days then oral aciclovir/valaciclovir/famciclovir for about 3 months. The time interval for therapy is based on the observation that ARN in the second eye most often occurs within 6 to 14 weeks of the initial symptoms in the first eye. ARN in healthy patients does not generally recur in the same eye after antiviral treatment. In those patients who are immunocompromised oral therapy will need to be continued for a longer period. Aciclovir reduces but does not completely eliminate the risk of fellow eye involvement. Bilateral involvement in ARN eventually occurs in up to 65% of patients. There is no correlation between the severity of ARN in the first eye and severity of the disease in the fellow eye. Involvement of the second eye may not be apparent initially; there may be a delay of several weeks. Thirty-four years is the longest reported interval for involvement of the contralateral eye.

Controversy exists about whether systemic corticosteroids should be given. They are normally reserved for those cases that have large amounts of vitreous debris limiting the fundal view and are usually commenced at least a few days after starting intravenous aciclovir. Topical steroid and mydriatic are given for the associated anterior uveitis.

Clinically, there may not be any obvious improvement for up to 5 days after starting therapy, then the lesions will become less white and more granular, eventually resulting in retinal atrophy. Argon laser photocoagulation is often performed in two rows anterior to the edge of the necrosis. This is a prophylactic measure and may wall off any detachment that could occur in the areas of retinal atrophy. If the retina does detach, as it does in about 50% of cases, then pars plana vitrectomy with silicone oil tamponade is the procedure of choice. The holes may be multiple, posterior and often associated with proliferative vitreoretinopathy.

Initial reports indicated that the long-term visual prognosis of ARN was poor with 60% of eyes having a final visual acuity of 6/60 or worse. Not all cases have a fulminant course and result in a poor outcome. Mild cases with limited peripheral retinitis and good visual outcomes have been reported, and some cases resolve spontaneously without treatment. In one study of eyes with limited retinal involvement at the time of diagnosis, final visual acuity was 6/12 or better in 50% and 6/120 or better in 92% of eyes after treatment with aciclovir and prophylactic laser photocoagulation.

Further reading

Crapotta JA, Freeman WR, Feldman RM, Lowder CY, Ambler JS, Parker CE, Meisler DM. Visual outcome in acute retinal necrosis. *Retina* 1993; **13:** 208–213.

Ganatra JB, Chandler D, Santos C, Kuppermann B, Margolis TP. Viral causes of the acute retinal necrosis syndrome. *American Journal of Ophthalmology* 2000; **129:** 166–72.

Holland GN. Standard diagnostic criteria for the acute retinal necrosis syndrome. *American Journal of Ophthalmology* 1994; **117:** 663–7.

ALBINISM

Alex V. Levin

Albinism is a condition in which there is a defect in melanogenesis or related processes. It is a disorder widespread throughout the animal kingdom. In ocular albinism, only the eye is affected. In oculocutaneous albinism, the eye and skin (as well as hair) are affected.

Problem

Although the severe forms of albinism make for easy diagnosis, more subtle forms of albinism can be difficult to recognize. Advances in molecular genetics have contributed to a redefinition of albinism accompanied by a new nomenclature that reflects the molecular basis of the disease.

Background

There are two types of melanin: eumelanin responsible for darker brown and black pigmentation, and pheomelanin which causes yellow, red and orange colouration. All melanin derives from tyrosine. The rate-limiting steps in melanogenesis are the first two, both of which are catalysed by the enzyme tyrosinase. If there is less than complete inactivation of tyrosinase, then there will be a preferential accumulation of pheomelanin. Melanin is contained in cells in melanosomes. If melanosome formation is impaired, then cells are unable to 'display' melanin properly and forms of albinism may result.

Melanin in the eye is located in the uveal tract and the retinal pigmented epithelial cells (RPE). Normal melanin in the RPE is required for proper induction of macular formation during embryogenesis. Likewise, proper pigmentation and retinal development are required for the normal decussation of ganglion cell axonal projections to the brain.

Melanin, in particular eumelanin, has a protective effect against ultraviolet-induced cancer formation. Albinism in Africa is a significant contributor to morbidity from skin cancer. Albinism can occur in any racial or ethnic population.

Albinism was previously classified as 'tyrosinase positive' or 'tyrosinase negative' based primarily on the external appearance of the patient. If the patient appeared to have some pigmentation they were called 'tyrosinase positive' under the assumption that they had at least some functioning tyrosinase enzyme. Sometimes classification was aided by the use of hair bulb analysis. Plucked hair was incubated with tyrosine to see if pigmentation occurred thus, presumably, indicating the presence of functioning tyrosinase. However, modern molecular studies have demonstrated that these methods of classification are not accurate and that mutations in tyrosinase ('tyrosinase related albinism') can allow residual activity and pigmentation that would have previously led to a classification of 'tyrosinase positive'. Forms of albinism which result from mutations in other genes, may now be referred to as 'tyrosinase unrelated albinism'.

Oculocutaneous albinism (OCA) is generally accepted to be an exclusively autosomal recessive disorder. However, although not yet proven by molecular genetics, there are rare pedigrees that seem to indicate the possibility of autosomal dominant disease. Digenic disease is another possibility that has yet to be ruled out. Ocular albinism (OA) is most commonly an X-linked recessive disorder although autosomal recessive forms of predominantly ocular albinism have now been demonstrated to be due to mutations in the tyrosinase or *p* genes.

Clinical features

The features common to almost all forms of albinism include nystagmus, iris transillumination, macular hypoplasia and fundus hypopigmentation. These features are present in virtually all cases. Although controversial, abnormalities of visual pathway decussation (over-decussation to the contralateral hemisphere), measured by multi-channel visual-evoked potential, are found in most but not all patients. Grey and mildly hypoplastic optic nerves may also be observed. Patients with albinism have a higher incidence of strabismus and refractive error. Most patients have subnormal vision although children can retain excellent near vision, perhaps through the use of convergence dampening of nystagmus plus accommodation, despite poor distance acuity. Some patients may also suffer from photophobia.

Type 1 OCA refers to tyrosinase related disease. Type 1A includes mutations which completely obliterate tyrosinase function thus resulting in the classic severe OCA with very poor visual acuity (usually ≤ 6/60), white hair and pale skin. Type 1B, also known as the yellow variant, and 1MP (<u>m</u>inimal <u>p</u>igment) have some residual tyrosinase activity that allows for pheomelanin pigmentation to accumulate. In 1B the clinical features in infancy may look very much like 1A but pheomelanin pigmentation gradually comes resulting in white-tipped yellow hair that, in both 1B and 1MP, might even eventually reach a 'sandy blond' or very light almost brown colouration. Vision tends to be better than it is in Type IA with better macular development, less nystagmus, and less iris transillumination. In Type 1TS (<u>t</u>emperature <u>s</u>ensitive) OCA, mutations in the tyrosinase gene result in enzyme activity that is reduced only in cellular environments with a temperature >35°C. As a result, the eyes show full signs of albinism and the hair on the head, axillae and groin is white. However, hair on the cooler chest and extremities is darkly pigmented. The tyrosinase gene is located on 11q.

Type II OCA is caused by abnormalities in the *p* gene located on 15q. The gene was in part discovered as a result of the association of hypopigmentation with two rare syndromes, Prader–Willi and Angelman, which result from abnormalities in a nearby region of 15q. The *p* gene product is thought to be involved in the transport of tyrosine into melanosomes. Patients with type II OCA have a wide variety of phenotypes, usually not as severe as type IA but often clinically indistinguishable from types IB and IMP.

The forms of Type III OCA are due to abnormalities in tyrosinase-related protein 1 (TRP1) on 9p. This would include rufous OCA, a form of albinism more common in Africa, and some forms of brown albinism. The term 'brown albinism' is used to describe a particular moderate phenotype that can occur in any racial population and may also be due to abnormalities in the *p* gene or other as yet undiscovered genes. In fact, perhaps many genes for isolated OCA have yet to be discovered.

Classic ocular albinism, also known as Nettleship–Falls albinism, is due to abnormalities in the *OA1* gene at Xp23 and represents 10% of albinism overall. Although affected males may have hair and skin that is slightly lighter when compared to their unaffected family members, their appearance is generally recognized to be within the normal range. However, their eyes are often quite severely affected. Skin biopsy in most affected individuals will demonstrate macromelanosomes, perhaps a reflection of the suspected role of OA1 in melanosome formation. Due to lyonization, female carriers may show hypomelanotic skin macules, mild iris transillumination, and a characteristic 'mud splattered' fundus appearance. Females may also have macromelanosomes on skin biopsy. Each of these signs represents clones of cells in which the unaffected X chromosome is inactivated. Rarely, if inactivation is particularly skewed in favour of the affected X chromosome, there may be sufficient cells expressing the abnormal X chromosome so that the female may appear to be affected with OA.

Both OA and OCA may also occur in combination with other disorders (e.g. contiguous gene deletion of Xp may result in OA1 plus ichthyosis) or in association with other findings caused by defects in the same gene. For example, pigment is required in the stria vascularis of the inner ear. The combination of hearing loss and albinism should always be considered. The two cardinal examples of multiple defects, including albinism, from the same gene defect are Hermansky–Pudlak syndrome (HPS) and Chediak–Higashi syndrome (CHS). Both appear to be disorders of intracellular vesicle formation (which includes melanosome formation). Macromelanosomes are seen in both disorders. Genes have been cloned. HPS is characterized by a very variable OCA (or even almost phenotypic OA in the same family) associated with a bleeding diathesis and ceroid lipofuscin deposition. It is particularly prevalent in Puerto Rico and Switzerland, but not exclusively so. Appropriate diagnostic investigations include platelet count, bleeding time, and platelet electron microscopy. The disorder should be considered in patients with albinism from these two countries or in the presence of a history of bleeding or gastrointestinal, renal, cardiac or pulmonary disease. CHS is characterized by OCA with a silvery metallic sheen to the hair and slate grey patches on the skin along with a defect in leukocyte chemotaxis. Other features may include optic nerve oedema (acceleration phase), a predisposition to lymphoreticular malignancy, and peripheral neuropathy.

Treatment

The ophthalmologist plays a key role in optimizing visual function for the patient with albinism through low vision interventions (in particular distance acuity aids such as a hand-held monocular), correction of refractive error, and eye muscle surgery to either correct strabismus, or in carefully selected cases, reduce nystagmus. For patients suffering from photophobia, the use of spectacles filtering in the 527 nm range can be very helpful. If this is too dark, some patients will prefer 511 nm lenses particularly for indoor use. In other patients, the darker 550 nm lens is needed outdoors. It is also important to educate the patient about the risks of sun exposure and the need for high protection factor sun block as well as appropriate clothing and avoidance behaviours.

The appearance of the patient with albinism presents a significant psychosocial challenge. The National Organization for Hypopigmentation and Albinism (NOAH) has many publications through which patients can find information and support.

Conclusion

Albinism is a term that describes a multitude of disorders that share in common pigment dysgenesis. The ocular effects may be isolated or seen in combination with cutaneous manifestations. Systemic signs may also be present. Understanding the molecular basis of these disorders allows us to appreciate their pathogenesis and approach possible therapeutic options for the future.

Further reading

Boissy RE, Nordlund JJ. Molecular basis of congenital hypopigmentary disorders in humans: a review. *Pigment Cell Res* 1997; **10**: 12–24.
Haefemeyer JW, Knuth JL. Albinism. *J Ophthalmic Nurs Technol* 1991; **10**: 55–62.
Imesch PD, Wallow IH, Albert DA. The color of the human eye: a review of morphologic correlates and of some conditions that affect iridial pigmentation. *Surv Ophthalmol* 1997; **41** (Suppl 2): S117–S123.
King RA, Hearing VJ, Creel DJ, Oetting, WS. Albinism. In: *The Metabolic and Molecular Bases of Inherited Disease* (Scriver CR, Beudet AL, Sly WS, Valle D, eds) 7th edn. New York, McGraw-Hill, Inc. 1995, pp. 4353–4392.

Related topic of interest

Nystagmus 1: nystagmus (p. 190).

ALKALI INJURIES

Anthony O'Driscoll, Stephen Ohlrich & Peter Shah

Ocular alkali injuries are potentially devastating. Patients may present after accidental injury in their working or domestic environment, or they may have been assaulted.

Problem

Three main problems exist in patients with alkali chemical injuries: (1) the assessment of the primary injury; (2) the initial management of the injury and limitation of limbal stem cell damage; and (3) the management of long-term complications. Evolution of damage continues after the initial insult, and the severity of these injuries should not be underestimated.

Background

Alkaline substances penetrate the eye rapidly and may damage the ocular surface tissues, corneal stroma and endothelium, deeper anterior segment structures and even the posterior segment.

Clinical features – assessment of the primary injury

As there is the possibility of rapid devastating tissue damage, first aid measures are the first concern with detailed assessment second. A detailed history of the circumstances of the injury is essential for both clinical and medico-legal reasons. The timing of the injury, exact chemicals involved and initial action taken should be recorded. Ammonia and sodium hydroxide have rapid corneal penetration. The penetration of calcium hydroxide in the form of 'lime' is less rapid, but retained particulate matter in the fornices may lead to prolonged exposure to the chemical.

Examination aims to document the extent of both corneal and conjunctival epithelial loss. Care should be taken when assessing corneal epithelial loss, as it is possible to miss total epithelial loss. If one suspects this, useful clues include the presence of a thin residual 'frill' of epithelium at the limbus and an inability to see distinct semicircular rings on applanation tonometry. The presence of stromal haze, anterior chamber activity and lens damage should also be recorded. The intraocular pressure should be measured in all patients, as it may be elevated. The degree of limbal ischaemia (blanching) correlates well with the severity of the injury and limbal stem cell damage, and should be carefully assessed. The skin of the lids and periorbital region should be examined for partial or full thickness chemical burns. The possibility of an associated inhalational injury should be considered in industrial accidents. Lid eversion and careful examination of the fornices is essential to identify retained granules.

Hughes' classification of chemical injuries relates clinical findings and prognosis:

Grade 1: no limbal ischaemia. Corneal epithelial damage only. Prognosis good.
Grade 2: less than one-third limbal non-perfusion, minimal corneal haze but iris details visible, prognosis good.

Grade 3: one-third to one-half limbal non-perfusion with total corneal epithelial loss, and corneal haze obscuring the iris details. Corneal scarring may reduce visual acuity to 6/60 or less. Guarded prognosis.

Grade 4: over one-half limbal non-perfusion and an opaque cornea. Prognosis is poor and corneal perforation possible.

Initial management

Speed is vital. Immediate irrigation with water at the place of injury is crucial, followed by copious irrigation at the referring unit prior to transfer for ophthalmic assessment. Irrigation should be continued until the conjunctival surface attains a neutral pH of 7.5 or the pH is equal to that in the non-exposed eye. Lavage should be instigated before a full history and examination. Double eversion of the lids should be performed, and any particulate matter removed from the fornices. Children with chemical injuries can be particularly difficult to assess, and may need an examination under anaesthetic in order to remove particulate matter. Initial irrigation should proceed even if restraint is needed. All severe alkali injuries should be admitted for intensive treatment. Initial treatment aims to limit limbal stem cell damage and restore an intact corneal epithelium, derived from those stem cells. This helps to reduce the complications of corneal scarring, vascularization, melting and perforation. The use of preservative-free preparations is preferred to reduce toxicity. Components of the regimen include:

1. Topical corticosteroids. Inflammatory changes delay epithelial cell migration, promote limbal cell death and cause cellular infiltration (e.g. neutrophil polymorphs), with an increase in local collagenase levels. High dose topical corticosteroids reduce inflammatory activity and, if used appropriately, do not have an adverse effect on epithelial healing. At about 2 weeks after the initial injury, the continued use of intensive topical steroids may compromise stromal repair and cause sterile ulceration. Therefore, after an initial period of frequent administration the steroid dose should be reduced. If the cornea has a persistent epithelial defect, the patient should be monitored closely for signs of stromal thinning.

2. Topical antibiotics. In the presence of extensive conjunctival and corneal epithelial defects, antibiotic cover may be of benefit as prophylaxis against secondary bacterial infection.

3. Topical cycloplegics. Patients with severe chemical injuries often have marked pain, and cycloplegia may help to reduce discomfort. Patients often require prolonged cycloplegia after these injuries.

4. Topical ascorbic acid (e.g. sodium ascorbate, 10% every hour). Ascorbate is an essential co-factor in the rate-limiting step of collagen formation, and is depleted in keratocytes and aqueous after chemical injuries. In the rabbit model, ascorbate has been shown to reduce the incidence of sterile ulcerations and corneal perforations, but does not alter the progression of a pre-existing ulcer. There is also evidence that ascorbate may act as a free-radical scavenger in the anterior chamber and perhaps limit damage in part through this mechanism.

5. *Oral ascorbic acid.* Many authorities supplement topical ascorbate with high dose oral ascorbate.

6. *Topical citric acid (e.g. sodium citrate, 10% every hour).* Sodium citrate is a calcium chelator that inhibits neutrophil polymorph chemotaxis and reduces collagenase activity. It has also been effective in inhibiting sterile ulcerations in the rabbit model. However, sodium citrate causes an extreme 'burning' pain on instillation (even more marked than ascorbate) and is therefore not widely used.

Management of long-term complications

Long-term corneal damage results from a combination of limbal cell dysfunction and ocular surface wetting problems. The ocular surface wetting is poor, due to diffuse damage to the conjunctiva and its goblet cells leading to reduced mucin production as well as damage to the lacrimal gland ductules. Cicatricial changes in the conjunctiva, resulting in poor lid globe apposition, further compound the surface wetting problems. Persistent corneal epithelial defects may be associated with progressive stromal melting. These patients are at risk of secondary bacterial infection.

Therapeutic options for managing epithelial defects and severe dry eyes include frequent topical lubricants, temporary or permanent punctal occlusion, tarsorrhaphy and the use of bandage contact lenses. Uninjured conjunctiva may be utilized to promote healing of persistent corneal epithelial defects, either as a Gunderson flap (same eye) or as a Thoft graft (fellow eye). Conjunctival epithelialization of the cornea should be prevented by removing conjunctival epithelium before it grows over the limbus. The patient with a vascularized, scarred cornea with conjunctivalization of the ocular surface presents a difficult surgical challenge, and requires specialist management by an anterior segment surgeon. In selected cases, a penetrating keratoplasty may be considered, but requires prior preparation of the local ocular surface environment.

Keratoepithelioplasty (autologous transplantation of limbal stem cells) to increase limbal stem cell function, and conjunctival auto-grafting, to restore the deep mucoid layer of the tear film, should be considered before keratoplasty. Despite these procedures to improve the recipient bed, the graft still has a substantial chance of developing problems. In bilateral cases, corneal grafting onto a dry, vascularized cornea with no capacity for epithelial regeneration carries a very poor prognosis. However, limbal stem cell allotransplantation usually requires systemic immunosuppression, with its associated problems.

Amniotic membrane has the potential to serve as a biological dressing, and to function as a medium for limbal stem cell culture.

In refractory cases, an alternative therapy which has a chance of regaining some useful vision is to insert a keratoprosthesis. Squamous metaplasia and keratinization of the ocular surface provide a source of long-term ocular irritation, which may be helped by the use of topical retinoic acid. Long-term control of intraocular pressure provides another difficult problem in severely damaged eyes.

Further reading

Chiou AG, Florakis GJ, Kazim M. Management of conjunctival cicatrizing diseases and severe ocular surface dysfunction. *Survey of Ophthalmology* 1998; **43**(1): 19–46.

Dua HS. The conjunctiva in corneal epithelial wound healing. *British Journal of Ophthalmology* 1998; **82**(12): 1407–11.

Pfister RR, Haddox JL, Yuille-Barr D. The combined effect of citrate/ascorbate treatment in alkali-injured rabbit eyes. *Cornea* 1991; **10:** 100–4.

Shimazaki J, Yang HY, Tsubota K. Amniotic membrane transplantation for ocular surface reconstruction in patients with chemical and thermal burns. *Ophthalmology* 1997; **104**(12): 2068–76.

Wagoner MD, Kenyon KR. Chemical injuries of the eye. *Principles and Practice of Ophthalmology* 1994; **1:** 234–43.

Related topic of interest

Stem-cell grafting (p. 295).

ANISOCORIA (UNEQUAL PUPILS)

Mike Burdon

Pupil size reflects the balance between parasympathetic drive to the constrictor pupillae muscle and sympathetic drive to the dilator pupillae muscle as well as the structural integrity of the iris.

Problem

The causes of pupil inequality range from simple physiological anisocoria to serious efferent pathway disease. It should be remembered that anisocoria is not caused by afferent disease because each eye innervates both Edinger–Westphal nuclei equally. An accurate clinical assessment is required to appropriately direct (and often to avoid unnecessary) investigation.

Background

The parasympathetic supply originates in the Edinger–Westphal nucleus, a midline structure situated posterior to the main third cranial nerve nucleus in the upper midbrain. On leaving the brainstem, the parasympathetic fibres are located in the superior medial portion of the third cranial nerve. They enter the orbit with the inferior division of the third cranial nerve and reach the ciliary ganglion via the nerve to the inferior oblique muscle. After synapsing within the ganglion, the parasympathetic supply arrives at the iris via the short ciliary nerves. The sympathetic supply to the iris is detailed in the Horner's syndrome topic.

The three essential steps in the assessment of anisocoria are firstly to determine the degree of pupil inequality in bright and dim light, secondly to observe pupil light and near responses, and thirdly to examine the iris and pupil on a slit lamp. If the anisocoria is worse in dim light then the smaller pupil is abnormal, if worse in bright light, the larger. A more general neurological examination is often required, playing particular attention to eyelid position and eye movements. A variety of pharmacological tests are available to confirm a clinical diagnosis.

The causes of anisocoria can be divided into two groups; those with a normal response to light and a normal slit lamp examination, and those with an abnormal response to light which may be associated with structural abnormalities of the iris.

Clinical features

Patients with anisocoria and a normal response to light have either a Horner's syndrome or physiological anisocoria.

A clinically detectable difference in pupil size is found in approximately one fifth of the normal population. The anisocoria is usually less than 0.5 mm, and is relatively the same in all illumination. The degree of anisocoria may vary or even reverse when an individual is observed over a period of days. Prior to diagnosing physiological anisocoria it is important to confirm that pupil reactions are symmetrically brisk and that there are no other neurological or ocular anatomic deficits.

Slit lamp examination is invaluable in the assessment of anisocoria with an abnormal response to light. The iris should be examined for a tonic contraction to light or a near target, vermiform movements, sphincter rupture, segmental or diffuse atrophy, and posterior synechiae. Anisocoria associated with iris abnormalities may be caused by Adie's syndrome, ocular disease or trauma.

Adie syndrome is a common cause of anisocoria with a prevalence of 2 per 1000. The condition usually affects women (70%). The mean age at presentation is 32 years but may even occur in childhood.

Most are unilateral initially, but become bilateral at a rate of 4% per year. The syndrome is due to damage to the ciliary ganglion with subsequent aberrant regeneration of postganglionic fibres. Adie pupils are characterized by poor but sustained (tonic) constriction to light, light-near dissociation, and segmental paralysis of the iris sphincter that produces vermiform movements most notable at the slit lamp. At presentation most are larger than the unaffected pupil. However, with time the Adie's pupil becomes miotic and eventually may become smaller than the unaffected pupil. Two-thirds of eyes have impaired or absent accommodation, and up to 90% of patients have reduced tendon reflexes (the Holmes–Adie syndrome). Denervation hypersensitivity develops in 80% of pupils and can be demonstrated with 0.1% pilocarpine. It is essential that Adie pupils are recognized to avoid patients being subjected to unnecessary and expensive investigation. Those with impaired accommodation may need reading glasses. Occasionally dilute pilocarpine may be required to treat excessive glare.

Posterior synechiae are well-known complications of anterior uveitis, and this condition may also promote a miosis, possibly from swelling of the iris and sphincter irritation. Corneal inflammation may also cause a miosis. Anisocoria due to diffuse or localized atrophy of the iris may be caused by angle closure glaucoma, herpes zoster ophthalmicus and anterior segment ischaemia. Traumatic mydriasis may be temporary or permanent because of damage to the iris or the ciliary nerves.

Anisocoria with an abnormal (usually absent) response to light but a normal ocular examination may be due to either an oculomotor nerve palsy or pharmacological mydriasis or miosis. A careful history of exposure to parasympatholytic or sympathomimetic medications or plants should be elicited, followed by an examination of eye movements and eyelid position. Where there is uncertainty, 1% pilocarpine can be used as a pharmacological test. It will constrict a dilated pupil caused by an oculomotor nerve palsy but not one caused by commonly available anticholinergic medications.

The clinical features of a third nerve palsy are discussed in the relevant topic.

Further reading

Lam BL, Thompson HS, Corbett JJ. The prevalence of simple anisocoria. *American Journal of Ophthalmology* 1987; **104:** 69–73.

Miller NR. Disorders of pupillary function, accommodation and lacrimation. In: *Walsh and Hoyt's Clinical Neuro-Ophthalmology*, 4th edn., Vol. 2. Baltimore: Waverly Press, 1985; 469–528.

Payne JW, Adamkiewicz J. Unilateral internal ophthalmoplegia with intracranial aneurysm. *American Journal of Ophthalmology* 1969; **68:** 349–52.

Thompson HS. Adie's syndrome: some new observations. *Transactions of the American Ophthalmology Society* 1977; **75:** 587–626.

Related topics of interest

Horner's syndrome (p. 133); Third (oculomotor) cranial nerve palsy (p. 306).

BEHÇET'S DISEASE

Philip I. Murray

Behçet's disease is a multisystem inflammatory disorder of unknown cause, that takes its name from the Turkish dermatologist Hulûsi Behçet who described the condition in 1937, although the clinical triad of uveitis with oral and genital ulceration was probably first recognized by Hippocrates.

Problem

Behçet's disease consists of a relapsing, acute (rather than chronic) inflammatory process of unknown aetiology, characterized by an occlusive vasculitis. Exacerbations and remissions are of unpredictable duration and frequency. Loss of vision is one of the most frequent and serious manifestations and total blindness may occur. There appears to be some debate as to the clinical classification system required for diagnosis, the efficacy of various treatment regimens and the causation of this condition.

Background

Cases of Behçet's disease cluster along the ancient Silk Road that extends from eastern Asia to the Mediterranean basin. Turkey has the highest prevalence: 80–370 cases/100000. The prevalence in Japan and Iran ranges from 13.5–20 cases/100000. In Western countries it is much less common, 0.64/100000 in the UK and 0.12–0.33/100000 in the USA. It affects mainly young adults (males > females in Middle Eastern countries but vice versa in Japan) and the mean age of onset is in the third decade. The frequency in families is 2–5% except in Middle Eastern countries where it is 10–15%. As there are no definitive laboratory tests to diagnose Behçet's disease, many sets of clinical criteria have been suggested in order to make a diagnosis. The most widely used classification has been proposed by the International Study Group For Behçet's Disease. This states that the main criterion is of recurrent oral ulceration either minor, major or herpetiform which recurs at least 3 times in one 12-month period *plus* two of: (i) recurrent genital ulceration: aphthous or scarring; (ii) eye lesions: anterior/posterior uveitis, cells in vitreous; *or* retinal vasculitis; (iii) skin lesions: erythema nodosum, pseudofolliculitis or papulopustular lesions; *or* acneiform nodules in postadolescent patients not on corticosteroid treatment; (iv) positive pathergy skin test with a sterile pustule seen 24–48 hours after oblique insertion of a 20-gauge needle. The prevalence of the HLA-B51 allele is high (up to 81%) among patients who live in areas along the Silk Road as compared to Caucasian patients living in Western countries (13%). In Japan, the incidence of HLA-B51 is significantly higher among patients with than without the disease (55% vs. 10–15%). The relative risk of the disease among carriers of HLA-B51 as compared to non-carriers is 6.7 in Japan and only 1.3 in the USA.

Vascular injuries, hyperfunction of neutrophils and autoimmune responses are characteristic of Behçet's. Levels of various cytokines have been found to be elevated, and there is clonal expansion of autoreactive T cells specific for the heat shock protein 60. Recent data suggest that Factor V Leiden may be an additional risk factor for the development of ocular disease and, in particular, retinal vaso-occlusion.

An infective cause, either herpesviruses or streptoccocus has also been suggested but no infectious agent has been proved to cause Behçet's disease.

Clinical features

The commonest ocular manifestation is a sight-threatening panuveitis and retinal vasculitis. This may result in macular oedema, retinal infiltrates, branch/central retinal vein occlusion, retinal haemorrhage and oedema, diffuse capillary leakage, retinal and optic disc neovascularization that can lead to vitreous haemorrhage and subsequent retinal detachment. An anterior uveitis with recurrent hypopyon is also well recognized. Secondary cataract results from the inflammatory process, use of steroids or a combination of both. Angle closure glaucoma or secondary glaucoma due to iris neovascularization or uveitis can occur. End-stage disease is characterized by retinal atrophy, associated with optic atrophy and often markedly attenuated and sclerosed retinal vessels and often blindness. Other less common manifestations are extraocular muscle palsies that may result from cranial nerve involvement, and papilloedema following cranial venous sinus thrombosis. The frequency of ocular manifestations is about 70% and it has been estimated that in those patients whose visual acuity deteriorated to 6/60 or less in both eyes, 90% reached this level within 5 years of onset. There appears to be a group of patients with grossly asymmetrical disease, in whom one eye appears to be preserved, while the other becomes blind. The development of sight-threatening disease can be unpredictable and may occur even in those patients on large doses of immunosuppressive drugs. Other clinical manifestations include: a mono- or polyarthritis that develops in about half of patients; vascular involvement with veins more commonly involved than arteries, leading to superficial thrombophlebitis, obstruction of superior/inferior vena cava; gastrointestinal symptoms of nausea, vomiting, pain, bloody diarrhoea; epididymitis; central nervous system involvement manifesting as meningoencephalitis, intracranial hypertension, or as signs and symptoms related to brainstem, cranial nerve, pyramidal, extrapyramidal, cerebellar, spinal cord or peripheral nerve involvement.

Treatment

The literature on Behçet's disease is full of uncontrolled studies of different modalities of drug therapy. The common mainstay of treatment is systemic corticosteroid but often this is given in combination with other agents. The other drugs used to control ocular disease include: cyclosporin A, azathioprine and until recently chlorambucil. All these drugs have potentially serious side-effects. There are only two randomized controlled treatment trials, one using cyclosporin and the other azathioprine. About one-third of patients respond well to treatment, and another third appear to have the disease stabilized but not improved. About one-quarter pursue a relentless course to blindness, irrespective of the treatment given. Other drugs used for extraocular manifestations include: thalidomide which is effective for severe oral ulceration, cyclosporin for mucocutaneous lesions and colchicine appears to have a role to play in preventing acute exacerbations of the disease. Recent trials of alpha interferon have shown encouraging results, particularly for ocular disease.

Further reading

Demiroglu H, Ozcebe OI, Barista I, Dundar S, Eldem B. Interferon alfa-2b, colchicine, and benzathine penicillin versus colchicine and benzathine penicillin in Behçet's disease: a randomised trial. *Lancet* 2000; **355:** 605–9.

International Study Group For Behçet's Disease. Criteria for diagnosis of Behçet's disease. *Lancet* 1990; **335:** 1078–80.

Masuda K, Urayama A, Kogure M. Double masked trial of cyclosporin in Behçet's disease. *Lancet* 1989; **1:** 1093–5.

Sakane T, Takeno M, Suzuki N, Inaba G. Behçet's disease. *New England Journal of Medicine* 1999; **341:** 1284–91.

Whallett AJ, Thurairajan G, Hamburger J, Palmer RG, Murray PI. Behçet's syndrome: a multidisciplinary approach to clinical care. *Quarterly Journal of Medicine* 1999; **92:** 727–40.

Yazici H, Pazarli H, Barnes CG, Tuzun Y, Ozazgan Y, Silman A, Serdaroglu S, Ogaz V, Yurkadul S, Lovatt GE, Yazici B, Somani S, Muftuoglu A. A controlled trial of azathioprine in Behçet's syndrome. *New England Journal of Medicine* 1990; **322:** 281–5.

BLUNT AND PENETRATING OCULAR TRAUMA

Anthony O'Driscoll & Peter Shah

Blunt and penetrating injuries to the eyes, adnexae and orbits are common. They arise as a result of trauma in five major instances: road traffic accidents, industrial accidents, sport and recreational activities, domestic accidents and assault. Careful evaluation is required to ensure accurate assessment of the injury. It is essential not to miss any sight- or life-threatening pathology.

Problem

Trauma to the eye presents the ophthalmologist with some challenging diagnostic and management problems. The patient may have concurrent or related injuries, they may be incapable of co-operating and have eyelids firmly apposed due to ecchymotic swelling. Patients are often in severe pain and may be nauseated and difficult to examine. Children present a particular problem in that the injury may not be witnessed or inaccurately reported. Examining children thoroughly is extremely difficult and requires considerable patience. They may also be the victims of non-accidental injury, and this possibility should always be considered.

Background

Obtaining a detailed history is essential. It is vital to ask about the situation in which the injury occurred. The injury may be due to high or low velocity trauma. Objects striking the globe may be blunt or sharp. If the patient was hammering, one should ask about the types of metal or other materials involved (e.g. steel hammer on copper nail) and whether any fragments were missing after the injury. The probability of wound contamination should be assessed. Previous visual acuity should be taken into account. Any changes in vision at the time of injury and subsequently, must be recorded. It should be noted whether protective eye wear was used at the time of the injury, car seat belts were fastened or an air bag was activated.

Clinical features

The patient must undergo a general examination to identify other bodily injuries, particularly in cases of severe trauma (e.g. road traffic accidents). Ophthalmologists should consult the appropriate trauma teams promptly where necessary. The overall condition of the patient should be noted as well as the presence or the absence of a head injury. The neurosurgical team should be called early if a skull fracture or intracranial trauma is suspected. One should exclude facial fractures and involve the maxillofacial team if appropriate. Midface (Le Fort) fractures should not be missed since they can cause problems for the anaesthetist during intubation. Crush injuries to the chest may cause Purtscher's retinopathy and fractures of long bones may cause retinal fat embolization.

Full ophthalmic examination is essential, and where it is difficult, modified techniques are necessary. Some assessment of visual acuity should be measured when possible. A near reading chart or some other text may be used in difficult cases. When the eyelids are impossible to open, a bright light directed through them may demonstrate light perception and possibly accurate projection. Visual fields assessed by confrontation help to identify retinal and neurological problems. Orbital fractures should be suspected when ocular movements are reduced or when the position of the globe has been altered. Examining for a relative afferent pupillary defect with a bright light is essential. Slit-lamp examination (stationary or hand-held) should be attempted in every patient. The Perkins tonometer, or a Tonopen, may be used in the case of the immobilized patient. Both pupils must be dilated at an appropriate time in all patients to facilitate fundus examination, even in the mildest of injuries. The time of instillation and the type of mydriatic used must be recorded clearly. The neurosurgeons should be contacted in those patients under neurosurgical observation prior to using any mydriatic agent.

CT and MRI are the optimal imaging techniques. However, if not readily available, plain skull and facial X-rays are the first line of investigation when necessary. Waters' view will demonstrate the maxillary sinus and orbital floor, the Caldwell view the orbit and Rhese view the optic foramina. They must be interpreted with caution and their limitations appreciated. One should always insist on viewing them personally and obtaining a radiologist's opinion. Ultrasound examination of the eye should be performed when the view of the fundus is obscured. Swabs taken from contaminated wounds will help to guide antibiotic therapy.

There are a wide variety of problems that may be encountered in patients who have sustained blunt or penetrating ocular trauma. Some of the more important problems are discussed below.

1.   *Eyelid lacerations.* A blunt injury may avulse a medial or lateral canthal ligament and repair will be required to establish the correct preorbital architecture. It is important to note whether the lid margin is involved in the laceration. An apparently simple eyelid laceration may overlie a much more serious injury, such as penetration of the globe, orbit or anterior/middle cranial fossae. The latter is particularly worrisome in puncture wounds of the upper lid. Special care should be taken to identify injuries to the canalicular system and lacrimal apparatus when the injury involves the medial canthal region. An experienced ophthalmologist or ocuplastic surgeon should undertake these repairs.

2.   *Tense orbital haemorrhage.* Severe periorbital haemorrhage will cause tight closure of the eyelids. If the haemorrhage is severe, differentiating it from an intraorbital haemorrhage is difficult. CT or MRI can be very useful in making this distinction. When an intraorbital haemorrhage develops, the eyelids are extremely tense, the globe may proptose and haemorrhagic and oedematous conjunctiva may prolapse through a narrow palpebral fissure. If the lids can be opened, useful information such as the visual acuity, ocular movements and the presence of a relative afferent pupillary defect can be obtained. Caution must always be taken not to apply pressure on the lids, because the globe may have been ruptured.

The effects of raised intraorbital pressure may be reduced by administering intravenous acetazolamide, or mannitol in more severe cases, to decompress medically the orbit. If medical treatment appears unsatisfactory then urgent surgical decompression will be necessary, either by lateral canthotomy or by trans-septal orbitotomy. An intraconal or intrasheath haemorrhage may require a lateral orbitotomy.

3.   *Subconjunctival haemorrhage.* Any subconjunctival haemorrhage may mask an underlying scleral rupture or perforation especially when 360°. Differentiation from a simple conjunctival contusion may be difficult. A penetrating injury must be suspected in the presence of an associated conjunctival laceration. If there is any doubt, surgical exploration is essential. A subconjunctival haemorrhage continuous with the inferior fornix may also be the only sign of an orbital blow-out fracture.

4.   *Corneal laceration.* Partial thickness wounds should be thoroughly examined to ensure that they are not perforating. Seidel test using fluorescein applied directly to the wound will help to expose occult penetrations. A focal defect on iris trans-illumination may indicate extension of the injury into the posterior segment. Primary repair under general anaesthesia must be performed urgently if the wound is not sealed. Where the corneal limbus is involved, peritomy is recommended to exclude scleral extension of the wound.

5.   *Traumatic hyphaema.* In cases of traumatic hyphaema, the ophthalmologist should examine for associated angle recession, iridodialysis, cyclodialysis, lens subluxation or dislocation and retinal dialysis. This will be difficult if blood obscures these structures. Gonioscopy should be delayed for 7 days to prevent further haemorrhage. If there is no fundal view, ultrasound examination is necessary to identify injuries to the posterior segment. Corneal blood staining may occur when the hyphaema is total and the intraocular pressure (IOP) exceeds 25 mmHg for 6 days. This may occur sooner with higher pressures.

The main advantages of mydriasis and cycloplegia are to facilitate early posterior segment examination and reduce the pain of associated traumatic uveitis. Once the pupil has been dilated it should be kept dilated to avoid undue movement of the iris.

Rebleeding usually occurs within a week, affecting about 5% of cases. Visual acuity of 6/60 or worse, raised IOP on presentation, an initial hyphaema greater than one-third and delayed presentation all have been shown to be associated with an increased chance of a rebleed. Patients who rebleed should be admitted to hospital. The value of bedrest has been debated. In some cases antifibrinolytics may decrease the chance of rebleeding. Patients in high-risk ethnic groups should be screened for haemoglobinopathies.

6.   *Drainage angle and iris injuries.* Angle recession must always be suspected in cases of blunt trauma. Deepening of the anterior chamber and iris recession are often associated with angle injuries. Corresponding sections of the drainage angles of each eye may be compared by gonioscopy. About 10% of patients with more than 180° of angle recession will develop secondary glaucoma, sometimes years later. However, patients who apparently have lesser degrees of damage may also develop raised IOP. Angle recession glaucoma is less common in children.

Traumatic mydriasis may result in reduced visual acuity or glare. Iridodialysis may be missed unless the iris is examined by transillumination.

7. *Low intraocular pressure.* When the IOP is low or there is an interocular difference in IOP, scleral perforation and retinal detachment must be excluded. Blunt trauma to the ciliary body with cyclodialysis or choroidal detachment may also cause a low IOP. One should not rely on a solitary IOP measurement, and if one is unsure the IOPs should be checked serially.

8. *Lens damage.* Phakodonesis, iridodonesis and a deepened anterior chamber are warning signs of lens subluxation. An anteriorly dislocated lens may cause pupil block and raised IOP. Traumatic cataract may occur immediately or may only become significant years later.

9. *Scleral perforation or rupture.* A thorough history and meticulous examination are required in all cases of ocular trauma, as occasionally a scleral perforation or rupture may occur in the presence of minimal clinical signs. Chemosis may be present with reduced extraocular movements. Ultrasound examination may assist diagnosis when there is a poor view of the globe or fundus. It should be done gently by an experienced operator so that prolapse of the uvea and vitreous may be avoided. Valsalva manoeuvres and periorbital pressure may also cause loss of globe contents. Anti-emetics may be given per rectum, iv or im but in children all efforts should be made to avoid upsetting the child. Rapid progression to examination under general anaesthesia is preferred. The eye and orbit should be protected with a shield but not a pad. A regimen of broad-spectrum systemic antibiotics should be considered. Surgical repair under general anaesthesia should be undertaken as soon as possible. A peritomy should be performed and the sclera examined thoroughly. The sclera is most likely to rupture at its thinnest points located at the corneo-scleral junction and posterior to the muscle insertions.

A double perforating injury may complicate any penetrating eye injury and should always be suspected even if a foreign body is located within the globe. A second perforation may be obscured by vitreous haemorrhage. A through-and-through injury of globe may also be accompanied by an orbital wall penetration. Failure to restore intraocular pressure at surgery may be a sign of an unrecognized posterior rupture.

10. *Intraocular foreign body.* An intraocular foreign body (IOFB) must be suspected in all cases of penetrating eye injury. Patients may present with IOFBs and yet may have minimal symptoms and signs, including normal vision after they have been using hammers or power tools. An IOFB may be missed if located in the iridocorneal angle, ciliary body or pars plana. Anteroposterior and lateral orbital X-rays (in up- and down-gaze) may be helpful to identify an IOFB although CT scan is preferred. Late presentation of IOFB may be with clinical features of siderosis or chalcosis.

11. *Vitroretinal injury.* Vitreous haemorrhage may either completely obscure the view of the posterior segment or may prevent a complete and thorough examination of the retina. Retinal detachment may occur initially or as a later event in the case of vitreous haemorrhage. The patient may not notice further visual deterioration and frequent clinical assessments are necessary to detect the development of a retinal detachment. Serial ultrasound examinations are useful until the retina can be adequately visualized. Thorough examination by indirect ophthalmoscopy with scleral indentation will be essential when the view is cleared. Particular attention should be paid to the inferotemporal and superonasal periphery, where most dialyses are located. Retinal holes or tears may be obscured by associated retinal haemorrhages, and follow up must be frequent until the haemorrhages have disappeared and retinal tears have been excluded by 360° scleral indentation. The presence of a choroidal rupture is also a sign of severe ocular trauma and may cause a serious permanent visual defect if the fovea or maculopapillary bundle are involved.

12. **Optic nerve injuries.** The optic nerve may be contused, avulsed, transected or compressed at the orbital apex. In cases of optic nerve avulsion it is important to examine the fellow eye for visual field defects that may result from chiasmal damage. Clinical diagnosis of an optic nerve injury is often difficult and CT or MRI is required to demonstrate the presence of a lesion. In some cases of traumatic optic neuropathy high-dose systemic steroids may be beneficial.

13. **Orbital foreign body.** Care should be taken to identify patients who may have an orbital foreign body. An orbital foreign body may be present with minimal external signs, perhaps just a small eyelid puncture wound. Radiolucent foreign bodies are difficult to detect on plain film X-rays and further investigations may be necessary. MRI may be helpful. Systemic antibiotics should be considered in all cases to prevent orbital cellulitis.

14. **Other sequelae.** Amblyopia may occur in children in whom prolonged hyphaema or corneal scarring has obscured the visual axis. Axial corneal scarring or astigmatism from penetrating wounds may have the same effect. Infectious endophthalmitis may follow any penetrating trauma and patients must be followed closely so that it will be detected at an early stage. Although rare, one should always remember the possibility of sympathetic ophthalmitis. Since early recognition is essential, both eyes should always be examined periodically. Patients should be instructed to report promptly any visual changes or redress in their good eye.

Conclusion

The importance of good management in ocular trauma cannot be over emphasized. A combination of detailed history, thorough examination and good clinical judgement are essential. The use of investigations should be well considered. Planned medical and surgical intervention will ensure that even severely injured eyes may obtain reasonable vision.

Further reading

Beatty RL (ed.) Ocular trauma. *Seminars in Ophthalmology* 1994; **9**: 143–228.

Eagling EM, Roper-Hall MJ. *Eye Injuries – an Illustrated Guide.* London: Gower Medical Publishing, 1986.

Fong LP. Secondary hemorrhage in traumatic hyphema. Predictive factors for selective prophylaxis. *Ophthalmology* 1994; **101**: 1583–8.

Levin LA, Beck RW, Joseph MP, Seiff S, Kraker R. The treatment of traumatic optic neuropathy: the International Optic Nerve Trauma Study. *Ophthalmology* 1999; **106**(7): 1268–77.

Ng CS, Sparrow JM, Strong NP, Rosenthal AR. Factors related to the final visual outcome of 425 patients with traumatic hyphaema. *Eye* 1992; **6:** 305–7.

Pavan-Langston D. Burns and trauma. In: Pavan-Langston D (ed.) *Manual of Ocular Diagnosis and Therapy*, 3rd edn. Boston: Little, Brown and Co., 1991; 31–45.

Pieramici DJ, Sternberg P Jr, Aaberg TM Sr *et al.* A system for classifying mechanical injuries of the eye (globe). The Ocular Trauma Classification Group. *American Journal of Ophthalmology* 1997; **123**(6): 820–31.

Related topics of interest

Orbital blow-out fractures (p. 222); Shaken baby syndrome (p. 285).

CAROTICO-CAVERNOUS FISTULA

Peter Shah

A carotico-cavernous fistula (CCF) results from an abnormal communication between the internal carotid arterial system and the cavernous sinus. The key to understanding the types and clinical manifestations of CCF is to consider the anatomy of the branches of the intra-cavernous internal carotid artery (ICA), and their anastomoses with neighbouring meningeal arteries.

The ICA enters the posterior dural cavernous sinus, arching upwards then forwards, grooving the medial wall of the sinus to exit superiorly just medial to the anterior clinoid process. The intra-cavernous ICA gives off three main branches, the cavernous, the hypophyseal and meningeal branches. The thin-walled secondary and tertiary branches of these vessels lie in the dural walls of the cavernous sinus. Some of these branches anastomose with the branches of the middle meningeal artery.

Any of these vessels may rupture and cause misdirection of the arterial blood into the cavernous venous sinusoids, with varying clinical effects.

Because of the potential connections between the right and left cavernous sinuses the ophthalmic features of CCF may be ipsilateral, bilateral or contralateral.

Ophthalmologists are confronted with the problems of diagnosing and identifying the types of CCF. The types of fistulae may be divided on the basis of aetiology, haemodynamics or angiographic findings.

- Aetiology: congenital, spontaneous or traumatic.
- Haemodynamics: high flow and low flow.
- Angiography: direct fistula and indirect (dural) fistula.

Direct, high-flow fistulae result when arterial blood from the main trunk of the ICA ruptures into the cavernous sinus. Indirect, low-flow (dural) fistulae result when arterial blood from one of the smaller branches of the ICA ruptures into the sinus.

> **1. Direct.**   High-flow fistulae often result from trauma with basal skull fractures and tend to occur in young men. High-flow fistulae produce a rapid onset of clinical features. Patients may present with pain, proptosis, diplopia and reduced vision.
>
> Signs include reduced visual acuity, chemosis, vessel engorgement, pulsatile proptosis, restriction of extraocular movement, raised intraocular pressure and the presence of an ocular bruit. Additional signs of anterior segment ischaemia with corneal oedema, anterior uveitis, iris rubeosis and lens opacity may be present. Orbital ultrasound and computed tomography may show dilated ophthalmic veins. Neurological referral is necessary and carotid angiography will demonstrate the abnormal anatomical communication.
>
> The fistula may close spontaneously but if treatment is necessary then various options exist. Ligation of the ipsilateral carotid artery in the neck, direct surgery on the cavernous sinus, and angiographically controlled embolization have all been used.
>
> **2. Indirect.**   Low-flow fistulae tend to occur more commonly in middle-aged women and are associated with medical conditions such as hypertension. Because

the arterial flow rate is slower, the onset of symptoms and signs may be more insidious. Features tend to be less dramatic than direct fistulae and hypoxic ocular sequelae are less common. The possibility of a low-flow fistula should be considered in patients who present with an insidious onset red eye. Patients may not have an audible bruit. Most cases will recover without the need for surgical intervention.

Hypoxic ocular sequelae affecting the anterior and posterior segments are the main ocular complications. Proptosis can lead to exposure keratopathy. Patients may also develop occlusive cerebrovascular complications after a CCF.

Further reading

Grove AS. The dural shunt syndrome. Pathophysiology and clinical course. *Ophthalmology* 1984; **91**: 31.
Leonard TJ, Moseley IF, Sanders MD. Ophthalmoplegia in carotid cavernous sinus fistula. *British Journal of Ophthalmology* 1984; **68**: 128–34.
Spector RH. Echographic diagnosis of dural carotid-cavernous sinus fistulas. *American Journal of Ophthalmology* 1991; **111**: 77–83.

Related topic of interest

Carotid artery disease (p. 30).

CAROTID ARTERY DISEASE

Graham Venables

In the population at risk of stroke, atheroembolic disease of the great vessels accounts for about 50% of all cases of ischaemic stroke. Disease of the heart, of which atrial fibrillation is the commonest, accounts for much of the remainder.

Problem

Atheromatous narrowing commonly occurs at the bifurcation of the internal and external carotid arteries, though atheromatous disease of the aorta and distal internal carotid artery is common and may also be responsible for stroke. Ischaemia may result from low flow when the stenosis is critical or there is complete occlusion. Alternatively, emboli may be discharged from biologically active atheromatous plaque. Their contents include cholesterol, calcific material and fibrin platelet aggregations. In younger patients either spontaneously or, not infrequently, as a result of trauma (e.g. following road traffic accident or neck manipulation), carotid dissection is responsible for symptoms.

Clinical features

Patients with carotid artery disease may have symptoms due to ischaemia of the eye or the brain or local damage to the artery.

(a) Transient cerebral ischaemia is a focal neurological deficit of ischaemic origin lasting < 24 h. Symptoms include a contralateral weakness involving the face and arm or leg and either a language disorder or other cortical deficits depending on the side. Episodes of hemiparesis or hemisensory loss involving the face, arm and leg are usually due to small vessel occlusion causing subcortical white matter ischaemia and are not usually related to large vessel occlusive disease.

(b) A stroke is an evolving clinical syndrome characterized by rapidly developing clinical symptoms and/or signs of focal (or global) loss of cerebral function with symptoms lasting more than 24 hours or leading to death with no apparent cause other than that of vascular origin. Minor stroke has symptoms lasting > 24 hours and < 7 days. Major disabling or non-disabling stroke has symptoms persisting more than 7 days.

(c) Transient monocular blindness (amaurosis fugax) which may be described as like a shutter falling, a curtain being drawn or vision dimming. Episodes usually last only a few minutes.

(d) Central retinal artery and branch retinal arteriolar occlusion may cause persisting visual loss.

(e) Retinal hypoperfusion with haemorrhages, microaneurysms, dilated veins, choroidal perfusion defects and neovascularization may occur.

(f) Horner's syndrome can be due to damage to the sympathetic nerves surrounding the internal carotid artery.

(g) Pain in and around the neck, face or eye is due to distension or damage to the ipsilateral internal carotid artery.

Patients with threatened stroke (i.e. those with transient retinal or neurological syndromes) may be at high risk of second, more devastating events. The presence or absence of a carotid bruit is no guide to those who might be at risk since patients with high-risk high-grade stenosis may only have a quiet high-pitched bruit which is often inaudible, and bruits not infrequently arise from other structures within the neck. Clues as to the presence of a carotid dissection occlusion may come from the presence of a Horner's syndrome, an absent carotid pulsation, low retinal arterial pressure, enlarged pulsatile superficial temporal and epitrochlear arteries.

Major risk factors for inflammatory and athero-embolic disease should be defined including: diabetes mellitus, hypertension, cardiac disease including ischaemic disease, valvular disease, atrial fibrillation or peripheral vascular disease.

Investigations should include: full blood count, differential white count, platelets and erythrocyte sedimentation rate, blood chemistry, glucose and cholesterol, tissue autoantibodies and tests for syphilis, electrocardiogram and chest radiograph. Non-invasive carotid artery imaging using either an ultrasound-based technique or magnetic resonance angiography depending on local availability, is essential.

Brain imaging should be undertaken in all those with focal neurological symptoms or signs to demonstrate haemorrhage or alternative confounding pathology as well as to define the distribution of the ischaemic lesion.

Treatment

All patients should be advised about lifestyle issues and risk factor modification to reduce the risk of all forms of vascular disease including: cessation of smoking, control of diabetes and blood pressure, cholesterol lowering if serum cholesterol > 6.0 mmol/l. Patients should be told not to drive for one month after their event and to notify the DVLA. A risk reduction of about 20% can be achieved using antiplatelet drugs, either aspirin 75 mg daily, or combination therapy with aspirin and modified release persantin 200 mg (Grade A recommendation) if attacks continue. Patients with minor stroke or retinal infarction in whom there is aspirin intolerance may also be considered for clopidogrel 75 mg daily (Grade A recommendation). Anticoagulants can be used to achieve a risk reduction of 66% only in patients in whom atrial fibrillation is thought to be the cause of the event and are not indicated in any other group of patients with stroke.

Patients with recently symptomatic high-grade carotid stenosis should be considered for urgent carotid intervention. Those with high-grade irregular stenosis and those having recent (within 2 months) cerebral events are at greater risk of stroke than those having ocular events. Carotid endarterectomy has been shown to reduce the risk of subsequent stroke and with appropriate selection as few as three patients need to be treated to prevent one stroke. Conversely, those with lesser degrees of stenosis and less recent events are at much less risk and many more operations need to be done to prevent a single stroke. An endovascular approach with angioplasty and stenting is an alternative method of treatment for patients unable to tolerate the risks of surgery, though, at present the procedure requires further evaluation of safety and efficacy. Patients with asymptomatic disease do not require surgery but should undergo risk factor modification and be offered antiplatelet therapy. It is customary to offer patients with carotid dissection anticoagulants until the arterial wall has healed. No randomized trials exist to support this view and at present this practice cannot be recommended on a routine basis.

Prognosis

Important independent predictors of stroke, myocardial infarction and vascular death include recent frequent cerebral (as opposed to ocular) events in older people, especially men, and those with peripheral vascular disease or left ventricular hypertrophy. Thus a woman of 75 with a single episode of transient monocular blindness within the previous three months, no other vascular disease or residual signs has a 1 year risk of stroke in the region of 3% rising to 8% in 5 years. A male of 55, however, with a minor stroke, left ventricular hypertrophy and intermittent claudication has a risk of 40% at 1 year and 80% at 5 years. Risk reduction and operative intervention therefore carries very different benefits in each of these groups and should be tailored to their individual needs.

Further reading

Warlow CP *et al.* 2000. *Stroke: a Practical Guide to Management.* Blackwell Science Ltd.

CATARACT SURGERY IN UVEITIS

Philip I. Murray

Cataract is a common complication of uveitis. It occurs at a younger age than the general population and is related to lens permeability changes resulting from chronic intraocular inflammation, systemic corticosteroid treatment or a combination of both.

Problem

Cataract surgery in these patients has always been undertaken with caution due to technical difficulties and risk of post-operative exacerbation of inflammation. Recent advances have contributed to safer and more successful surgical intervention in these eyes. These advances include a better understanding of the pathogenesis of the various uveitis syndromes, use of systemic drugs other than corticosteroids to control inflammation, improved microsurgical techniques, and new designs and materials of intraocular lenses. The indications for cataract surgery in patients with uveitis are visual disability or lens opacities obscuring visualization of the posterior segment. Pre-existing macular pathology should not necessarily be a contraindication for surgery. There are a number of important factors that must be considered before surgery is undertaken. These are: the timing of surgery, the pre- and post-operative medical management, the choice of surgical procedure and the type of intraocular lens to be implanted.

Background

Establish an accurate diagnosis as prognosis may depend on the type of uveitis syndrome, e.g. Fuchs' heterochromic cyclitis (FHC) patients are more likely to have a better visual outcome. Draw up a plan of management and manage each patient according to their individual circumstances. Explain this plan and the potential risks of surgery to the patient. It is important that the patient understands that surgery needs to be performed under the best possible circumstances. In those cases where visualization of the fundus is difficult, B scan ultrasound and electrodiagnostic testing may be of value. In some patients the latter may allow a prediction of outcome of surgery. Decide on the type of anaesthesia – many younger patients prefer a general anaesthetic.

Maximum control of the intraocular inflammation (less than 1 + anterior chamber cells) is critical and should be achieved for a minimum period of three months prior to cataract surgery. In patients with chronic inflammation, it may be almost impossible to eradicate all anterior chamber activity, as residual flare may be present as a result of chronic blood-aqueous barrier breakdown rather than active inflammation. To control inflammation prior to surgery introduction of systemic therapy such as oral steroids or other immunosuppressives may be necessary. In cases with co-existing glaucoma the intraocular pressure should be adequately controlled before proceeding to cataract surgery.

Immediately prior to surgery, it is usual for patients to have an increase in medical therapy to protect against any increase in inflammatory activity in the per-operative, immediate and early postoperative periods. This additional therapy may depend on the type of uveitis the patient has. In patients with history of recurrent inflammation of the anterior segment that has been quiescent for several years then intensive topical steroids for one to two weeks prior to surgery may be sufficient. In patients with chronic inflammation of the posterior segment such as intermediate uveitis, panuveitis with or without retinal vasculitis who already require systemic immunosuppression an increase of the maintenance steroid dose (to 40 mg/day) or introduction of oral prednisolone (40 mg/day) 2 weeks prior to surgery is an option. The use of non-enteric coated prednisolone is preferred as absorption may be erratic with the enteric-coated preparation. Care must be taken in patients also suffering with diabetes mellitus as the increase in steroid dose is likely to upset their diabetic control. Other authors suggest a combination of prednisolone (1 mg/kg/day) and oral diflunisal (500 mg twice daily) for 2 days prior to surgery, or 0.5 mg/kg/day oral prednisolone for 3 days pre-operatively or a pulse of i.v. methyl-prednisolone 500 mg–1 g in the immediate pre-operative period. Patients with FHC usually do well following cataract surgery and it is not usually necessary to suppress the inflammatory response for 3 months prior to surgery or to give any additional topical or systemic steroid just before surgery.

Clinical features

As with any type of cataract surgery pupil dilation is important. Apart from the standard preoperative dilating drops, the addition of a topical non-steroidal may be useful in maintaining mydriasis throughout surgery. Adrenaline in the infusion will also be advantageous. Adhesions between the iris and lens, and pupillary membranes can often be dissected mechanically: synechiolysis with a micro-spatula and the use of viscoelastics, disposable iris hooks (retractors) or pupil stretching also offer a relatively atraumatic approach particularly in combination with a high viscosity viscoelastic. Sphincterotomies or a sector iridotomy (following a peripheral iridectomy) can be performed but may result in a greater post-operative inflammatory response.

Phakoemulsification is the procedure of choice. A clear corneal incision may be a better approach than a scleral tunnel, particularly in patients with associated scleral thinning from scleritis. It may also facilitate future drainage surgery if required as there is no conjunctival or episcleral scarring.

A well-centred capsulorhexis with a minimum diameter of 5–6 mm is recommended. Too small a rhexis may result in phimosis postoperatively. Meticulous aspiration to remove all cortical material is important to avoid postoperative lens-induced inflammation, fibrotic capsule contraction and posterior capsule opacification. A sub-conjunctival injection of steroid is given at the completion of surgery.

Choice of intraocular lens

Many papers have shown that it is safe to implant intraocular lenses (IOL) in adults with uveitis. There is some evidence to show that a rigid heparin-surface-modified implant may have better biocompatibility in an uveitic eye. However, one recent study has shown that phakoemulsification with a foldable implant can give excellent results in these eyes. Using an acrylic, hydrogel or silicone foldable, at final follow-up

56/60 eyes (93.3%) had an improvement in visual acuity compared to pre-operative levels, 34 (56.6%) achieved an improvement of ≥ four Snellen lines and 44 eyes (73.3%) achieved 6/9 or better. No real differences were identified between the types of biomaterial implanted.

Postoperative management

The most common complications after cataract surgery are an exacerbation of inflammation, fibrin membrane formation, posterior synechiae formation, rise in intraocular pressure, inflammatory deposits on the optic of the IOL, and posterior capsule opacification. Post-operative or exacerbation of pre-operative cystoid macular oedema is also more common in patients with uveitis. Anterior capsular contraction syndrome has been reported. Unfortunately, some eyes will develop post-operative complications whatever implant material is used, whether it is rigid or foldable.

Intensive topical steroids, often with a short-acting mydriatic at night, are recommended and may be required for several months according to the individual response. It is important not to reduce the topical therapy too quickly as this may result in a rebound increase in anterior segment inflammation which could lead to inflammatory deposits on the optic of the IOL and posterior synechiae formation. Systemic steroids are also tapered according to the inflammation (usually decreased by 5–10 mg/week) until they are either stopped (if they were initiated pre-operatively) or reach the preoperative maintenance dose.

Raised intraocular pressure should be managed medically. Examination of the angle is mandatory to try and ascertain the reason for the rise in pressure.

YAG laser can be used to remove foreign body and giant cells on the optic but in the majority of cases these cells return and 'polishing' of the optic may need to be undertaken on numerous occasions.

Posterior capsular opacification occurs more frequently in uveitic eyes (up to 80% in one series) but this does not mean that all these eyes require YAG laser capsulotomy. Although laser capsulotomy is a common procedure it is not without its possible (occasionally sight-threatening) complications. It is not a procedure that should be undertaken lightly in uveitic eyes. Indications are eyes that see 6/12 or worse or occasionally 6/9 and are symptomatic, or where visualization of the posterior segment is difficult. As laser treatment may exacerbate anterior segment inflammation it is usual to wait at least 6 months following surgery. Laser capsulotomy should not be performed in an eye with active inflammation and the eye should usually be quiet for a minimum of 2 months prior to laser. All eyes should receive intensive topical steroid for at least 2 weeks following laser. Prophylactic topical α-2 agonist or oral acetazolamide can also be given to prevent a pressure rise. The smallest amount of energy possible should be used and techniques may need to be altered according to the type of implant. If a silicone lens has been implanted then great care must be taken not to crack the optic.

Conclusion

One of the most important factors influencing the visual outcome following cataract surgery in patients with uveitis appears to be the meticulous control of inflammation both pre- and postoperatively. By having a planned approach, timing the surgery appropriately, using the most appropriate techniques and choice of IOL, the majority of uveitis patients will benefit greatly from cataract extraction. Phakoemulsification is preferred. The use of foldable IOLs in eyes with uveitis does not appear to add more risk, but the optimal biomaterial has yet to be found.

Further reading

Akova YA, Foster CS. Cataract surgery in patients with sarcoidosis-associated uveitis. *Ophthalmology* 1994; **101**: 473–9.

Barton K, Hall AJH, Rosen PH, Cooling RJ, Lightman S. Systemic steroid prophylaxis for cataract surgery in patients with posterior uveitis. *Ocular Immunol Inflamm* 1994; **4**: 207–16.

Foster CS, Fong LP, Singh G. Cataract surgery and intraocular lens implantation in patients with uveitis. *Ophthalmology* 1989; **96**: 281–8.

Hooper PL, Rao NA, Smith REP. Cataract extraction in uveitis patients. *Surv Ophthalmol* 1990; **35**: 120–44.

O'Neill D, Murray PI, Patel BC, Hamilton AMP. Extracapsular cataract surgery with and without intraocular lens implantation in Fuchs heterochromic cyclitis. *Ophthalmology* 1995; **102**: 1362–8.

Rauz S, Stavrou P, Murray PI. Evaluation of foldable intraocular lenses in patients with uveitis. *Ophthalmology* 2000; **107**: 909–19.

Rojas B, Foster CS. Cataract surgery in patients with uveitis. *Curr Opin Ophthalmol* 1996; **7**: 11–16.

Stavrou P, Murray PI. Heparin surface modified intraocular lenses in uveitis. *Ocular Immunol Inflamm* 1994; **2**: 161–8.

CENTRAL SEROUS RETINOPATHY (CSR OR CENTRAL SEROUS CHORIORETINOPATHY)

Ben Burton & Peter Shah

Central serous retinopathy (CSR) also known as central serous chorioretinopathy, is a neurosensory retinal detachment attributed to fluid leakage at the level of the retinal pigment epithelium.

Problem

This diagnosis is easily missed if a careful history and detailed fundus examination are not performed (preferably with a 60D lens or a fundus contact lens). In particular it can be confused with optic neuritis if there is little subretinal fluid, as the patient will often notice colour desaturation and a central or paracentral scotoma. Other symptoms are blurred vision and metamorphopsia (which can suggest macular disease) and hence choroidal neovascularization (CNV) also needs to be excluded. The management of patients with CSR is still an area of some controversy. Laser treatment has a role only in selected cases and steroids should be avoided.

Background

There is usually no obvious cause for the leakage. It typically occurs in the 20- to 45-year-old age group with males 8 times more likely to be affected than females. Patients are more likely to have type A personalities and conversional neurosis than non-affected individuals and are more likely to use psychopharmacologic medication. A disturbing psychological event was reported to precede the onset of CSR in 90% of patients. Recently systemic hypertension has also been shown to be associated with CSR. Pregnancy is known to increase the risk for CSR. Systemic and inhaled steroids have also been implicated as a cause for some cases. Solid organ transplantation has rarely been reported in association with CSR.

Elevated catecholamine levels are thought to be important in the pathogenesis as are nitric oxide, prostaglandins and free radicals which could induce anomalous autoregulation of choroidal blood flow resulting in ischaemia. Indocyanine green angiograms show delayed choroidal arterial filling, capillary and venous dilatation and vascular hyperpermeability. This may be due to thrombotic occlusion of the choroidal veins. Retinal pigment epithelium (RPE) dysfunction has also been postulated as an important factor although this may be secondary to the choroidal blood flow changes.

Clinical features

Symptoms usually develop acutely and patients present with mild blurring of vision or metamorphopsia. Most patients have relatively well preserved visual acuity at about 6/9 but it can fall to as low as 6/60. In some cases a +1.00 D lens in front of the affected eye may improve acuity as this corrects the acquired hypermetropia caused by elevation of the retina. Contact lens examination using a moving, thin bright slit of light can make the retinal elevation more obvious. Red free light may also make examination easier and aids the detection of retinal haemorrhages. The presence of haemorrhages alerts one to the possibility of choroidal neovascularization. A relative afferent pupillary defect favours optic neuritis over CSR but it can rarely occur in CSR as well.

The typical clinical appearance is of a well-demarcated round, shallow serous retinal detachment found at the macula with loss of the foveal reflex. The serous fluid can be cloudy. There may also be an underlying RPE detachment with pigment migration particularly in chronic cases. Occasionally multiple small serous detachments may occur in the mid-periphery of the retina. Detachments vary in size from being barely detectable to several disc diameters across. There is no evidence of ocular inflammation and the condition is usually unilateral (80%).

When examining patients it is important to look for an optic disc pit as the management of CSR is different in these patients. Other reported causes and associations of serous retinal detachments include tilted discs, disc coloboma, choroidal tumour, malignant hypertension, eclampsia and inflammatory conditions such as Vogt–Koyanagi–Harada syndrome (particularly if bilateral), Systemic lupus erythematosis (SLE) and scleritis. Hence it is essential to perform a thorough examination of the anterior and posterior segments and to check the patient's blood pressure.

A fluorescein angiogram can give much useful additional information. The classic finding is the 'smoke stack' appearance of a focal leak through the RPE; the dye slowly filling the space of the serous retinal detachment. However, 90% of cases do not show a classical 'smoke stack' but instead have a slow diffuse filling of the serous detachment through one or more focal leakage points. In chronic CSR, atrophy and pigment mottling of the RPE may be present with areas of granular hyperfluorescence and this may be referred to as diffuse retinal pigment epitheliopathy. Some authorities consider chronic CSR to be a different condition to acute or recurrent CSR. In some cases it may be difficult to tell whether the diagnosis is CNV or CSR in which case sequential clinical examinations and repeat angiography should be performed over a period of several weeks.

Fortunately many cases of CSR resolve spontaneously. Spontaneous resolution of the serous detachment usually occurs by 4 months and visual acuity can continue to improve for up to a year after that. The vision usually recovers to near normal levels (about 6/9), hence many patients require no treatment. However, 50% of all patients suffer recurrences and a few patients develop a chronic form of CSR. Patients with chronic CSR do not respond well to laser treatment and usually follow a slowly progressive course with the vision deteriorating to around 6/36 over several months. No medication has conclusively been shown to be effective in this condition, although acetazolamide and beta-blockers have been tried without convincing results. The recent association of hypertension with CSR suggests that active control of hypertension may be beneficial.

Laser photocoagulation directly to the site of leakage may hasten the resolution of the serous detachment, but the effects on recurrence rate and long-term visual outcome are debated. Laser can be considered if the patient has persistently reduced visual function on follow up, although the optimum time for intervention has not been determined. It is reasonable to consider treating CSR which is not resolving spontaneously after 4 to 6 months, or which is characterized by recurrent episodes when previous episodes have resulted in permanent decrease in visual acuity in either eye and when chronic changes, such as cystoid macular oedema appear to be developing. Laser photocoagulation of CSR is a specialist area and an evolving area of practice. The risk of developing CNV following laser treatment is 2–5% which may be a little higher than the risk in non-treated patients.

Vitrectomy, gas tamponade and barrier laser treatment (between the optic disc and the fovea) have been used to treat CSR associated with optic disc pits. In these patients the subretinal fluid is thought to come from the vitreous through a tiny hole in the diaphenous tissue overlying the disc pit rather than from abnormal RPE and choroidal function. Very few patients have been treated in this way as it is a very rare condition. However initial results have been encouraging.

Inferior hemisphere retinal detachment can sometimes be found in association with CSR. If the detachment has spontaneously reattached then RPE atrophy and occasionally bone spicules may be seen. Of these few patients with evidence of a previous inferior hemisphere detachment, 25% will be left with acuity of 6/60 or worse in the affected eye. Other causes of visual loss in CSR include cystoid macular oedema or the development of CNV which may progress to disciform scarring. Excessive laser treatment has the potential to cause CNV formation or visual loss from direct retinal damage when treating lesions near the fovea, or damage to the papillomacular bundle.

Further reading

Ficker L, Vafidis G, While A, Leaver P. Long-term follow-up of a prospective trial of argon laser photo-coagulation in the treatment of central serous retinopathy. *British Journal of Ophthalmology* 1988; **72**: 829–34.

Iijima H, Iida T, Murayama K *et al.* Plasminogen activator inhibitor 1 in central serous chorioretinopathy. *American Journal of Ophthalmology* 1999; **127**(4): 477–8.

Postel EA, Pulido JS, McNamara JA, Johnson MW. The etiology and treatment of macular detachment associated with optic nerve pits and related anomalies. *Transactions of the American Ophthalmology Society* 1998; **96**: 73–88. Discussion 88–93.

Tittl MK, Spaide RF, Wong D *et al.* Systemic findings associated with central serous chorioretinopathy. *American Journal of Ophthalmology* 1999; **128**(1): 63–8.

CHILD ABUSE

Alex V. Levin

Millions of children are victims of child abuse each year throughout the world. This epidemic has been taking place for centuries and cuts across all cultural, ethnic, socioeconomic, gender and racial groups. Almost all countries have laws, which require physicians to report their suspicion of child abuse to the appropriate agencies to ensure the protection of potential child victims. Child abuse is usually divided into four sub-types: physical abuse, sexual abuse, child neglect and emotional abuse.

Problem

The ophthalmologist may be faced with situations in which findings suggest possible abuse. Although the examining eye doctor has an obligation to report their suspicion of abuse, there is also a desire to avoid unnecessary and inaccurate reporting. If the child has been abused, then the physician may be called upon to provide documentation, or even legal testimony, as to the medical findings that support the diagnosis.

Background

In all forms of abuse, there is a wide spectrum of behaviour some of which may be considered acceptable by some elements of the population, and other behaviours that are in a 'grey zone'. However, there is always clearly an end of the spectrum in which abuse is easily recognized by the majority. There are many segments of society (this author not included) who believe that spanking is an acceptable form of child discipline. Yet discipline which results in fractures or death is clearly unacceptable. Child abuse may represent an act of omission or commission. Failure to appropriately ensure the safety of a child can result in physical injury as a form of child neglect. Child neglect may also encompass delays in seeking medical attention or medical non-compliance that results in injury. The ranges of child neglect include psycho-emotional failure to thrive and even starvation to death. Emotional abuse is perhaps the most difficult form of abuse to define. This would include constant belittling, extreme threatening and harsh forms of emotional punishment.

It has been estimated that ophthalmic findings are present in 4–6% of abused children. The head and neck are particularly vulnerable sites to physical abuse as the caretaker responds to the crying or difficult child. Perhaps over 90% of perpetrators do not actually intend to harm their child. Rather, child abuse is a behaviour that represents, in general, a loss of control that may be brought on by many stresses in the caretaker's life. Yet, this loss of control, with subsequent injury to a child, is punishable by law in most jurisdictions. The goal of interventions however, is usually to preserve family unity wherever possible as long as the safety of the child can be guaranteed. Reporting of child abuse does not necessarily mean that the parents will go to jail, the family will be separated, the child will be placed in a strange foster home, or the physician will have to testify in court. It is the latter concern that has led many ophthalmologists to avoid reporting for fear that the time commitment and subsequent involvement will be too demanding. Ophthalmologists will be asked to testify in less than 1% of the cases in which they are involved. Reporting can be potentially life saving for the child.

In evaluating a case of possible child abuse, it is important that the physician clearly document the nature of the interactions with the family and child as well as all physical findings that are observed. Photography is particularly useful. Physicians should willingly collaborate with investigators and lawyers representing governmental agencies. The principles of informed consent may apply differently in cases of abuse as the child's protection is paramount to the parental concerns. However, where possible, parents should be informed that reporting is planned. Most perpetrators will not resist reporting, as they indeed are regretful that the child has been injured. However, confrontations between parent and physician are also a potential concern and are best dealt with by the involvement of multi-disciplinary personnel including, nursing, social work and physicians especially trained in the field.

Clinical features

1. Physical abuse. Any physical injury to the eyeball or adnexa could have been caused by an abusive mechanism. Factors which might help the physician to recognize the possibility of non-accidental injury include a history which is inconsistent with the injury, a history which is inconsistent with the developmental level of the child, a changing history offered by one or multiple caretakers, or the absence of a history of trauma in the presence of an injury which is clearly traumatic. Perhaps the most common form of physical abuse with ocular findings is the Shaken Baby Syndrome, which is covered elsewhere in this book.

Periorbital ecchymosis can be caused by both accidental and non-accidental means. The physician should be very cautious in trying to date the age of these bruises as the loose skin around the eyeballs allows for more accumulation of blood than other sites of the body from where dating recommendations were generated. In addition, one should remember that a blow to the forehead could result in bilateral periorbital ecchymosis. Injuries that imply that trauma has indeed occurred include avulsion of the vitreous base, commotio retinae, and laceration of the globe. One should also consider the possibility of trauma in cases of unilateral optic atrophy, cataract, ectopia lentis and hyphema. Infantile retinal detachment may also be a presenting sign of abuse.

Another form of physical abuse is Munchausen Syndrome by Proxy (also known as Factitious Disorder by Proxy) in which the caretaker, most often the mother, causes the child to have the appearance of an illness by direct covert physical injury (e.g. suffocation), falsification of laboratory specimens (e.g. spitting into urine taken for culture) or falsification of historical information. Ophthalmic manifestations might include subconjunctival haemorrhage in the case of smothering, neurophthalmic findings as a result of covert poisoning or damage to the conjunctiva and cornea as a result of direct covert installation of chemical substances. The reader is referred elsewhere for a more complete description of this syndrome. Physicians should have an index of suspicion for this disorder particularly when a chronic illness is presenting in unusual fashions, without clear explanation, with inappropriate responses to therapy, and when the parent, particularly the mother, has visited multiple physicians and appears to be the 'perfect parent' with overly attentive if not pathologically enmeshed behaviour with the child.

2. Sexual abuse. Sexual abuse of children, unlike other forms of abuse, is indeed an intentional act which is chronic, non-violent, secretive and rarely results in physical injury. Activities may range from excessive fondling, to exposure, and even full penetration of the vagina or rectum. The perpetrator is usually well known to the child and takes advantage of their position of relative power to coerce the child into these activities while preventing the child from disclosing the nature of the activities either by confusing the immature child or threatening them.

Ophthalmic manifestations can result from sexually transmitted diseases. However, one must be sure that the presence of a sexually transmitted disease in a child is not due to transmission through normal birth. In addition, adolescents may acquire sexually transmitted diseases through consensual sexual activity with their peers. Outside of these situations, sexual abuse must be considered. In those situations, syphilis always represents sexual transmission. Interestingly, although gonorrhea of the anus, vagina, throat or urethra is always sexually transmitted, there is some evidence that suggests that non-sexual transmission to the conjunctiva may occur. The same may also be true for chlamydia and pubic lice. Further research is necessary. Herpes and molluscum infection on or around the eyeball is most often non-sexual, however sexual transmission can occur. HIV infection may also be acquired as a result of sexual abuse.

3. Child neglect. Although actual ocular injury from child neglect is uncommon, the ophthalmologist is more likely to run into circumstances where medical non-compliance (e.g. failure to patch) results in permanent visual loss. It may be helpful, when repeated patterns of non-compliance are observed, to bring your concerns to the family's attention including the possibility of reporting to protective agencies. A helpful step is to write a brief 'contract' in the chart indicating your intention to report should continued non-compliance be observed. This can be signed by the physician, the caretaker and a witness. Should the next appointment be missed or further non-compliance be observed, then this written document may help the appropriate agencies to intervene more effectively as it demonstrates that the caretaker understood the potential outcome. However, one must be sure to use social work resources to rule out 'acceptable' explanations for non-compliance such as financial concerns, poor education by the physician, an inability of the caretaker to understand the instructions, child care issues which prevent attendance at visits or transportation issues.

4. Emotional abuse. A well recognized scenario is the parent who becomes emotionally abusive and threatening towards their child in the ophthalmologist's waiting room. Although this is not acceptable, it may be a manifestation of the stress induced by waiting too long for the physician. If a parent demonstrates such behaviour, it would be appropriate to take them out of turn, and call for the appropriate social worker or nursing support, to help diffuse the situation. However, it is important not to overtly challenge the inappropriateness of the caretaker's behaviour as they would be likely to respond with only greater fervor. Rather, the physician should open the dialogue by acknowledging the frustrations that the parent might be feeling in the care for their child in this stressful situation.

One might also consider inappropriate viewing as a form of ophthalmic 'emotional abuse'. Should a child be allowed to view their caretakers engaging in sexual activity, violent crime or drug abuse? What effect will this have on the psychosocial development of the child?

Functional visual symptoms or other related disorders in children (e.g. blinking) can rarely be a manifestation of covert abuse going on in the home. In approximately 50% of functional ophthalmic signs in children, there is a known stressor in their life. The physician should consider enquiring about the presence of violence or abuse in the home where appropriate.

Treatment

Multi-disciplinary care is the cornerstone of child abuse treatment. The primary concern is protection of the child and their siblings from further harm. The suspicion of abuse, especially physical abuse, should lead to further physical examination looking for other signs. In cases of sexually transmitted disease, it is important for the ophthalmologist to directly notify the child's primary physician or a child abuse physician, as a full sexual abuse history by trained personnel, examination of the genitalia, and culturing of all other relative orifices is essential to determine whether sexual abuse may have occurred. Contact with the primary care physician is also important in cases of child neglect and emotional abuse as long-standing patterns may go otherwise unrecognized.

There is a wide body of literature which can assist physicians in preparing themselves for expert testimony if required. In general, it is important for physicians to allow themselves to give expert testimony only when they are indeed experts. The physician should remember that they are not on trial in the courtroom and should avoid emotional responses or verbal battling with the attorneys. Rather, simple explanations that are understandable by the lay judge and jury, as well as a calm enunciation of the facts of the case, are most useful.

Conclusion

Dealing with child abuse is uncomfortable and unpleasant for most ophthalmologists. Yet, it is one of the few areas in our field that allows us to protect children from further injury if not death. The ophthalmologist therefore has an important mandate to recognize and report any reasonable suspicion that abuse may have occurred.

Further reading

Catalano RA, Simon JW, Krohel GB *et al.* Functional visual loss in children. *Ophthalmology* 1986; **93:** 385–90.

Kempe CH, Silverman FN, Steele BF *et al.* The battered-child syndrome. *Journal of the American Medical Association* 1962; **181:** 17–24.

Levin AV. Ophthalmologic manifestations of child abuse. *Ophthalmology Clinics of North America* 1990; **3:** 249–64.

Levin AV. The ocular findings in child abuse. *American Academy of Ophthalmology, Focal Points: Clinical Modules for Ophthalmologists* 1998; **16**(7): 1–8, 13.

Levin AV, Sheridan M, eds. *Munchausen Syndrome by Proxy: Issues in Diagnosis and Management.* New York: Lexington Books, 1995.

Lewis L, Glauser T, Joffe MD. Gonococcal conjunctivitis in prepubertal children. *American Journal Disease of Childhood* 1990; **144:** 546–8.

Ludwig S, Kornberg A, eds. *Child Abuse: A Medical Reference,* 2nd edn. New York: Churchill Livingston, 1992, pp. 191–212.

CHILD WITH STRABISMUS: WORK-UP

Robert H. Taylor

Strabismus occurs in about 3% of children. Amblyopia is present in approximately 5% of children. Strabismus is a cause of amblyopia and amblyopia is a cause of strabismus. Strabismus may be associated with a neurological or visual pathway abnormality, but more commonly reflects a refractive problem, usually hypermetropia or anisometropia, or is idiopathic. Despite the complexity of strabismus management, it cannot be overstressed that accurate diagnosis and exclusion of ocular and systemic conditions (e.g. cranial nerve palsies) are mandatory. Detection and treatment of refractive error and management of amblyopia are important goals. Surgery for the ocular deviation is approached only after these issues have been addressed.

Problem

The pathophysiology of strabismus is complex and poorly understood. A great deal of information has to be gathered from each patient before a diagnosis can be reached and a treatment plan implemented.

Background

Most cases of poor visual function or ocular deviation present to an ophthalmologist between the ages of 3 months and 4 years old. Any ocular deviation at any age needs a full work up although temporary ocular misalignment is often seen before 2 months of age. It may be appropriate to involve a paediatrician or geneticist if a systemic disorder is suspected. Combined care with an orthoptist may be beneficial.

Clinical features

1. History.   Ocular deviation is usually initially intermittent, particularly when tired or studying close objects. Ask about any previous history of occlusion therapy or strabismus surgery. A family history of refractive errors and strabismus should be documented. An obstetric and neonatal history should be taken. Prematurity, birth trauma and the achievement of developmental milestones should be noted. If the child has developed a recent onset headache or has become clumsy or irritable, one has to be particularly vigilant to exclude intracranial pathology. Previous photographs may show strabismus or a compensatory head posture.

2. General examination.   It is important to look for dysmorphic features and hydrocephalus. Document any abnormal head posture before commencing examination of the eyes. To do this it is important to ask the child (if old enough) to read the lowest line on a Snellen chart, without them knowing why, as they may correct the posture if they do. It may be relevant to carry out a full neurological examination with particular attention to the cranial nerves.

3. Visual function.   The visual performance is measured in each eye. Some information may be obtained from uniocular fixation, but binocular assessments (e.g. stereopsis) should be done first as covering one eye to test acuity may cause binocularity to be lost if fusion is tenuous. Forced-choice preferential looking can be carried out in pre-verbal children with grating cards or Cardiff cards. A crude approximation to Snellen visual acuity is possible and charts are available for comparison with a normal population. These tests do not detect the crowding phenomenon. For verbal children, matching pictures (Kay, Allen or Lea) or Snellen letters are appropriate. It is important that the occlusion of each eye is complete to ensure that each eye is tested separately. When comparing visual acuity measurements separated in time remember to note if different tests have been used.

4. Binocular status. This is best tested early in the examination as disruption of binocularity may occur with the dissociating tests that follow. A finding of normal stereopsis is extremely important, and suggests that any strabismus is intermittent. A variety of tests are available for all ages. Tests that do not involve wearing glasses are particularly important for the younger patient (e.g. Frisby, Lang). Demonstration of a fusion range gives an assessment of the strength of any fusion. Some degree of stereopsis may be present with a small angle strabismus, e.g. in the monofixation syndrome or microtropia. In cases where there is no measureable stereopsis, the Worth 4 dot test carried out at either distance or near can offer information about suppression.

5. Ocular alignment. Most childhood strabismus is concomitant. Incomitant deviations may occur with certain childhood conditions (e.g. Brown and Duane syndrome), but it is important to exclude a cranial nerve palsy. Ocular alignment is tested by carrying out a cover/uncover test, and an alternate cover test both in the distance and for near, to accommodative targets. Note if one eye tends to be strabismic, or if the two eyes freely alternate. If appropriate, testing is carried out with and without spectacles. A simultaneous prism cover test quantifies any manifest deviation (i.e. when the eyes are not dissociated). An alternating prism cover test (APCT) quantifies the deviation with the eyes dissociated. The tests may be carried out in the nine positions of gaze where indicated. This can be obtained by asking the child to fixate on a distance target and moving the head approximately 25° to the right for left gaze, 25° to the left for right gaze and so on. The measurements should be repeated until a reproducible and stable measurement is obtained for the purpose of surgical planning.

A or V patterns and any dissociated vertical deviation (DVD) need to be documented. A horizontal strabismus with a V pattern is defined as having more than 15 prism dioptres difference in the APCT between up- and down-gaze, with the visual axes more divergent in up-gaze. In an A pattern, there is more than 10 prism dioptres difference between up- and down-gaze, with the visual axes being more divergent in down-gaze.

The accommodative convergence/accommodation ratio (AC/A) can be assessed where there is a large disparity between the angle for distance and near fixation.

Any torsion can be assessed using a double maddox rod mounted onto a trial frame if the patient can appreciate double vision. An objective assessment can be obtained using fundus examination.

The synoptophore is used for the measurement of ocular deviation and can be useful for measuring torsion, for example from a superior oblique palsy. The synoptophore is also used to investigate binocular function and retinal correspondence.

6. Ocular rotations. The versions and ductions need to be assessed. In small children it may not be possible to bring the eyes into all areas adequately. In patients with large eso-deviations, full abduction of each eye must be demonstrated if at all possible to exclude lateral rectus weakness. Occlusion of an eye for a short period (up to an hour) or use of the vestibulo-ocular system may help in persuading the child to abduct the eye. Overacting muscles (e.g. the inferior oblique muscle) or underacting muscles (e.g. superior oblique) are also documented. Convergence is tested by bringing a target close to the nose.

Nystagmus may be present and needs to be carefully assessed. A convergent strabismus may be present as part of the nystagmus blockage syndrome. Manifest/latent nystagmus occurs in association with esotropia (possibly as part of a primary infantile esotropia syndrome with DVD and inferior oblique overaction).

7. Refraction. This is carried out under cycloplegia in children and even young adults (to exclude latent hypermetropia). In general, cyclopentolate 1% is adequate. It is advised to wait 40 minutes from the administration of the drug to allow for full cycloplegia. A post-cycloplegic subjective test may be possible in older children. There is a debate about the use of cyclopentolate, and some ophthalmologists recommend atropine for initial refractions or in those with heavily pigmented irides.

8. Ocular examination. Undertake a full ophthalmic examination. The pupil reflexes are checked for a relative afferent pupil defect. The fundi are examined once the pupils are dilated. Young children can be difficult to examine and if initial examination is inadequate, the fundi must be re-examined at a later date. This cannot be overemphasized, as conditions such as retinoblastoma and hydrocephalus with papilloedema may present with strabismus.

9. Other tests. In those children in whom there is visual loss with or without strabismus, electrodiagnostic examination may provide further useful information. It is indicated if there is reduced vision bilaterally, and the diagnosis is not made from examination in the clinic. Neuroimaging may be indicated in cases of a cranial nerve palsy or where a structural abnormality is suspected, for example in cases of large colobomas or optic disc hypoplasia.

Further reading

Mein J, Trimble R. In: *Diagnosis and Management of Ocular Motility Disorders*, 2nd edn. Oxford: Blackwell Scientific Publications, 1991; 1–147.
Tongue AC. Acquired esotropia. In: Cibis GW, Tongue AC, Strass-Isern ML (eds). *Decision Making in Pediatric Ophthalmology*. St Louis: Mosby Year Book, 1993; 224–7.
Wilson ME, Buckley EG, Kivlin JD, Ruttum MS, Simon JW, Magoon EH. *Pediatric Ophthalmology Section 6*. American Academy of Ophthalmology 1999; 45–73.

Related topics of interest

CHILDHOOD CATARACT

Robert H. Taylor & Tina Kipioti

Congenital cataract is a major cause of blind and partially sighted children, with an incidence of 1 per 4000–10 000 live births. In particular, neonates with bilateral dense lens opacities are particularly at risk of long-term visual deprivation and warrant urgent surgical intervention, within the first 6 weeks of life whenever possible. Amblyopia is the main limiting factor of the final visual outcome and its management important. To this end parental education about visual prognosis and surgery, and their key role in post-operative refractive correction and occlusion therapy, is crucial.

Problem

Important aetiologies of congenital cataract need exclusion as they may require attention. Treatable causes should be eliminated as the development of some metabolic cataracts can be reversed if discovered early. Although a variety of approaches to manage cataracts in children have been studied no consensus exists on the indications, optimum approach, and choice of IOL implantation.

Background

There are many causes of congenital cataract.

1. Sporadic. No cause is found in 30–50% of congenital cataracts. This is particularly true of unilateral cases. Some of these may be new mutations.

2. Heritable. About a third of congenital cataracts are inherited, most with an autosomal dominant pattern, with variable expressivity. Autosomal recessive and X-linked recessive patterns may also occur. Autosomal recessive cataract is more likely in cases of parental consanguinity.

3. Ocular disorders. It is important to exclude persistent hyperplastic primary vitreous, microphthalmia, aniridia, trauma, retinopathy of prematurity (ROP), retinal detachment and uveitis. Cataract has also been reported following laser treatment for ROP.

4. Intrauterine infections. The most important is rubella. This can cause a unilateral or bilateral dense cataract. The cataract results from direct invasion of the lens by the virus, which can be cultured from lens aspirates. Infants with congenital rubella shed the virus for several weeks after birth. Other examples of maternal infections causing cataract include varicella zoster, herpes simplex, cytomegalovirus, polio, influenza, hepatitis, toxoplasmosis gondii and syphilis.

5. Metabolic disorders. Galactokinase deficiency is a autosomal recessive condition causing bilateral lamellar cataracts. The child is otherwise well. It is different from galactosaemia (galactose-1-phosphate uridyl transferase deficiency), also autosomal recessive, causing oil drop cataracts, failure to thrive, hepatosplenomegaly, jaundice and mental retardation. Both have reducing substances in the urine and can be separated by enzyme studies. Galactosaemic cataracts may reverse if galactose is withheld from the diet. Hypocalcaemia secondary to hypoparathyroidism or pseudohypoparathyroidism creates a cataract with punctate cortical dots, and the child may have fits and fail to thrive. Infantile hypoglycaemia is associated with transient or persistent lamellar cataracts.

6.   Chromosomal and other syndromes.   Some degree of cataract is found in up to 60% of Down syndrome infants. These are often lamellar, which may be compatible with reasonable vision. Dense cataracts also occur. However the most common form of cataract is visually insignificant 'snowflake' opacities. Other examples include trisomy 18, trisomy 13 and deletion of the short arm of chromosome 5 (cri-du-chat). Lowe's syndrome is an X-linked condition, manifesting in infancy with dysmorphic facies, mental and psychomotor retardation, failure to thrive, aminoaciduria and cataracts, usually present at birth. Female carriers may have radiating dot lens opacities. Cataracts may also be the presenting sign of the Hallermann–Streiff–François syndrome comprising dyscephaly, short stature, dental anomalies, hypotrichosis and blue sclerae. There are many other syndromes associated with cataract. In general, if a child has two malformations in addition to the cataract, consideration should be given to genetics consultation.

7.   Low birthweight.   Transient vacuolated cataracts have been described with low birthweight babies. These usually resolve after 2 months of life.

8.   Toxic/radiation.   It is important to exclude maternal drug ingestion or radiation injury during pregnancy.

9.   Systemic disease.   There are a number of systemic conditions that can be associated with cataract. Juvenile chronic arthritis is associated with cataract due to the uveitis. Neurofibromatosis type 2 patients may have juvenile posterior subcapsular cataracts and any form of steroid therapy can induce cataracts.

Clinical features

The age at diagnosis and family impression of the visual function should be documented at the first visit. Ask about any rashes, infections or febrile illnesses during the pregnancy. Was there any exposure to drugs or toxins or ionizing radiation? In case of positive family history or dysmorphic features a consultation with a geneticist may be helpful. It is always advisable to involve a paediatrician in the assessment and care of these patients. The examination of parents and siblings can be very informative even if they are asymptomatic.

Assessment of vision is most important, as it influences the timing of surgery. The presence of nystagmus is a poor prognostic indicator. Pupil reflexes are recorded and an attempt should be made to evaluate the integrity of the retina and optic nerve. If the cataract prevents adequate examination the ultrasound should be performed.

Examination of the red reflex before dilatation can give an idea of the density of the cataract and its effect on vision. Cataracts more likely to affect vision are posterior, denser, axial and greater than 3 mm across. The morphology of persistent hyperplastic primary vitreous, galactosaemic, rubella and hypocalcaemic cataracts may be characteristic on slit lamp examination. Blue dot cataracts are usually inherited.

Investigations may include serology for intrauterine infections (toxoplasma, rubella, cytomegalovirus, herpes simplex virus types 1 and 2), urine analysis for reducing substances and amino acids, biochemistry profile and chromosome analysis in the presence of dysmorphology. Electrodiagnostic investigations may complement the clinical information. However, in an otherwise well child with a normal physical examination and no risk factors or history, extensive lab testing is likely to be non-informative.

Treatment

Parental education is essential before treatment commences. In many cases, management with contact lenses and patching following surgery will be a new concept. It may be necessary to predict a limited visual outcome in those with unilateral cataract, late presentation or poor initial vision.

It is known from animal studies that reduced visual input from birth to 3 months leads to reduced connections of cortical cells to the affected eye and a reduced number of binocularly driven cells. These changes are reversed if there is early restoration of the vision. For humans, the sensitive period may be slightly longer. The visual outcome may still vary even though the treatment appears ideal.

Surgery is not usually necessary for lens opacities confined to the centre of the anterior capsule or the anterior cortex. Early surgery is indicated for cataracts profoundly reducing vision. For bilateral cases the second eye is operated on a few days after the first, to reduce the risk of amblyopia.

The procedure of choice remains controversial. Lensectomy-vitrectomy using a cutter is usually favoured for infants and children under 2 years of age particularly if bilateral lens implantation is not intended immediately. In older children a limbal approach may be used, a curvilinear capsulorhexis made in the anterior capsule and the lens aspirated either manually or with an automated aspiration device. However, due to the relatively strong and elastic nature of the paediatric capsule, many surgeons prefer mechanical capsulotomy. Use of some form or anterior chamber irrigation may be beneficial. This helps to wash out pigment and prostaglandins and helps to keep the pupil dilated.

Management of the posterior capsule in paediatric cataracts is crucial as opacification is universal. Elective posterior capsulotomy with an anterior vitrectomy is suggested if no IOL is to be inserted. A clear visual axis and a generous vitrectomy aim to significantly reduce both the posterior capsule re-opacification rate and the amount of post-operative uveitis. It also eliminates the risk of vitreous causing a pupil block. If an intraocular lens is to be inserted, this can be placed on the posterior capsule. A pars plana approach is then used for an anterior vitrectomy and posterior capsulotomy. This has the advantage of leaving the anterior chamber undisturbed and minimizing any possibility of vitreous becoming involved with the IOL or wound. An alternative is to fashion a posterior caspulorhexis before IOL implantation. Posterior subluxation of the optic through this posterior capsule opening offers further insurance against posterior capsular re-growth.

Unlike the common practice in adults, wounds in children are not self-sealing and require closure with an absorbable suture.

The choice of IOL and the selection of lens dioptric power remain controversial issues especially in infants under 2 years of age. However, primary lens implantation seems to be the optimal management for children older than 2 years. If the eye is rendered emmetropic at the time of surgery, a myopic shift typically occurs later, requiring correction with spectacles, contact lenses and rarely IOL exchange. For this reason most surgeons will aim to under-correct aphakia at the time of implantation, hoping the residual refractive error will resolve with age and relying on glasses in the interim. When correcting the residual refractive error one should take into account the well documented spontaneous reduction of astigmatism post-operatively continuing up to 5 months after surgery.

Contact lenses remain the standard method of optically correcting aphakia following cataract surgery in infancy. Soft daily wear, extended wear, gas permeable or silicone lenses have all been used successfully. Parental education and support is very important. As the eye grows frequent changes of contact lens power are needed.

Over-refractions should be part of the examination at nearly every visit. Desired values are −2.00 to −4.00 up to 1 year old, −1.00 to −2.00 from 1–2 years old, 2nd plane (with bifocal near correction) from 2 years old on.

Visual rehabilitation only starts with surgery and must be continued throughout childhood. Visual outcomes have been improving over the last decade. These have been related to early surgery in bilateral cases as well as occlusion of at least 3 hours a day in unilateral cases.

Complications

Paediatric cataract surgery is considerably more challenging than its adult counterpart. In addition to the complications encountered in adult cataract extractions a florid anterior uveitis may follow any intra-operative procedure especially if complicated (e.g. iris prolapse). Retinal detachment may occur 10–30 years later. A high proportion of children operated on for congenital cataract will develop strabismus, and up to 30% develop aphakic glaucoma. Unilateral cataracts are associated with a poorer visual outcome than bilateral cataracts. Problems associated with the use of contact lenses are also common and include microbial keratitis and frequent loss or change of lenses due to alteration of the refractive status and contact lens loss. The use of spectacles may provide an alternative in cases of contact lens intolerance but the cosmetic result is poor and induced optical aberration may compromise the visual outcome. Complications of IOL implantation include adverse refractive outcome, vigorous inflammatory response, IOL decentration, and iris capture. Intensive steroid treatment, even parenterally, may be required.

Further reading

Ainsworth JR, Cohen S, Levin AV, et al. Pediatric cataract management with variations in surgical technique and aphakic optical correction. Ophthalmology 1997; 104(7): 1096–101.

Asrani S, Freedman S, Hasselblad V, Buckley E, Egbert J, Dahan E, Gimbel H, Johnson D, McClatchey S, Parks M, Plager D, Baselli E. Does primary intraocular lens implantation prevent 'aphakic' glaucoma in children? Journal of AAPOS 2000; 4(1): 33–9.

Dahan E. In Yannof M, Duker JS (eds.): Ophthalmology. 1st edition. Mosby Publications 1999; 30: 1–6.

Isenberg SJ. *The Eye in Infancy.* 1994, Second Edition; Year Book Publishers, Inc., Chicago.

Lambert S. In Taylor D (ed.) *Paediatric Ophthalmology.* 2nd edition. Blackwell Science Ltd., 1997; 445–76.

Lewis TL, Maurer D, Brent HP. Development of grating acuity in children treated for unilateral or bilateral congenital cataract. *Investigative Ophthalmology and Visual Science* 1995; **36**(10): 2080–95.

Lloyd IC, Goss-Sampson M, Jeffrey BG, Kriss A, Russell-Eggitt I, Taylor D. Neonatal cataract: Aetiology, pathogenesis and management. *Eye* 1993; **6**(2): 184–96.

Russell-Eggitt I, Lightman S. Intrauterine infection and the eye. *Eye* 1993; **6**(2): 205–10.

Young TL *et al.* The IOLAB, Inc. pediatric intraocular lens study. AAPOS Research Committee, American Association for Pediatric Ophthalmology and Strabismus. *J AAPOS* 1999; **3**(5): 295–302.

Zwaan J *et al.* Pediatric intraocular lens implantation. Surgical results and complications in more than 300 patients. *Ophthalmology* 1998; **105**(1): 112–18; discussion 118–19.

Related topic of interest

Congenital nystagmus (p. 69).

CHLAMYDIAL CONJUNCTIVITIS

Robert H. Taylor

Chlamydial infection (inclusion conjunctivitis) may present at any age. In tropical countries children and adults may contract trachoma. Patients may present many years later as a result of symptoms generated by the long-term sequelae of trachoma. Infection of the conjunctiva is sometimes known as inclusion conjunctivitis after the cytoplasmic inclusion bodies seen in conjunctival epithelial cells.

Problem

Adult chlamydial conjunctivitis may be difficult to diagnose and missed unless specifically examined for and appropriate tests undertaken. Chlamydial infections are difficult to treat and may require repeated courses of antibiotics.

Background

Chlamydia trachomatis types D–K are the most common causes in the Western world. A microbiology profile is mandatory and can be done at the same time as the examination. Gram staining is carried out on a conjunctival swab to look for gram negative diplococci (*N. gonococcus*) as well as other organisms. A bacterial culture is taken. Traditionally *Chlamydia trachomatis* is grown on McCoy cell culture. However, this has been largely superseded by either direct immunofluorescence antibody staining, polymerase chain reaction analysis or enzyme immunoassay. These more modern tests have a higher sensitivity and are quicker than culture. It is advisable to avoid administering fluorescein to the conjunctiva before taking a scrape for immunofluorescence staining.

Trachoma is caused by *C. trachomatis* types A, B and C. It is endemic in Africa, India, Asia and South America. It is estimated that 500 million are affected, with up to 2 million being blind. Initial infection is a chronic conjunctivitis in children. It is contagious and transferred by insect vectors, person to person contact and materials used for wiping the eyes.

Clinical features

*1. **Newborn conjunctivitis.*** This form of chlamydia conjunctivitis usually occurs in the first 28 days of life but may present up to 4 years later. During the second stage of labour there is direct contact between the ocular tissues and the cervix causing transmission of maternal genital infections. In the United Kingdom it is a notifiable disease. A notification form, issued by the local authority (city or county council), is sent to the environmental health department who informs 'the proper officer' – normally the consultant in communicable disease control (CCDC).

Babies usually develop a mild conjuctivitis but may rarely develop the rapid preseptal cellulitis (including conjunctivitis and mucopurulent discharge) and systemic illness more common with gonorrhoea. It is particularly important to exclude a corneal opacity or ulcer. Care must be taken on opening the lids, as pus may be present under pressure. Chlamydial pneumonitis may subsequently develop during the first 6 weeks of life. It is characterized by a nasal discharge, cough, and tachypnoea.

2. Non-neonatal inclusion conjunctivitis. Chlamydia trachomatis types D–K primarily cause urethritis in men and cervicitis in women which is sexually transmitted. Characteristic features include an age range of 15 to 40 years old, a chronic disease course, unilateral or asymmetric disease, ptosis, a combined follicular/papillary conjunctival response, coarse epithelial keratopathy with peripheral corneal infiltrates and regional lymphadenopathy. A superior corneal pannus may develop after several months. Questions should be directed to elicit genito-urinary symptoms. Patients and all recent partners should be referred for genito-urinary examination. It is important that the microbiological investigations carried out in the genito-urinary clinic are completed before systemic treatment is initiated.

3. Trachoma. The disease stages have been classified as follows:

- Stage I.   Active trachoma. There is a mild conjunctivitis with follicular and mild papillary response and a superficial keratitis.
- Stage II.   Active trachoma. Marked conjunctivitis with tarsal follicles and papillae, upper limbal follicles, a superior corneal pannus and subepithelial infiltrates. Necrosis of superior limbal follicles lead to Herbert's pits, a sign pathognomonic of trachoma.
- Stage III.   Inactive trachoma with scarring. This is characterized by advanced scarring seen on the superior tarsus as a horizontal line (Arlt's line).
- Stage IV.   Inactive trachoma with advanced scarring. Severe scarring causes trichiasis and cicatricial entropion, characteristically affecting the upper lids; a dry eye, corneal vascularization and scarring also occur.

The active conjunctivitis is often complicated by secondary bacterial conjunctivitis. The chronic cicatricial changes that make this disease blinding only occur with repeated infections. The corneal complications tend to occur with the later stages but may occur earlier. The ultimate complication of trachoma infection is bilateral blindness.

Treatment

Newborn conjunctivitis is treated with systemic erythromycin and topical tetracycline. Systemic tetracycline is contraindicated in young infants as it stains developing teeth yellow. Debate exists about the necessity of admission to hospital for chlamydial newborn conjunctivitis although pre-septal and orbital cellulitis may develop rapidly in a young child – it is unusual. The mother should be asked if the baby is feeding well and pyrexia excluded. One should have a low threshold for consultation with a paediatrician regarding admission. The parents must attend for a genito-urinary assessment and treatment.

Treatment of adult inclusion conjunctivitis is usually systemic tetracyline or a related compound, or erythromycin for those who are allergic to tetracycline. Topical treatment with tetracycline ointment (four times a day for 3 weeks) may be given in addition, although systemic treatment alone is usually sufficient. Repeated courses are sometimes required. Complications of long-term genito-urinary infections (which may be asymptomatic) include prostatitis in men and salpingitis and infertility in women.

Treatment of trachoma is aimed at reducing cross-infection by improving living conditions, educating the population, chemotherapy and surgical correction of the lids. Systemic treatment may be used such as erythromycin in children and tetracycline in adults, but topical tetracycline twice daily for 2 months is usually sufficient. Surgical correction of lid malposition and trichiasis is important to reduce corneal scarring. Tear supplementation may help to reduce long-term symptoms.

Further reading

Lambert S. Conjunctivitis of the newborn. In: Taylor D (ed.) *Paediatric Ophthalmology*. London: Blackwell Scientific Publications, 1997; 167–70.
Sandford-Smith J. *Eye Diseases in Hot Climates*, 2nd edn. Northampton: Wright Publishers, 1990; 79–92.

Related topics of interest

Cicatricial conjunctivitis (p. 56); HIV and the eye (p. 127).

CICATRICIAL CONJUNCTIVITIS

Helen Devonport & Robert H. Taylor

Cicatricial conjunctivitis is a potentially blinding form of conjunctival inflammation caused by physical or chemical injury, infection, immunologic oculocutaneous disorders, drugs and associated systemic disease. Visual loss is attributable to corneal scarring resulting from complications such as dry eye, entropion, symblepharon and trichiasis. Constant ocular irritation may further diminish quality of life. Optimal management comprises early, accurate diagnosis and effective treatment to arrest disease progression and prevent blinding complications.

Problem

There are many possible causes of cicatricial conjunctivitis. Early diagnosis is often difficult as initial symptoms can be non-specific. Treatment may require immunosuppression with significant risk of adverse effects, making accurate diagnosis essential. Conjunctival biopsy can be useful in reaching a diagnosis but has the potential to exacerbate disease activity.

Clinical features

1. Injury. Scarring can occur following thermal, ionizing radiation and chemical injury. Severe scarring follows severe or untreated alkali injury (see separate topic). Significant conjunctival scarring can be present following surgery for strabismus, retinal detachment and dermoid removal. This is more so following multiple operations.

2. Staphylococcal blepharitis. Some degree of keratinization or scarring adjacent to the meibomian glands may occur in staphylococcal blepharitis. The lid border may become rounded or notched. Altered meibomian gland function and bacterial lipases combine to destabilize the tear film and cause irritation.

3. Infective conjunctivitis. Worldwide, *Chlamydia trachomatis* infection is the most common cause of conjunctival scarring. Repeated infection and secondary bacterial infection enhance the cicatrization. Other forms of membranous and pseudomembranous conjunctivitis, either bacterial or viral, may also result in subepithelial scarring. True membranes are associated with *Streptococcus pneumoniae* and diphtherial infections. Pseudomembranes can be associated with gonnococcal or adenoviral conjunctivitis, though conjunctival scarring is rare in adenoviral infection.

4. Immunologic oculocutaneous disorders. A number of acquired conditions affecting skin and mucous membranes are associated with conjunctival scarring. They include cicatricial pemphigoid (CP) (also known as benign mucous membrane pemphigoid), erythema multiforme, Stevens–Johnson syndrome, toxic epidermal necrolysis, dermatitis herpetiformis, linear immunoglobulin A (IgA) disease, chronic atopic keratoconjunctivitis and porphyria cutanea tarda. Bullous pemphigoid and pemphigus vulgaris have less commonly been associated with a cicatricial conjunctivitis.

Cicatricial pemphigoid (CP) is generally more common in women and characteristically presents over the age of 60. Any mucosal or skin surface may be involved in the inflammatory process, which is thought to be initiated by linear deposition of immunoglobulin and/or complement components at the basement membrane. The early ocular presentation is characterized by a bilateral, often asymmetric chronic papillary conjunctivitis. Symptoms are of non-specific ocular irritation. With disease progression conjunctival vesicles appear and rapidly ulcerate. Cicatrization of the conjunctiva occurs with loss of the plica semilunaris, symblepharon formation and loss of the fornices. Diagnosis is confirmed by biopsy, preferably of affected buccal mucosa. In the absence of buccal involvement, inflamed bulbar conjunctiva should be taken from the intrapalpebral fissure adjacent to the limbus, minimizing the risk of further symblepharon formation. Direct immunofluorescence will detect anti-basement membrane antibody.

Erythema multiforme, Stevens–Johnson syndrome (SJS) and toxic epidermal necrolysis (TEN) are thought to represent a spectrum of the same disease process. They affect younger age groups than CP. Onset is acute and follows either drug ingestion or infection. Erythematous or bullous skin eruption may be accompanied by bullous eruption of the conjunctiva, lips, oro-pharynx and respiratory mucosa. A localized autoimmune vasculitis causes infarction, membrane formation and subsequent cicatrization.

Dermatitis herpetiformis is characterized by IgA and complement deposition at the epidermal basement membrane. When the IgA deposition is linear it is known as linear IgA disease. Although mucosal involvement is rare, both conditions may affect the conjunctiva, resulting in less severe cicatrization than that seen in CP.

Chronic atopic keratoconjunctivitis is frequently associated with asthma and eczema. Chronic ocular inflammation may lead to subconjunctival scarring and shortening of the fornices.

Porphyria cutanea tarda, the most common form of porphyria may be associated with sun-induced skin lesions and vesicular conjunctivitis leading to scar formation.

5. *Drug related.* Cicatricial changes of the conjunctiva have been associated with the use of both topical and systemic medications. Drug-associated conjunctival changes vary from mild subclinical inflammation to drug-induced cicatrizing conjunctivitis (DICC), which is clinically indistinguishable from ocular CP. Chronic follicular conjunctivitis has been described with topical pilocarpine, adrenaline and dipiverine. Medications associated with DICC include systemic practolol and penicillamine and topical adrenaline, pilocarpine, timolol, idoxuridine, trifluridine, gentamicin and guanethidine. DICC is usually non-progressive although occasionally progression occurs despite withdrawal of the causative agent. It is not clear whether the drugs mimic, promote or trigger CP.

6. *Inherited conditions.* Conjunctival scarring can be present as a primary finding in ectodermal dysplasia. Other conditions such as epidermolysis bullosa and ichthyosis (Harlequin baby, collodian baby) cause an upper and lower lid ectropion, exposure and corneal problems. A variety of inheritance patterns occur including X-linked, autosomal dominant and autosomal recessive.

7. Systemic disorders. Rosacea and Sjögren's syndromes may be associated with modest cicatrization caused by chronic inflammation. Inflammatory bowel disease, chronic graft-versus-host disease and paraneoplastic syndromes may also cause mild cicatrization.

Treatment

Treatment can be divided into correction of the aetiological factor causing the scarring and correction of the effects of the scarring itself.

For staphlococcal blepharitis appropriate treatment of the infection and lid margin disease may alleviate symptoms. This may include local or systemic antibiotics, such as minocycline. Local lid cleaning regimes and replacement tears where appropriate also help. For infective conjunctivitis appropriate antibiotic therapy is indicated based on the bacteriology.

For cicatricial pemphigoid, systemic immunosuppression is required during the active phase, with dapsone recommended for mild to moderate cases with slow progression and cyclophosphamide for moderate to severe inflammation or scarring that is progressing more rapidly. Local treatment comprises tear substitutes, topical steroids and antibiotics which where possible should be preservative-free. Other approaches include punctal occlusion, tarsorrhaphy, upper lid botulinium and lid cryotherapy. Surgical approach to trichiasis and entropion is possible but division of symblepharon is not advised.

In erythema multiforme systemic treatment with corticosteroids is recommended by some, but remains controversial. Topical steroids and antibiotics may be used in the acute phase. Early surgical intervention to correct lid malposition and trichiasis is advised.

In general correction of lid malposition should be delayed until inflammation is quiescent as surgery may accelerate cicatrization. Supportive measures for the cornea include lubrication, punctal occlusion, meticulous atttention to lid margin disease, bandage contact lens wear (with careful follow up) and easy access to specialist help.

Other therapeutic avenues may include surgical correction of trichiasis and lid margin malposition, conjunctival grafting, mucous membrane transplantation, limbal stem cell transplantation, amniotic membrane transplantation, penetrating keratoplasty and in severe cases, keratoprosthesis for visual rehabilitation.

Conclusion

Cicatricial conjunctivitis can be a devastating disease. Loss of goblet cells and accessory lacrimal glands as well as occlusion of the secretory lacrimal and meibomian gland orifices result in severe dry eye and diffuse keratinization. Trichiasis occurs due to lid margin scarring and cicatricial entropion. Symblepharon formation can result in lagophthalmos and subsequent exposure keratopathy. Involvement of the limbus may decrease the stem cell population resulting in corneal epithelial breakdown, delayed healing or vascularization.

The compromised ocular surface is at increased risk of secondary bacterial infection that may lead to corneal ulceration or perforation.

Further reading

Bernauer W, Broadway DC, Wright P. Chronic progressive conjunctival cicatrization. *Eye* 1993; **7**(3): 371–8.

Chiou AGY, Florakis GJ, Kazim M. Management of conjunctival cicatrizing diseases and severe ocular surface dysfunction. *Survey of Ophthalmology* 1998; **43**: 19–46.

Holsclaw DS. Ocular cicatricial pemphigoid. *International Ophthalmology Clinics* 1998; **38**(4): 89–106.

Liesegang TJ. Conjunctival changes associated with glaucoma therapy: implications for the external diseases consultant and the treatment of glaucoma. *Cornea* 1998; **17**(6): 574–83.

Wagoner MD. Chemical injuries of the eye: current concepts in pathophysiology and therapy. *Survey of Ophthalmology* 1997; **41**: 275–313.

Related topics of interest

Alkali injuries (p. 12); Chlamydial conjunctivitis (p. 53); Sjögren's syndrome (p. 292); Toxicology: drugs for non-ocular diseases (p. 319).

CLINICAL COLOUR-VISION TESTING

Scott E. Brodie

Effective evaluation of colour vision abnormalities remains an important task, in steady demand by patients, their families and employers. This topic will outline the common forms of colour vision deficiency, and provide an annotated summary of the standard tools for colour-vision testing.

Problem

Abnormality of colour vision affects upwards of 5% of the male population (as well as a very small proportion of females), and thus constitutes one of the most prevalent visual disorders. Acquired dyschromatopsia is often tested for in clinical practice although generally a rare complaint. Evaluation of colour vision attracts little interest among practising ophthalmologists, perhaps because the disorder is seldom amenable to therapy, or perhaps because the available tools remain obscure. The clinical tests used for acquired dyschromatopsia are often inappropriate.

Background

Human photopic (light-adapted) vision is mediated by the cone photoreceptors. The cones usually contain one of three 'visual pigments', each of which absorbs light over a fairly broad spectral band. The so-called 'blue cones' are rather few in number, and absorb light primarily of short wavelength (S cones). The 'green' and 'red' cones absorb medium and longer wavelength light, respectively (M & L cones), but in fact their absorption curves greatly overlap. The colour perceived in any visual stimulus is determined only by the effective absorption of the light from the stimulus by the three types of cones. Subsequent neural mechanisms 'compare and contrast' the responses of the different cones. Since absorption of light is an essentially linear process, this implies that the 'front end' of the mechanism of colour perception functions as a linear device. This allows colour sensations to be depicted on a two-dimensional graph (such as the 'CIE Colour Diagram') so that each chromatic sensation can be represented as a weighted sum of vectors corresponding to the stimulation of the individual cones. In particular, if one type of cone is inactive or defective, the affected individual will be unable to differentiate between colours that differ only along vectors corresponding to the stimulation of the abnormal cone. These indistinguishable colours will lay along straight lines on the CIE Colour Diagram ('lines of confusion'), which radiate from a point, characteristic of the abnormal cone type.

Clinical features

In practice, a colour-normal individual is unable to distinguish the very similar colours that lie in a small neighbourhood surrounding any given colour. This small patch of colour space is referred to as the 'MacAdam ellipse'. A person with abnormal colour vision will typically exhibit a decidedly larger elliptical region of indistinguishability. The longer axis of the ellipse lies on the line of confusion through the given colour. The orientation of this ellipse indicates the nature of the defective cone type.

Near the centre of the CIE colour diagram is a point where a normal individual finds the component colour signals 'in balance' so as to produce a grey 'achromatic' stimulus. The confusion ellipses about this point indicate the hues that a colour-abnormal individual is unable to distinguish from various shades of grey. The most common cases are abnormalities of the 'red' cone pigment, which cause confusion of greys with reds, and abnormalities of the 'green' cone pigment, which cause confusion of greys with purples. In either case, the abnormal input to the mechanism which compares the absorption of the 'red' and 'green' pigments impairs the differentiation between reds and greens, causing the typical 'red–green' colour-vision abnormalities commonly inherited as an X-linked trait.

Deficiencies of the 'red' or 'green' pigments can be complete or only partial. Total failure of the 'red' cones is known as 'protanopia'; total failure of the 'green' cones is known as 'deuteranopia'. These conditions result in colour-vision based on only two remaining cone types, and are thus known as 'dichromatic' colour-vision abnormalities. Incomplete deficiencies of the 'red' and 'green' cones are known as 'protanomaly' and 'deuteranomaly', and are referred to as 'anomalous trichromatic' conditions.

The visual system appears to combine the output of the 'red' and 'green' cones into an internal 'yellow' signal, which is then compared with the response of the 'blue' cones. Abnormalities in this blue/yellow axis are referred to as 'tritanopic' colour vision deficiencies. These occur only rarely on an inherited basis, but are more frequently encountered as acquired disorders in patients with cataract, glaucoma or other optic nerve diseases.

Diagnosis

Demonstration of colour vision abnormalities usually requires the use of carefully chosen colour stimuli. Most patients with colour vision deficiency are readily able to correctly identify the colours of everyday objects. This is because very few individuals are truly 'colour-blind', with no colour discrimination, and because the world is a very redundant place – most people learn soon enough that it is generally understood that the grass is 'green' and the sky is 'blue'. Effective tests provide subjects the opportunity to confuse either very similar colours (tests of 'colour discrimination'), or to confuse quite disparate colours ('confusion tests'). In either case, the colours lie along the lines of confusion for individuals with one or the other type of colour vision deficiency, and are chosen from within the appropriate MacAdam ellipses. In practice, it is desirable to control for variations in apparent brightness. This is not difficult in discrimination tests, where the subjects attempt to sort nearly identical colours. However in confusion tests, it is often useful to deliberately introduce a random variation in the brightness of the colour samples, so as to confound any apparent correlation between the hue and the perceived brightness of the colours.

Most definitive colour vision tests are supplied as colour samples on paper discs, or printed pages. The need for stringent quality control in the reproduction of the colours accounts for the high price of these materials. In order for the tests to perform as designed, it is necessary to specify the light by which they are to be viewed. The usual source constitutes an attempt to replicate the slightly bluish light scattered by the sector of the sky opposite the sun on a clear day, referred to as 'CIE Illuminant

"C"', which can be produced by using an ordinary incandescent lamp with a suitable filter. Colour vision testing with printed materials viewed under other illumination (such as unfiltered tungsten light bulbs or fluorescent lights) cannot be relied upon to realize the intentions of the test authors, as printer inks will exhibit different patterns of contrast and similarity when viewed under different lights, a phenomenon known as 'metamerism'.

Reproductions of these colour-testing materials in other media (such as lantern slides) are seldom calibrated against the genuine materials, and are frequently unreliable. In particular, the dyes used in lantern slides are unstable and will fade with time, further reducing the reliability of these tests. Computer simulations of the colour targets are currently research tools. It is unclear to what extent the variations between commercially available computer monitors may degrade the utility of computer-based colour vision tests. Even if unsuitable for definitive testing, they may be suitable for low-cost screening.

Discrimination tests

1.   Farnsworth-Munsell 100-Hue test.   The prototype discrimination test is the Farnsworth-Munsell 100-Hue test. Eighty-five colour samples are mounted in black holders resembling bottle-caps, and are presented to the subject in boxes of 21 or 22 caps, one box at a time (the name '100-Hue' describes an earlier version of the test, but remains in universal use). The caps in each box are scrambled, and the subject is asked to arrange them in order 'by colour' so as to span the colour range between two fixed reference colours. The hues are of medium saturation, and were chosen so that the contrast between adjacent colours approximates the 'just-noticeable difference' between colours as perceived by the best observers with normal colour vision. The colours trace out a complete circle on the CIE diagram. An individual with normal colour vision typically makes a small number of minor transpositions. Individuals with abnormal colour vision are typically unable to distinguish among several similar colours that lie within their MacAdam ellipses, and their lines of confusion will run tangent to the circle of the test colours. In these sectors, the subjects have no choice but to randomly arrange the indistinguishable colour caps.

The test is scored by assigning to each cap the absolute difference between its cap number and the numbers of the caps placed on either side of it. A perfect arrangement assigns to each cap a value of 2. The cap scores are plotted on a polar plot, and the sum of all the scores, less 170 (the minimal possible score) is recorded. As zones of confusion, if any, are typically found on opposite sides of the circle, typical plots for colour-abnormal individuals show two lobes, roughly opposite each other across the circle. The orientation of these lobes indicates the type of the colour vision abnormality, readily distinguishing between protan, deutan and tritan confusion axes. Dichromats typically produce much higher error scores than anomalous trichromats.

The 100-Hue test was developed to identify individuals with superior colour discrimination for industrial applications, such as mixing paints or matching textile dye-lots. It is also popular as a 'gold-standard' for evaluation of candidates for jobs where colour-vision abnormalities are disqualifying.

2. Hardy-Rand-Rittler plates. The 'H-R-R' plates also function as a test of discrimination. Figures (X O and a triangle) are formed in dots of the various test colours, to be viewed against a background of similar dots in various shades of grey. Failure to perceive the figures indicates enlargement of the 'neutral zone' in the indicated direction. Targets are provided to test the protan, deutan and tritan axes, at varying levels of saturation, allowing a crude gradation of the severity of the colour-vision defect.

The H-R-R plates were originally published by the American Optical Company using silk-screen technology. After the initial press run was exhausted, AO declined to reproduce them. A new reproduction of the H-R-R plates, produced with laser-printer technology has recently become available, though no definitive data calibrating them against the original plates have been published.

3. Nagel anomaloscope. The definitive test for the differentiation between dichromats and anomalous trichromats is the Nagel anomaloscope, an instrument that relies on the 'Rayleigh equation' – the equivalence of a spectral yellow to the superposition of a spectral red and spectral green. The observer is allowed to adjust two knobs: the first varies the intensity of a patch of pure yellow light; the second varies the ratio of the red and green components which are superimposed to produce an adjacent patch of colour. A colour-normal individual will perceive as a match only a very narrow range of the red/green mixture against a single intensity of the pure yellow. Dichromats accept a broad range of red/green mixtures as a match to yellow. Protanopes perceive the redder mixtures as dimmer, adjusting the pure yellow to lower intensities. Deuteranopes match the range of red/green mixtures to a constant intensity of yellow. Dichromats always accept the match of a normal observer. Anomalous trichromats reject the normal match, but usually accept a slightly expanded range of anomalous matches. Protanomalous trichromats require extra red. Deuteranomalous trichromats require extra green. The Nagel anomaloscope is no longer produced commercially. While it is the definitive test for classifying red/green abnormalities, it has no provision for evaluating the tritan axis.

4. City University colour vision test. This test uses a series of selected paper colour samples. The centre circle is surrounded by four circles of slightly different colours. Each page has a correct circle and three incorrect ones, each incorrect one being consistent with a protan, deutran or tritan deficit.

Confusion tests

1. Farnsworth D-15 panel. The Farnsworth D-15 panel was developed as a screening test for military use. It consists of 15 caps chosen from the FM 100-Hue colour circle, so as to trace out most of the circle of colours. The caps are scrambled, and the subject is asked to find the cap which best matches a blue reference cap. He is then asked to find the best match from the remaining caps to the cap just selected. He continues in like fashion until he has placed all 15 caps in order. This presentation offers the opportunity for dichromats and severely anomalous trichromats to confuse colours that lie across the colour circle, along their confusion lines. In most cases, the confusions lie along nearly parallel lines. The predominant orientation of this crossing pattern characterizes the patient as protanopic, deuteranopic or tritanopic. As the MacAdam ellipses of most anomalous trichromats do not extend all the way across the circle defined by the D-15 colours, most anomalous trichromats make at most one or two crossing errors on this test, allowing them to be identified as suitable candidates for most jobs which do not require perfect colour-vision.

The D-15 panel is rapidly and easily administered. It detects and classifies both red/green and blue/yellow defects. It is calibrated to a level of difficulty suitable for most occupational screening purposes. While the test requires a degree of subjective interpretation, this is seldom difficult.

2. Lanthony desaturated D-15. The Lanthony desaturated D-15 is a modification of the Farnsworth D-15 panel intended to facilitate the detection of extremely subtle colour vision defects. The test is similar in design to the Farnsworth D-15, except that the colour chips are taken from a much smaller circle on the CIE diagram, which lies very near the central neutral zone. The colours are thus highly desaturated, resembling the pale tints used in wall-paint. The procedure is identical to that used in the Farnsworth D-15. In practice, the Lanthony desaturated D-15 is a very difficult test, requiring excellent colour vision, as well as patience and care in order to achieve a normal arrangement of the colours. With suitably selected subjects, very subtle colour vision disturbances can be detected.

3. Ishihara plates. The Ishihara plates are perhaps the most widely used colour vision test. Figures, most commonly Arabic numerals, are depicted in coloured dots against complex backgrounds of coloured dots. In many cases, the colours are chosen so that those with normal colour vision see one numeral, while those with red/green abnormalities see little contrast defining the 'normal' image, but more prominent contrast (scarcely noticeable to the normal observer) indicating a different number. Positive and negative controls are provided. A few plates also present numerals in red or purple against a background of grey and black dots; these plates are intended to separate the subjects with red/green defects detected with the previous plates into protan or deutan classes. Protans miss the red numbers but see the purple ones; deutans see the red numbers but miss the purple ones. There is no provision for detecting blue/yellow defects.

The Ishihara plates are very easy to use, and are available in editions with various numbers of plates, and even editions with geometric objects instead of numerals for use with children or illiterate adults. The luminance 'noise' created by the backgrounds of dots of varying colours, sizes and intensities is extremely effective, allowing the Ishihara plates to identify many individuals with extremely mild red/green colour vision abnormalities. This extremely high sensitivity is useful clinically, but is often excessive for occupational purposes.

4. Other plates. Many other sets of colour vision testing plates have been published over the years. Most of these are less well designed than the Ishihara or H-R-R sets, and are not recommended. In particular, the 'AO PIP' (or 'Pseudoisochromatic Plates') set is a compilation of plates from many different sources, and has little coherent rationale.

5. *Screening slides.* Compact vision screening systems, such as the AO 'TeleBinocular' or the various versions of the 'Titmus Vision Screener' typically include one or more lantern slides containing simulations of the Ishihara plates. As discussed above, the quality control of these colour samples is poor, and the dyes are unstable. These slides typically screen only for red/green defects, and rarely include a classification target. If they are used, abnormal results should be re-checked using genuine Ishihara plates or other well-calibrated materials.

6. *Lantern tests.* Special purpose lanterns, intended to simulate the appearance of signal lights, have been developed over the years, primarily for occupational purposes. The Farnsworth Lantern was developed for use by the American military, and is still required by many military agencies. It is very expensive, and is no longer commercially available. These lantern tests are usually calibrated against the visibility of actual signal lights, and are not designed for classification of colour vision abnormalities in clinical terms.

Conclusion

There is no one colour vision test that is suitable for all purposes. Clinicians using only one or two tests should be aware of the design goals of the tests, their strengths and their limitations.

CLINICAL GENETICS

Kevin Gregory-Evans

Genetic abnormality is the commonest cause of blindness in the Western world. In the UK, genetic eye disease accounts for 24% of the 1 million adults and 23–50% of the 10 000–25 000 children considered legally blind or partially sighted. Age-related macular degeneration, glaucoma and diabetic retinopathy are all examples of common eye diseases with a clear genetic influence. Patients who are most likely to attend genetic eye clinics however usually express simple Mendelian conditions, such as retinitis pigmentosa and other retinal dystrophies, congenital cataract, congenital glaucoma and ocular disease in association with systemic malformations (e.g. Marfan's syndrome).

Problem

Patients with genetic eye disease generally ask three questions: What disease do I have? Is it treatable? Will it affect my children? Often there is no positive family history at the first consultation.

Background

The first requirement in any genetic consultation is to establish a precise diagnosis. A diagnosis reported by a patient should never be taken at face value. This is especially so in genetic patients where there are implications for family members other than the patient. Detailed clinical examination and appropriate investigations should be undertaken in the proband (the first family member to attend clinic) and may be helpful in other family members who attend for counselling.

Over the last decade a large number of ocular genetic diseases have been linked to specific regions of the human genome and disease genes subsequently identified. Molecular genetic diagnosis is now available for many diseases. In cases where only a genomic localization is available, linkage analysis can be used for diagnosis. In such cases, DNA needs to be collected from about 12 affected and unaffected family members. In cases where the disease gene is known, a number of techniques can be used to identify specific mutations in a single affected individual. Single-base mutations within coding sequences (exons), or regions required for the processing of a transcript (splice sites), are the commonest causes of genetic eye disorders. These may take the form of missense mutations, in which the triplet codon for one amino acid is exchanged for that of another (e.g. CAC-TAC changes a histidine to a tyrosine): nonsense mutations which introduce a pre-mature stop codon into the transcript, leading to truncation of the resultant polypeptide; frameshifts induced by small insertions or deletions that alter the codon reading frame and often lead to truncation of the protein due to introduction of a stop codon or splice-site mutations result in abnormal processing of the transcript also leading to truncated or no protein product. Genes containing repeated sequences can be unstable either because of a tendency for repeat expansion of the region or because they may be more prone to deletions as a result of mis-pairing between repeated sequences in meiosis. The most widely used techniques to identify mutations are SSCP (single-strand conformation polymorphism) analysis, DGGE (denaturing gradient gel electrophoresis) and heteroduplex analysis. The gold standard technique is direct sequencing.

Genetic ocular disease is often seen in association with systemic defects. In such patients, karyotyping should be undertaken. Most chromosomal deletions and translocations are not passed on to future children. Parents of an affected individual should however be screened to detect rare inherited cases or balanced translocation carriers.

All these molecular techniques can be used for prenatal diagnosis. Although this is undertaken in retinoblastoma, it is infrequently used for most genetic eye diseases in the UK and few molecular laboratories offer a diagnostic service.

Assessing risk to children and future generations is mostly based on determining the manner of inheritance in the family of interest. A detailed and extensive family pedigree is required, accurately documenting relationships between affected family members and any consanguineous unions. It is common at the initial consultation for an affected patient to deny that any other family member is also affected. Such patients should be given the opportunity to re-assess this by contacting family members in the knowledge that they may be affected.

An autosomal dominant trait often presents with affected members in each generation and male to male transmission. This would imply a 50% risk to each offspring of affected individuals. Spontaneous mutations may also occur. In such cases the family history will be normal. Variable expression (differences in severity of disease) and incomplete penetrance (patients with the genetic abnormality but no clinical disease) are particular problems in counselling dominant cases. Although the risk of getting the particular gene defect is 50%, such a child may not be as severely affected as the proband. This should especially be taken in to account when prenatal diagnosis is requested.

In autosomal recessive disorder the proband's parents are usually normal. In such families the risk of any other child being affected is 25% irrespective of the number of children already affected. An affected individual with an autosomal recessive disease has a small risk of having an affected offspring depending on the frequency of carrier state in the population. If there is a tradition of consanguinity within the family however, this risk increases. A union between an affected individual and a heterozygote has a 50% risk of producing an affected child and may give rise to a pedigree suggestive of dominant transmission. In families where consanguinity is common, there is also risk to grandchildren. This is called a pseudodominant pattern of inheritance.

Classically, in X-linked recessive traits only affected males (hemizygotes) are symptomatic. However, female carriers of X-linked retinitis pigmentosa, ocular albinism or choroideraemia for example, can be symptomatic and demonstrate fundus abnormalities. The variability and spectrum of clinical expression in x-linked carriers is attributed to lyonization, the random inactivation of one of the two X chromosomes in every cell, with the extent of disease dependent upon the relative proportion of active paternal X chromosomes. Affected males cannot transmit the abnormal X chromosome gene to their sons, but all daughters will be carriers (obligate heterozygotes).

Other types of inheritance may also be seen. Mitochondrial inheritance is seen in Leber's optic neuropathy and mitochondrial myopathy. In such cases inheritance is always through the maternal line. Complex traits, e.g. diabetes mellitus, involve inheritance of a number of predisposing genetic abnormalities which interact to cause disease with or without environmental influences. Risk cannot be as precisely calculated as for Mendelian traits. Without a clear pedigree, the risk of glaucoma in the first-degree relatives of affected patients, for example, is estimated to be 10 times that for the general population.

The assessment of risk to offspring in simplex cases where there is no family history of disease is a common problem. As many as 40% of retinitis pigmentosa patients will not have a positive family history. These cases may represent new mutations which will be inherited as autosomal dominant, recessive or X-linked traits. Unless a family history is found at a later date, without further information, it is assumed that the overall risk to offspring is small (i.e. < 5%) unless the parents relationship is consanguineous or the phenotype is known to be classically dominant (e.g. lattice corneal dystrophy) or X-linked (e.g. choroideraemia).

Conclusion

A major fallacy in the management of genetic disease is the common assertion that these conditions are untreatable. In fact it is more accurate to say that they are incurable. A patient with retinitis pigmentosa, for example, could well benefit from careful refraction and low vision aids, cataract extraction or treatment with acetazolamide for macular oedema. It should not be forgotten that helping the patient to become adjusted to their disease through supplying useful information and support can do a great deal of good. During consultation, patients often raise difficult questions about unconventional therapies that have been promoted in the lay media. Such regimens usually have little scientific basis for their claims and often lead to great disappointment for patients. Ophthalmologists involved in the care of patients with genetic disease are obliged to dissuade them from subjecting themselves to the risks of unsubstantiated therapies and should warn patients that the pursuit of false hope can lead to significant emotional trauma and economic loss.

Further reading

http://www.ncbi.nim.nib.gov/omim/

Baraitser M, Thompson E. Ophthalmic Genetics. In *Pediatric Ophthalmology*, 2nd edn. Oxford: Blackwell Science, 1998; 122–31.

Evans K, Gregory CY, Fryer A *et al*. The role of molecular genetics in the prenatal diagnosis of retinal dystrophies. *Eye* 1995; **9**: 24–8.

Traboulsi EI. *Genetic Diseases of the Eye*, 1st edn. Oxford: Oxford University Press, 1998.

CONGENITAL NYSTAGMUS

Robert H. Taylor & Peter Shah

There are many systems for classifying nystagmus which is present at birth or noted in early infancy. The use of the term 'congenital nystagmus' to describe nystagmus seen in this period is disputed, and the terms 'early onset' and 'infantile' nystagmus may be encountered. Some authors include manifest latent and latent nystagmus as forms of congenital nystagmus (see separate topic). Congenital-infantile nystagmus (CN) has an approximate incidence of 1 in 6550 live births, and a consistent pattern of clinical features. It may be classified as:

(a) Idiopathic (no identifiable underlying ocular pathology). This is sometimes termed congenital motor nystagmus, or congenital benign idiopathic nystagmus.
(b) Secondary or sensory (degraded visual input and secondary sensory deprivation).

These can be broadly divided into:

(i) anterior segment abnormality (e.g. corneal opacity, lens opacity, aniridia or glaucoma);
(ii) a posterior segment abnormality (e.g. retinopathy of prematurity, retinal dysplasia, retinochoroidal coloboma, macular scarring, albinism, optic nerve hypoplasia and optic atrophy);
(iii) posterior segment pathology but normal fundus exam (e.g. Leber's amaurosis, achromatopsia, early cone dystrophy, and blue cone monochromatism).

Problem

Of those children who present to a paediatric ophthalmologist, a large percentage will have secondary nystagmus due to a degraded visual input and sensory deprivation. There are two key problems which must be addressed:

(a) to differentiate those with a degraded visual input from idiopathic motor nystagmus;
(b) to identify the small group of children in whom there is an acquired ocular oscillation secondary to either intracranial or systemic disease.

Background

1. Idiopathic congenital-infantile nystagmus. Typical idiopathic CN is not usually present at birth but develops around the age of 2 months. Strabismus is present in 30% of cases. There is an evolution of the wave form in the early years. From 2–4 months of age the wave form is triangular large amplitude (45°) and low frequency (1 Hz). From 6–8 months the nystagmus becomes symmetric, pendular and low amplitude (3°), with a higher frequency wave form (3 Hz). From 18–20 months the more characteristic jerk nystagmus evolves, but elements of the first two may persist. The wave form in older children characteristically shows a slow phase with increasing velocity (the slow phase in latent nystagmus has a decreasing velocity).

The characteristic nystagmus is bilateral, conjugate and uniplanar, usually horizontal in all positions of gaze. Although it may have a rotatory component it is rarely vertical. The amplitude of the nystagmus increases with gaze in the direction of the fast phase 'gaze modified'. It may be better or worse with occlusion and is often dampened by convergence (fusional or voluntary convergence – not accommodative), with near acuity better than distant acuity. Attempted distance fixation increases the intensity of the nystagmus. There is frequently a null zone (a field of gaze in which the nystagmus is less), and the child may develop a compensatory head posture with associated benefit for vision. Patients do not complain of oscillopsia. An associated head oscillation may be present. The nystagmus is abolished in sleep and anaesthesia. Disruption of the optokinetic reflexes occurs in about two-thirds of patients in the horizontal plane, but is usually preserved in the vertical plane, which provides a useful tool for visual assessment.

Idiopathic CN can occur as autosomal dominant, autosomal recessive, or an X-linked recessive pattern of inheritance, with some female carriers showing evidence of nystagmus. Latent nystagmus may co-exist. Congenital forms of see-saw nystagmus and periodic alternating nystagmus also exist albeit uncommon.

2. Sensory nystagmus. The wave form is often more erratic and more commonly vertical, particularly with achromatopsia and cone dystrophy. The severity of the nystagmus depends on the age of onset of the visual loss (worse if young), the site of the pathology (worse if anterior) and the degree of visual loss (worse if severe). There may be an overlay of searching eye movements.

Clinical features

When confronted with an infant with nystagmus, one must start with a careful history and examination of the child and parents. A detailed neuro-developmental assessment is essential, and one should ensure that the child is not losing abilities already acquired. Parents will often have valuable views on whether their child can see. Ask about photosensitivity. Oscillopsia is not usually present, but may be noted in older children in eccentric gaze positions or in acquired nystagmus.

Examination should include a search for iris transillumination (albinism) in all cases as well as an assessment of the visual field to confrontation. A thorough dilated retinal examination looking for retinal disorders and optic atrophy is also essential. The use of a cycloplegic refraction is mandatory.

On the basis of the clinical findings, one must decide on appropriate further investigations and management of the child. The combined management with a paediatrician has many advantages, especially when one is considering the possibility of visual pathway space occupying lesions. Features which should increase suspicion of possible systemic disease include asymmetry of nystagmus, acquired nystagmus occurring after the age of 3 months, a changing plane of nystagmus in different gaze, see-saw nystagmus, optic disc pallor, deteriorating vision and loss of developmental milestones or other neurologic signs.

Many conditions which degrade the visual input are clinically obvious; however, electrodiagnostic testing provides information necessary to make the diagnosis of certain retinal conditions in which the retina may appear remarkably normal. Electroretinography performed under photopic and scotopic conditions differentiates congenital stationary night blindness, Leber amaurosis, achromatopsia and cone dystrophies. Hemi-field visually evoked cortical responses may suggest abnormal chiasmal decussation suggestive of albinism. Neurodiagnostic imaging techniques, such as MRI may be required when the ophthalmic and/or systemic features suggest the possibility of organic nervous system disease.

Once again, it is emphasized that 'idiopathic' motor nystagmus is a diagnosis of exclusion. One should be prepared to reconsider the diagnosis in the light of changing clinical information. The clinician should have a low threshold for undertaking electrodiagnostic tests or repeating previously normal imaging studies.

Treatment

Optimal visual function can be achieved by correction of refractive errors and strabismus. Spectacles may be useful but contact lenses may give superior vision if the refractive error is large. Optical correction can be combined with tints if photophobic. The use of prisms to move the image the patient sees into their null zone, correct strabismus or induce convergence may rarely improve image quality. Full use should be made of low vision aids. Medical therapy with drugs is rarely useful. Rectus muscle surgery to modify the null point (Kestenbaum/Anderson type) or to reduce the power of the muscles (four muscle recession), may be appropriate but is usually delayed until older (around 8 years of age) to avoid inducing amblyogenic strabismus.

Conclusion

The visual potential of the child will depend on the underlying pathology. Children with typical 'idiopathic' nystagmus often have a final visual acuity of 6/9 to 6/36. It is important to emphasize that vision usually improves, patients do not have oscillopsia, and the amplitude of the nystagmus reduces with time. It is also important to parents to state that most babies with idiopathic congenital nystagmus grow up healthy, go to normal schools, are of normal intelligence and live a full and productive life. If appropriate, genetic counselling may be offered to the parents of children in whom inherited disease is detected.

Further reading

Casteels I, Harris CM, Shawkat F, Taylor D. Nystagmus in infancy: mini review. *British Journal of Ophthalmology* 1992; **76:** 434–7.

Dell'Osso LF, Ellenberger C Jr, Abel LA. The nystagmus blockage syndrome. Congenital nystagmus, manifest latent nystagmus, or both? *Investigative Ophthalmology and Visual Science.* 1983; **24:** 1580–7.

Harris C. Nystagmus and eye movement disorders. In: Taylor D (ed.) *Paediatric Ophthalmology*, 2nd edn. Blackwell Science Ltd, 1997; 869–924.

Lambett SR, Taylor D, Kriss A. The infant with nystagmus, normal appearing fundus, but an abnormal ERG. *Survey of Ophthalmology* 1989; **34:** 176–87.

Leigh RJ, Zee DS. Clinical features of ocular motor nerve palsies. In: *The Neurology of Eye Movements*, 3rd edn. New York, Oxford University Press, 1999; Section 10; 405–82.

Reinecke RD. Idiopathic infantile nystagmus: Diagnosis and treatment. *JAAPOS* 1997; **1**(2): 67.

Related topics of interest

CORNEAL GRAFT FAILURE

Rajesh Aggarwal

Credit for the first corneal graft with some degree of clarity goes to Edward Zirm (1906). Since then, advances in microsurgical techniques, suture materials and the screening of donor material by spectromicroscopy (for endothelial cell density and morphology) has vastly reduced the incidence of corneal graft failure.

Problem

It is of paramount importance to identify those patients at risk of graft failure and recognize the symptoms and signs of failure early. Although corneal graft survival is approximately 90% at 12 months this drops to 60% by 10 years. The most common cause of failure is irreversible immunological rejection. Corneal graft failure may occur as a result of early or late post-operative complications, infection or corneal graft rejection. The cause of the failing graft needs to be identified and appropriate early and aggressive treatment can make the difference between the success and failure of the graft.

Background

The avascularity of the cornea, the absence of classic antigen-presenting cells (APCs) in the centre of the cornea, inhibitory factors in the aqueous humour, the blood–ocular barrier and the phenomenon known as anterior chamber-associated immune deviation (ACAID) are the main factors thought to render the cornea its immune-privileged status. Breakdown in any one or more of the above may contribute to corneal graft rejection.

Graft rejection is more likely if there is pre-existing corneal vascularization as this reduces the relative immune-privilege. The graft size and position also affect the probability of rejection. The optimum graft size appears to be 7–8 mm. Large grafts are more likely to reject as they lie nearer to the limbus and hence nearer the limbal vessels and host antigen-presenting cells. Grafts which are too small are also more prone to failure due to insufficient endothelial cells to maintain function. Iris–graft interface adhesions promote graft rejection as does post-operative ocular inflammation including that induced by loose or broken sutures. Repeated grafts have a higher probability of rejection due to sensitization. A similar mechanism applies to previous pregnancies and blood transfusions. Rejection is also influenced by the primary pathology requiring grafting (e.g. keratoconus has a good prognosis, whilst herpes simplex keratitis has a poor prognosis).

Clinical features

Rejection episodes tend to occur soon after surgery with > 50% in the first 6 months following surgery and 65% of the total rejections within the first year. Rejection occurring in the second year accounts for 20% and in the third year 15%.

In early graft failure, symptoms include reduced visual acuity, photophobia, ocular discomfort and red eye. The patient must be educated to appreciate the importance of these symptoms and report them urgently so that they can be assessed and treated as required.

The patient may be found to have epiphora, conjunctival injection and graft oedema with or without signs of intraocular inflammation.

Late failure is defined as greater than 10 days after surgery for the first graft. The above causes of early graft failure may also present late. However the most important diagnosis to consider is corneal graft rejection. Patients with symptoms and signs suggestive of rejection should be treated for this until proved otherwise.

Symptoms are similar to early graft failure and include ocular irritation, photophobia, blurred vision and red eye. Signs include peri-limbal injection, increased graft thickness (often an early sign), diffuse keratic precipitates, anterior chamber activity, sub-epithelial infiltrates (resembling adenovirus keratitis), an epithelial rejection line (raised linear aggregates of lymphocytes), an endothelial rejection line or 'Khodoudoust line' (aggregates of lymphocytes on endothelium arranged in linear fashion) and graft oedema.

Both epithelial and endothelial rejection lines start in the periphery of the graft and move centrally, the latter destroying endothelial cells thus contributing to the corneal oedema.

Treatment

The treatment of early graft failure depends on the aetiology. Primary endothelial cell dysfunction, now a rare cause of graft failure due to the screening of donor tissue for endothelial cell density and morphology, usually requires re-grafting once ocular inflammation has settled. Surgical trauma is also uncommon since the advent of modern microsurgical techniques and newer suture materials. Treat initially with topical corticosteroids to control inflammation, followed by re-grafting if the cornea does not clear. Pre-existing or persistently raised intraocular pressure after grafting must be controlled medically and if necessary surgically. Likewise, pre-existing ocular inflammation requires control prior to surgery and careful monitoring post-operatively. The initial approach to vitreo-endothelial touch in aphakic keratoplasty is aimed at attempting to reduce the touch by reducing intraocular pressure and inducing mydriasis. If unsuccessful, anterior vitrectomy should be considered. Otherwise, chronic endothelial irritation can lead to retrocorneal fibrous membrane (between Descemet's membrane and the endothelium) formation resulting in permanent graft dysfunction. Lastly, infection within the graft with or without associated inflammation needs aggressive early treatment to optimize the chances of graft survival.

Rejection episode must be recognized early, the stimulus for rejection treated when possible (e.g. loose or broken sutures) and corticosteroids initiated. The dose and route of administration of steroids will depend on the degree and intensity of rejection. Most episodes of rejection can be controlled using intensive topical steroids (e.g. 1 hourly prednisolone 1%). More severe episodes may require additional local steroids (subconjunctival injection) and/or the addition of parenteral steroids. Rarely, additional immunosuppression may be required. Topical cyclosporin-A has little beneficial effect, however systemic administration can effectively reverse or stop a rejection episode. It must always be remembered that use of systemic immunosuppressive drugs can have significant adverse side effects and requires close monitoring by a physician experienced in their use.

After penetrating keratoplasty topical steroids need to be gradually reduced and stopped over 9–12 months. Some patients require long-term low-dose topical steroid therapy. Any cause of inflammation should be corrected immediately. Loose or broken sutures must be removed immediately as they would otherwise act as a nidus, not only for infection, but also for inflammation. Both of these can stimulate rejection. Each episode of suture removal must be covered by an increase in the frequency of administration of topical steroids. The patient must be informed how to recognize the symptoms of graft failure and advised to seek medical attention promptly.

Further reading

The immunology of corneal graft rejection. *Critical Reviews in Immunology* 1998; **18**: 305–25.
Niederkorn JY. The immune privilege of the corneal allografts. *Transplantation* 1999; **67**(12): 1503–8.
The Australian graft registry 1990–1992 report. *Australian and New Zealand Journal of Ophthalmology* 1993; **21**(2): supplement.
The collaborative corneal transplantation studies research group. Effectiveness of histocompatibility matching in high-risk corneal transplantation. *Archives in Ophthalmology* 1992; **110**(10): 1392–1403.

Related topics of interest

Alkali injuries (p. 12); Corneal opacity (p. 75).

CORNEAL OPACITY

Adam P. Booth & Robert H. Taylor

The optical function of the cornea is to refract and transmit light. The maintenance of corneal transparency is therefore of paramount importance.

Problem

It can be difficult to determine the cause of a corneal opacity from its appearance, especially in view of the vast number of potential aetiologies. In the acute phase of corneal disease other signs may be present that have diagnostic significance. In chronic opacification the diagnostic clues may be limited.

Background

The cornea remains transparent because of its relative dehydration, absence of blood vessels and pigment, and regular arrangement of stromal layers and collagen fibrils. Almost all corneal diseases can interfere with corneal transparency, so leading to corneal opacification and a concomitant deleterious effect on corneal function. The cause of a corneal opacity may be obvious from the history. A full-slit lamp examination should employ the techniques of direct illumination, scleral scatter and retro-illumination. One should describe the corneal opacity in terms of its location, size, shape, thickness, depth, colour and vascularization as well as any associated features. Both eyes should be examined as some opacities are characteristically bilateral or unilateral. The detection of reduced corneal sensation is important. Neighbouring structures need careful examination, including the conjunctiva and lids. Systemic examination for conditions such as acne rosacea or rheumatoid disease may be required.

Clinical features

(a) The corneal dystrophies are a group of rare, bilateral but often asymmetrical disorders, characterized by abnormal deposition of substances that alter corneal architecture, resulting in varying degrees of opacification. Vascularization is not a feature. Most show autosomal dominant inheritance, except macular corneal dystrophy, which is autosomal recessive. Determining the anatomical position of the dystrophy is the key to diagnosis.

The anterior dystrophies involve the epithelium and Bowman's layer. Cogan's dystrophy results in a microcystic or 'map dot fingerprint' appearance. Meesman's dystrophy is characterized by clear epithelial microcysts, Reis–Bücklers dystrophy affects the epithelium, Bowman's layer and anterior stroma, giving a central honeycomb appearance with progressive scarring of Bowman's layer.

The stromal dystrophies initially affect the anterior stroma but later the whole stroma. Lattice dystrophy appears as branching, criss-crossed lines, later replaced by a general haze. In granular dystrophy the mid-stromal opacities are axial with a clear corneal periphery. Each opacity is separated by clear cornea. In contrast, the opacities in macular dystrophy involve the entire stromal thickness, including the periphery. The stroma between the opacities is diffusely cloudy.

The main endothelial dystrophy is Fuchs' endothelial dystrophy. It is characterized initially by Descemet's membrane excresences and endothelial protuberances. Later, stromal oedema and bullous keratopathy develop. Eventually the stroma can become opacified and vascularized. Posterior polymorphous dystrophy is another endothelial dystrophy. Mild cases may be asymptomatic with only subtle vesicular, geographical or band-like opacities on the posterior corneal surface. More severe cases may be associated with corneal stromal haze and/or glaucoma. In Schnyder's dystrophy the deposits are yellowish and occur as a ring-like opacity in the anterior central stroma.

(b) Infections are an important cause of corneal opacification. Predisposing factors include exposure, dry eyes, anaesthetic cornea, contact lens wear, lid abnormality (e.g. blepharitis, trichiasis) or other corneal disease. Bacterial infections often result in corneal opacities. *Streptococcus pneumoniae* infection can cause a crystalline keratopathy. Viral keratitis (e.g. adenovirus) may be associated with small subepithelial opacities which fade with time. This needs differentiating from Thygeson's superficial punctate keratitis. Herpes simplex keratitis may form a central or paracentral disciform scar in the mid-stroma with vessel in-growth and associated keratic precipitates. An anaesthetic cornea is often an associated feature. Fungal keratitis should always be considered in the differential diagnosis of bacterial and viral keratitis, particularly when subacute or chronic and unresponsive to antibiotics or anti-fungals.

Acanthamoeba keratitis, characterized by a central or paracentral ring abscess, is often related to poor contact lens hygiene. Trachoma is the leading cause of preventable blindness in the world. Superior limbal pannus or stromal opacification is seen along with Herbert's pits and conjunctival scarring. Interstitial keratitis, a stromal inflammation, is characterized by deep stromal opacification with ghost vessels. Herpes simplex virus, rather than congenital syphilis, is now the commonest cause. Chlamydia keratoconjunctivitis may cause peripheral corneal infiltrates.

(c) Peripheral corneal opacities often have an inflammatory aetiology. Marginal keratitis, characterized by marginal corneal opacities with clear cornea peripherally, is due to an immune response to staphylococcal exotoxins from the lid margin. Blepharitis is often an associated finding. Rosacea keratitis has a characteristic, often inferior, 'thumb print' appearance. Meibomianitis and acne rosacea are associated findings. Phlyctenulosis, also an immune response to staphylococcal antigens, causes limbal nodules, which can extend centrally often with a clear or vascularized zone between the corneal opacity and the limbus. Mooren's ulcer initially causes peripheral corneal ulceration in the horizontal meridian, but later can spread centrally. The differential diagnosis is Terrien's marginal degeneration which starts in the vertical meridian peripherally. A number of the collagen vascular disorders can cause peripheral ulceration and opacification, including rheumatoid arthritis, systemic lupus erythematosus, polyarteritis nodosa and Wegener's granulomatosis.

Vernal keratoconjunctivitis may result in sub-epithelial opacification. Pemphigoid, Stevens–Johnson syndrome and epidermolysis bullosa can all cause corneal exposure secondary to cicatricial conjunctival changes, leading to opacification.

(d) The corneal degenerations are a group of slowly progressive, bilateral, degenerative disorders, whose distribution is the key to diagnosis.

A pterygium invades Bowman's layer from the limbus in the horizontal meridian, usually nasally. Spheroidal degeneration consists of subepithelial, spherical, extracellular deposits of degenerative collagen initially peripheral and later central. Arcus senilis is a peripheral, circumferential opacity separated from the limbus by clear cornea. The mosaic shagreen of Vogt is central and in the anterior stroma, while Vogt's limbal girdle degenerations (types I and II) are peripheral, in the interpalpebral space.

Band keratopathy represents calcium deposition at the level of Bowman's layer. Lipid keratopathy is usually eccentric with large vessels leading into it. Salzmann's nodular degeneration, characterized by multiple subepithelial grey-white nodules, develops in eyes that have had chronic corneal inflammation e.g. trachoma. Lipid keratopathy, due to extracellular deposition of lipid, occurs adjacent to areas of corneal vascularization. Amyloid can be deposited at Bowman's layer in some chronic eye diseases.

(e) Ectasias are characterized by corneal thinning. In early keratoconus, Vogt's vertical striae, which disappear on gentle pressure, may be seen in the posterior stroma. There may be reticular scarring of Bowman's layer with fine central fibrillary opacities and prominent corneal nerves. In advanced disease or after acute hydrops (also seen in keratoglobus and pellucid marginal degeneration) a dense central scar often develops.

(f) Metabolic disorders can result in the deposition of excess metabolites in the cornea. All of the mucopolysaccharidoses, except Hunter's and Sanfilippo, cause corneal deposition of mucopolysaccharides. The most severe deposition occurs in Hurler disease and Scheie syndrome, in which corneal clouding can be present at birth. Wilson's disease results in the corneal deposition of copper, which is seen as a brown/green ring in the peripheral part of Descemet's membrane (Kayser–Fleischer ring) usually first recognized in the superior temporal quadrant. Fabry's disease, another cause, is an X-linked recessive sphingolipidosis which causes a vortex keratopathy. Cystinosis is a rare metabolic disorder characterized by tissue deposition of pine needle-like cysteine crystals in the corneal stroma and iris.

(g) Many drugs can affect the cornea. Vortex keratopathy is characterized by the bilateral symmetrical build-up of epithelial opacities in a swirling vortex pattern. Drug causes include amiodarone, chlorpromazine, chloroquine, hydroxychloroquine, gold, indomethacin, pethidine, tamoxifen and clofazamine. Other drugs causing corneal opacification include thiomersal (pannus formation) and epinephrine (black pigmentation at Bowman's layer).

Red/purple deposits of gold (chrysiasis) can also be seen in the deep inferior stroma after prolonged administration of gold compound. Other metabolic and systemic causes of corneal deposits include hyperuricaemia, argyrosis, oxalosis, multiple myeloma, Waldenström's macroglobulinaemia and lymphoma.

(h) Epithelial iron deposition can occur for a variety of reasons, the Hudson–Stahli line with ageing, Ferrier line inferior to a drainage bleb, Stocker line anterior to an advancing pterygium, and Fleischer ring at the base of the cone in keratoconus. Stromal iron deposition may occur in siderosis or following a complete hyphaema. Iron deposits may also be found as a result of corneal scarring following trauma or surgery.

(i) Mechanical trauma causes opacification only if Bowman's layer is breached, or Descemet's layer ruptured. Chemicals, heat and ionizing radiation can also result in opacification.

(j) The use of excimer and holmium lasers in refractive surgery can result in corneal opacification, as can any other surgical procedure involving the cornea.

(k) Corneal graft. The original pathology for which a graft was performed can recur in the graft (e.g. stromal dystrophies, herpes simplex keratitis). The graft is also at risk of opacification from many of the other disease processes already mentioned in this chapter. During graft rejection there may be epithelial or endothelial rejection lines and stromal opacification with vascularization.

(l) Prominent corneal nerves can be found in keratoconus, Fuchs' endothelial dystrophy, leprosy, buphthalmos, Refsum's disease, icthyosis acanthamoeba and multiple endocrine neoplasia, neurofibromatosis type I or as an idiopathic normal variant.

(m) Congenital anomalies can also cause corneal opacification, including limbal dermoids, anterior segment dysgeneses, sclerocornea, Peter's anomaly and corneal ectasia. Breaks in Descemet's membrane with or without overlying acute oedema or chronic haze can be seen as Haab's striae in buphthalmos (horizontal breaks) or following a traumatic forceps delivery.

Further reading

Committee on Ophthalmic Procedures Assessment. American Academy of Ophthalmology. Excimer laser photorefractive keratectomy (PRK) for myopia and astigmatism. *Ophthalmology* 1999; **106**: 422–37.

Kaufman HE, Brown BA, McDonald M. *The Cornea.* Oxford: Butterworth-Heinemann, 1997.

Krachmer JH, Palay DA. *Cornea Colour Atlas.* St Louis: Mosby, 1995.

Leibowitz HM, Waring GO. *Corneal Disorders: Clinical Diagnosis and Management.* Philadelphia: WB Saunders, 1998.

CYSTOID MACULAR OEDEMA

Andrew S. Jacks & Peter Shah

Cystoid macular oedema (CMO) is a clinical feature of a range of conditions affecting the retina. CMO is a common cause of visual loss in, for example, diabetic retinopathy, retinal vein occlusion and uveitis. CMO may be difficult to manage and is both a diagnostic and a therapeutic challenge.

Problem

CMO is a diagnosis based on the clinical appearance of the macula and intravenous fundus fluorescein angiography features. Prompt diagnosis is valuable as early treatment may result in resolution of the oedema and restoration of macular anatomy and function. Late diagnosis results in permanent distortion of the anatomy with an associated reduction of retinal function. Treatment may not be effective and in some cases involves significant side effects. In some diseases there is debate about management protocols for CMO.

Clinical and pathological features

CMO is best diagnosed using a 78D, 60D or contact fundus lens. Initially macular oedema is seen as retinal thickening with dulled light reflection from the inner limiting membrane. In more severe cases the appearance becomes cystic (hence the name) with collections of fluid surrounding the fovea in a petaloid appearance. The visual acuity may not be reduced especially in mild cases and where resolution occurs. However, the cystic changes alter the retinal anatomy and can lead to chronic changes in retinal function. Decompensation or loss of the non-permeable characteristics of the perifoveal capillaries and retinal pigment epithelium occurs resulting in fluid leakage into the retina. Initial fluid accumulation may be within the Müller cells, eventually the fluid collects in cystic spaces in the fibre layer of Henle. As this fibre layer radiates in a spoke-like fashion from the fovea the cystic spaces assume a petaloid appearance seen histologically as clear cystoid spaces. Eventually the spaces may coalesce to form a lamellar hole.

The diagnosis of CMO may be difficult to make for example in diabetic retinopathy and uveitis where the view of the retina may be poor due to cataract or the retinal oedema may be difficult to identify from other retinal pathology such as laser scars. Fluorescein angiography can be of great benefit here as the macula oedema can be seen as leakage of fluorescein from the retinal vessels into the extravascular tissue corresponding to the clinical picture confirming the diagnosis.

Differential diagnosis

CMO is a feature of diabetic retinopathy, central and branch retinal vein occlusion, uveitis and retinal vasculitis, following ocular surgery, choroidal neovascular membranes, retinal telangiectasia and retinitis pigmentosa. A cystoid macular appearance can be seen in Goldman–Favre syndrome, juvenile retinoschisis and nicotinic acid maculopathy but these are not caused by leakage from the retinal vasculature.

1. Diabetic retinopathy. Macular oedema is a common cause of visual loss in diabetic patients. It can be divided into focal, diffuse, ischaemic and mixed. CMO may also be associated with proliferative changes resulting in fibrosis and traction on the macula. Panretinal photocoagulation can cause or exacerbate macular oedema, particularly if applied heavily.

Treatment involves early identification and appropriate laser treatment according to guidelines described in the diabetic retinopathy trials, the aim being to balance resolution of the oedema and damage from the laser with establishment of CMO and resultant reduction in visual acuity. Discriminating between macular oedema which requires laser treatment and changes associated with laser burns in a previously treated macula or ischaemia can be difficult. Fluorescein angiography can help to identify areas of retina which require laser treatment. Oedema due to macular traction may resolve after vitrectomy.

2. Central and branch retinal vein occlusion. Macular oedema is a common finding in both of these conditions. The management and outcome of the macular oedema has been well described by the central and branch retinal vein occlusion study groups. Essentially laser treatment to macular oedema in central retinal vein occlusion may result in resolution of the oedema but with no improvement in the vision. Attempts have been made to reduce macular oedema using chorioretinal venous anastomoses, the results of this treatment are the focus of much debate. The macular oedema in branch retinal vein occlusion may resolve spontaneously and laser treatment is only indicated if it persists and there is no ischaemia of the macula on the fluorescein angiogram.

3. Uveitis and retinal vasculitis. Cystoid macular oedema is a significant problem in this group of patients. The oedema may be difficult to diagnose as the view of the macula may be obscured by cataract and vitritis. The clinician should have a low threshold for suspecting macular oedema and if there is difficulty with the diagnosis a fluorescein angiogram or optical coherence tomography may help. The macular oedema is controlled by treating the patient with immunosuppressants. These may be given locally in the form of orbital floor or posterior subtenons injections of short-acting and depot steroid or systemically. Systemic immunosuppression involves the use of systemic steroids and other potent immunosuppressants. There is debate about the use of vitrectomy in patients with macular oedema secondary to uveitis. The idea being that the imflammatory mediators (which might cause the oedema) present in the vitreous are removed by the vitrectomy, and thus the CMO should resolve.

4. Following ocular surgery. Macular oedema is a possible outcome after any form of intraocular surgery. The most commonly performed intraocular procedure is cataract surgery and in this situation is called the Irvine–Gass syndrome (originally described in patients after intracapsular cataract extraction). Typically the patient undergoes uneventful surgery and initially has good vision. The vision may drop 1 to 3 months postoperatively (but has been described years postoperatively). The oedema accumulates from leakage from perifoveal capillaries. The cause of this leakage is not fully understood and may be due to vitreous traction or to action of inflammatory mediators such as prostaglandins. The Irvine–Gass syndrome is more common in patients with diabetes and hypertension. The incidence is highest in intracapsular cataract patients, and increases with significant postoperative uveitis, and complications such as vitreous loss and iris prolapse.

The majority of these patients will do well with the oedema settling spontaneously in 75% of uncomplicated cases. Treatment involves prostglandin synthetase inhibitors, acetazolamide and topical steroids. CMO may be associated with vitreous adhesions to the iris and corneal wound. Cutting these with vitrectomy or NdYAG laser may be helpful. Prophylaxis for the second eye with prostaglandin synthetase inhibitors, and topical and systemic steroids is recommended.

5. Choroidal neovascular membranes.   CMO is present with choroidal neovascular membranes but is not the primary feature, and not a main diagnostic feature. If CMO is seen and no obvious cause is noted a juxtafoveal choroidal neovascular membrane may be present and should be looked for. This may be treated with laser to the area of neovascularization if appropriate.

6. Juxtafoveal telangiectasia.   The signs in juxtafoveal telangiectasia may be subtle and will vary according to the type of telangiectasia present. Treatment will also depend on the exact diagnosis of subtype. The telangiectasia may be most easily seen with fluorescein angiography.

7. Retinitis pigmentosa.   The CMO in retinitis pigmentosa may be a cause of reduced visual acuity. It is understood to be due to loss of polarity of retinal pigment epithelial cells. Treatment with acetazolamide may well re-establish this polarity and hence reduce the CMO resulting in increased vision.

Further reading

DCCT Research Group. The effect of intensive treatment of diabetes on the development and progression of long-term complications in insulin dependent diabetes mellitus. *New England Journal of Medicine* 1993; **329:** 977–1034.

ETDRS report No 2. Early Treatment Diabetic Retinopathy Study Research Group: treatment techniques and clinical guide-lines for photocoagulation of diabetic macular oedema. *Ophthalmology* 1987; **94:** 761–74.

Keenan J, Kritzinger E, Dodson P. Management of retinal vein occlusion. *British Journal of Hospital Medicine* 1993; **49:** 268–73.

Tso MOM. Pathology of cystoid macular oedema. *Ophthalmology* 1982; **89:** 902–15.

DERMATOLOGY AND THE EYE 1: LOCAL LID DISEASE

Farida Shah & Peter Shah

There are many diseases in which the fields of ophthalmology and dermatology overlap. Dermatological conditions may present to the ophthalmologist with involvement of the eyelid alone, or in association with other skin lesions. There are also many systemic diseases which have both ophthalmic and dermatological manifestations. The advice of a dermatologist may be useful in the management of these ophthalmic problems, particularly in patients with external eye disease.

Management

It is important to have a systematic approach to dermatological problems. Accurate assessment requires a detailed history and thorough description of the lesion. In the history it is important to elucidate how long a skin lesion has been present, whether it has changed in size, whether it is symptomatic (e.g. itching/bleeding) and whether it is present constantly or intermittently. A history of contact with cosmetics, topical medications or the use of eye drops is important when an allergic contact dermatitis is suspected. A history of aggravating factors (e.g. sunlight) should be taken.

Local lid involvement in dermatological disease

1. Dermatitis. The eyelid is a frequent site of dermatitis which may be atopic, irritant, contact or seborrhoeic dermatitis. The most common causes of a contact dermatitis affecting the eyelids are cosmetics (especially nail varnish), nickel, topical skin medications and eye drops. Sensitization may occur to either the drug or preservative in topical drops. The affected eyelids are usually dry, scaly, red, oedematous and thickened due to frequent rubbing. Itching of the skin is an important symptom to elicit.

2. Rosacea is another primarily dermatological condition with ocular manifestations. Skin involvement is characterized by telangectasia, pustules and papules typically occurring in the malar area, nose, chin and forehead. The patient may report marked facial erythema after ingestion of alcohol and coffee. In less obvious cases the patient may describe intermittent swelling of the eyelids due to lymphoedema. About one-third of patients with rosacea have a chronic blepharoconjunctivitis and meibomitis. Corneal problems include marginal keratitis, vascularization (initially inferior) and less commonly, a progressive ulceration. Oral acetazolamide has been reported to exacerbate rosacea. Both the ophthalmic and dermatological aspects of rosacea usually respond well to treatment with oral tetracyclines, which need to be used for 3–6 months initially. Tetracycline use is contraindicated in pregnant women and breast-feeding mothers.

3. Discoid lupus usually causes a rash in a malar distribution, but may present as eyelid lesions. It is usually a relatively benign, chronic cutaneous condition which most frequently affects sun-exposed areas. It is characterized by well-defined red, scaly patches with subsequent pigmentary changes, atrophy and scarring.

4. Angio-oedema is a severe form of type 1 allergic reaction with gross eyelid swelling. It may be part of a generalized anaphylaxis, but is usually short-lived and self-limiting. Familial angio-oedema may be due to a deficiency of C1 esterase inhibitor. Angio-oedema responds well to oral anti-histamine therapy. In severe disease, recurrent problems may lead to dermatochalasis.

Vascular and pigmentary lesions of the eyelids

1. Oculodermal melanocytosis (naevus of Ota) is a condition of unilateral hyper-melanosis, in which ocular melanosis is seen in combination with ipsilateral melanosis of the peri-orbital skin and eyelids. The condition is more common in dark-skinned races and is usually present at birth, but features may occasionally be delayed until puberty or early adult life. Although malignant change in the skin is very rare, a few cases have been reported of malignant melanoma developing in the choroid, iris or orbit.

2. Infantile haemangioma is a common developmental vascular tumour which presents within the first weeks of life, undergoes a proliferative phase in the first year and characteristically involutes, so that by the age of 5 years involution of most lesions is virtually complete. The prevalence of infantile haemangiomata is approximately 10% at 1 year and is increased in babies born prematurely. Periocular lesions are not uncommon and are important because of the risk of amblyopia. Amblyopia is most often secondary to monocular astigmatism caused by the mass effect of the lid lesion on the globe. If the lid lesion is very large, then amblyopia may result from stimulus deprivation. As infantile haemangiomas resolve spontaneously, treatment is often not necessary, however the risk of visual loss with periocular lesions is an indication for active management. Options include the use of systemic and intralesional steroids, interferon, laser therapy or surgery.

3. Port wine stain (PWS) is a vascular malformation characterized clinically by persistent erythematous macules often involving the superior and middle branches of the trigeminal nerve. It differs from a haemangioma in that there is no endothelial proliferation, and pathologically there is ectasia of dermal capillaries. Whilst the lesions are usually macular in infancy they may become raised in adulthood. Unlike haemangiomas there is no spontaneous resolution. Eye and brain abnormalities are found in 8–15% of patients with facial PWS. Sturge–Weber syndrome is the association of PWS with vascular malformations in the eye and leptomeninges and radiological evidence of calcification in the brain. Ocular problems associated with PWS include dilated conjunctival vessels, glaucoma, tortuous retinal vessels and choroidal haemangioma. Around 10% of patients with PWS around the eye have leptomeningeal involvement and of these 30–60% will develop glaucoma. The risk of developing glaucoma is not confined to patients with Sturge–Weber syndrome. Laser treatment with the pulse dye laser is effective in treating PWS.

Tumours of the eyelids

Almost any neoplastic skin disease can affect the eyelid. Precancerous lesions such as actinic keratoses and Bowen's disease should be treated aggressively because of the risk of future malignancy.

The most common malignant tumour of the eyelid is basal cell carcinoma and 70% occur on the lower eyelid. If left untreated, these lesions can invade the orbit and sinuses, with devastating results. Squamous cell carcinoma and malignant melanoma also occur on the eyelids.

A sebaceous cell carcinoma arising from a meibomian gland may present with a persistent unilateral lid swelling, which may be mistaken for a recurrent chalazion. Any chalazion which does not behave in a typical manner should be considered to be a neoplastic lesion until proven otherwise.

Keratoacanthomas are single dome-shaped nodules with a central crater containing keratin. They grow very rapidly and may achieve a size of 1–2 cm in several weeks. The natural history of the lesion is to regress spontaneously after several weeks or months. If the behaviour of the lesion is atypical, care should be taken as it may be a squamous cell carcinoma, the appearance of which can sometimes be mistaken for a keratoacanthoma.

Local infections

1. *Molluscum contagiosum* virus may cause small, painless, grey/white nodules on the eyelids. The nodules are characteristically umbilicated, and can be missed unless specifically looked for. Necrotic debris from the skin lesion can cause a recurrent follicular conjunctivitis, sub-epithelial opacities and in rare instances may lead to corneal pannus formation and scarring.

2. *Dacroadenitis* may present with painful lateral lid swelling and an S-shaped lid contour. The possibility of an underlying malignancy in the lacrimal gland should be remembered.

3. *Herpes simplex* virus is a common cause of ocular problems. Primary ocular infection often occurs in childhood. The initial lesions are erythematous papules which rapidly progress to small clusters of clear vesicles. These vesicles often become pustular and have superficial crusts. Healing occurs without scarring. In patients with eczema, the virus may cause particularly severe disease (eczema herpeticum).

4. *Cellulitis* affecting the eyelids needs to be differentiated into preseptal and orbital cellulitis. It must be remembered that orbital cellulitis is a potentially life-threatening condition. Orbital cellulitis is usually differentiated from preseptal cellulitis on the basis of signs of orbital involvement. These include: proptosis, chemosis, restriction of ocular movements, reduced visual acuity and swelling of the optic disc.

5. *Necrotizing fasciitis* is a particularly dangerous infection, often due to streptococci. The patient usually has systemic signs of infection including pyrexia, tachycardia and a neutrophil leukocytosis. When it involves the eyelids there is a spreading purple discoloration of the skin with subsequent blistering and ulceration. Treatment is with high-dose intravenous antibiotics, and early debridement.

The surgery may need to be quite extensive as this is a potentially life-threatening condition.

6. *Erysipelas*   is a common skin infection which may affect the eyelids. The rash has the appearance of well-demarcated erythema and vesicles, often with gross lid swelling. Facial involvement may spread to the orbit and be complicated by cavernous sinus thrombosis. The causative organism is usually a group A streptococcus and treatment is with intravenous benzylpenicillin.

DERMATOLOGY AND THE EYE 2: SYSTEMIC DISEASES

Farida Shah & Peter Shah

There are many diseases in which ophthalmological and dermatological signs coexist. Some of these are primarily dermatological conditions with involvement of the eyes, and some are conditions in which there are characteristic dermatological features which may help make the diagnosis. Behçet's syndrome (see p. 19) is a classical example of one of these diseases.

1. ***Xanthelasma*** are yellow-brown plaques found on the eyelids. They begin as flat yellow lesions at the inner canthal regions of the upper lids and often become symmetrical on all four lids. They are of importance because they are often associated with hyperlipidaemia. A patient with xanthelasma should be carefully examined for other signs of hyperlipidaemia, such as arcus lipidus, lipaemia retinalis, tendon xanthomas and eruptive cutaneous xanthomata. A careful family history should be taken, with particular emphasis on early deaths due to cardiovascular disease. Serum cholesterol and triglycerides should be measured. Xanthelasma may be found in association with other medical conditions, such as hypothyroidism and primary biliary cirrhosis.

2. ***Dermatopolymyositis*** is an inflammatory, systemic connective tissue disease which is more common in women and presents between 30 and 60 years of age. An underlying malignancy is present in a proportion of cases (20–70%) and is more common in older males. The classical involvement of the eyelids is by a violaceous (heliotrope) periorbital rash. Rarely there may also be weakness of the extraocular muscles. The condition may be fulminant, with a lethal outcome in a few days, or may have a prolonged course. Treatment is with systemic steroids.

3. ***The amyloidoses*** are a group of conditions characterized by deposition of an abnormal protein in various organs. Amyloid deposition may occur in the skin of the eyelid. The lesions are macular or papular and often demonstrate purpura after minor trauma. Amyloid may also be deposited in the orbit, the cornea or at the limbus.

4. ***In the Vogt–Koyanagi–Harada syndrome*** the ocular findings of a granulomatous panuveitis with exudative retinal detachments are associated with central nervous system and dermatological features. Patients develop vitiligo, patchy alopecia and poliosis, which are usually not present when the patient presents with ophthalmic problems, but develop subsequently.

5. ***Systemic lupus erythematosus*** is a multisystem, autoimmune connective tissue disease which may affect the eyes. The characteristic cutaneous lesion is a photosensitive, erythematous butterfly rash found in the malar area. A cutaneous vasculitis and scarring alopecia may also be found. There may be features of retinal vasculitis and ischaemic changes (cotton wool spots). Optic atrophy, uveitis, keratitis, conjunctivitis and dry eyes are also features.

6. Thyroid eye disease may be associated with skin disorders. Patients with Graves' disease may have pretibial myxoedema (a chronic, erythematous, oedematous swelling of the anterior aspect of the lower legs). The association of Graves' disease with finger clubbing is termed thyroid acropathy. In hypothyroid patients the skin is often dry and there may be loss of the lateral third of the eyebrow.

7. The Stevens–Johnson syndrome is characterized by erythema multiforme with associated mucous membrane involvement. The mucosae of the mouth, genitalia and eyes may be involved in a severe ulcerative process. In extremely severe cases internal organs (e.g. kidney/lung) can be affected. Stevens–Johnson syndrome may be a life-threatening condition. Common causes include infection with herpes simplex and mycoplasma, and drugs such as sulphonamides, phenytoin, barbiturates and penicillins. The typical rash of erythema multiforme consists of target lesions, which are usually symmetrical and most common on the distal aspect of the limbs. Acute conjunctival involvement may be either catarrhal, purulent or pseudomembranous. Corneal involvement can result in ulceration and perforation. Chronic cicatricial ocular disease can result in severe keratoconjunctivitis sicca and lid abnormalities.

8. Human immunodeficiency virus (HIV) infection may have various dermatological features, including Kaposi's sarcoma, oral hairy leukoplakia and multiple facial mollusca contagiosa. Kaposi's sarcoma is a vascular tumour. The lesions are usually purple in colour and in the early stages may look ecchymotic, however, they are almost always palpable and of a firm consistency. There may be marked lymphoedema in the surrounding tissues, and the hard palate is a very common site for their first presentation. Other dermatological manifestations of HIV infection include infections with herpes simplex, herpes zoster, Candida and other opportunistic organisms, all of which may be more severe in HIV disease.

9. Tuberculosis may manifest in the skin in a variety of ways. Ulcerative lesions may occur at the site of percutaneous innoculation with the mycobacterium, but the classical signs are associated with endogenous spread. Lupus vulgaris describes the condition in which patients develop a reddish/brown, slightly scaly plaque which exhibits an apple-jelly (yellow-brown) appearance on diascopy (pressing on the lesion with a glass slide). A chronic granulomatous uveitis is the most common ophthalmic manifestation of disease. Posterior segment involvement usually consists of a focal or multifocal choroiditis.

10. Syphilis.   The lesion of primary syphilis is a painless chancre which is usually, but not always, found on the genitalia. There is usually an associated regional lymphadenopathy. Secondary syphilis occurs 2–6 months after the primary infection. The skin rash (which lasts several weeks) consists of macules and papules which are copper-brown in colour and located on the trunk and, specifically, on the palms and soles. There may also be condylomata lata on the genital and perineal skin. Secondary syphilis may present with an acute anterior uveitis, which may become chronic. A diffuse chorioretinitis can also occur and is bilateral in about 50% of cases. Neuroretinitis results from primary involvement of the optic nerve and retina. The classical skin lesion of tertiary syphilis is the gumma, which is a painless, rubbery lesion in the subcutaneous tissue. Diffuse chorioretinitis, optic atrophy and Argyll Robertson pupils may be seen in neurosyphilis and its sequelae.

11. Leprosy.   There are two main types of infection with *Mycobacterium leprae*. In tuberculoid leprosy the skin lesions consist of a few well-defined, hypopigmented, anaesthetic macules. Thickened peripheral nerves may be palpable. In lepromatous leprosy there are usually many small erythematous, anaesthetic papules and nodules. The skin is often diffusely thickened and the patient may lose the hair of the eyebrows and lash hairs. Ophthalmic features of leprosy include acute and chronic anterior uveitis, interstitial keratitis, thickened and beaded corneal nerves, corneal scarring, iris pearls, lens opacity and scleritis. Visual loss most commonly results from complications of uveitis.

The genodermatoses

A number of inherited disorders of the skin have ophthalmological manifestations. These include epidermolysis bullosa, some ichthyoses (e.g. KID syndrome; Keratitis, Ichthyosis and Deafness) and many of the neurocutaneous disorders. A few of the genodermatoses with ophthalmological features are discussed in more detail.

1. Xeroderma pigmentosum   is an inherited condition with defective DNA repair. Patients present at an early age with grossly sun-damaged skin and the development of pre-malignant and malignant skin lesions. The eyes are involved in over 80% of cases, with photophobia and conjunctival inflammation. Later changes include severe keratitis, symblepharon and corneal vascularization. Patients with this condition often develop ectropion. Basal cell and squamous cell carcinomas are commonly found. Malignant melanomas may also develop. These patients need careful dermatological and ophthalmological follow-up. In addition to strict avoidance of sun exposure, these patients benefit from the use of oral retinoids, which do seem to reduce the number of new epithelial cancers.

2. Pseudoxanthoma elasticum   is an autosomal recessive disorder of connective tissue involving the elastic tissue of the skin, eyes and blood vessels. The classical dermatological signs are loose folds of skin, most commonly in the neck, and axilla, with a yellow chamois leather or plucked chicken skin appearance. Angioid streaks are seen on fundal examination, and may be associated with choroidal neovascularization. The associated involvement of the elastic tissues in blood vessels means that these patients also suffer with cardiac disease, gastrointestinal bleeding, hypertension and intermittent claudication.

3. Incontinentia pigmenti (Bloch–Sulzberger syndrome)   is a disorder inherited as X-linked dominant and is therefore usually lethal for affected males. Patients present with vesicles and verrucous lesions in a linear or whorled distribution in the neo-natal period. These usually resolve over a period of months leaving linear hyperpigmented lesions, which may be quite subtle. Thirty percent of affected patients have ocular abnormalities. The most typical abnormality is retinal detachment of a dysplastic retina. Other abnormalities include microphthalmos, uveitis, cataract, optic atrophy, pigmentary retinopathy and chorioretinitis. Other features of incontinentia pigmenti are dental abnormalities (common) and neurological complications (rare).

4. Ectodermal dysplasia encompasses a large group of disorders with abnormalities of one or more of the structures of ectodermal origin i.e.: hair, nails, teeth and sweat glands. A number of the ectodermal dysplasia syndromes have ophthalmic features, which include abnormalities of the lacrimal system, photophobia, strabismus and cataract. Patients may also have skeletal abnormalities e.g. ectrodactyly-ectodermal dyplasia-clefting (EEC) syndrome.

The ophthalmic and dermatological manifestations of the phakomatoses, sarcoidosis, cicatricial pemphigoid and albinism are considered separately in the appropriate topics.

Further reading

Barrett GH, Karcioglu ZA, Gordon RA, Pechous BP. Capillary hemangioma (infantile periocular hemangioma). *Survey of Ophthalmology* 1994; **38:** 399–426.

The skin and the eye. In: *Rook, Wilkinson, Ebling – Textbook of Dermatology.* RH Champion (ed.). Oxford: Blackwell Scientific Publications, 1998.

Related topics of interest

Albinism (p. 8); Behçet's disease (p. 19); Cicatricial conjunctivitis (p. 56); Neurofibromatosis (p. 180); Phakomatoses (p. 230); Sarcoidosis (p. 276); Thyroid eye disease (p. 315).

DIABETES MELLITUS: MEDICAL ASPECTS

Paul Dodson

Diabetes mellitus is a group of conditions characterized by chronic hyperglycaemia secondary to absolute or relative insulinopaenia. It is a common condition, affecting 3–7% of the adult population in the Western world.

The WHO classification divides diabetes into Type I (insulin-dependent diabetes mellitus) and Type II (non-insulin-dependent diabetes mellitus). The classification also includes malnutrition-related diabetes, gestational diabetes and diabetes related to other conditions such as pancreatic disease, drug-induced diabetes and certain genetic conditions. There are wide geographical variations in the prevalence of diabetes. Type I is the most common type of diabetes in young people (<30 years of age) in the Western world and is rare in the developing world. However, Type II accounts for 85% of diabetes in the developed world, and it is particularly common in Asian (Indo-Pakistani) migrants, of whom up to 35% of elderly adults may be affected.

Problem

Diabetes and its complications are a major cause of morbidity and mortality in the community. It is a major risk factor for cardiovascular disease, with the risk of myocardial infarction or cerebrovascular accident two to three times that of the general population. Diabetes mellitus is still a leading cause of blindness in young people in the developed world. Accurate diagnosis and careful management are essential to reduce the long-term complications.

Diagnosis

In the patient with classic symptoms of diabetes (thirst, polyuria, weight loss) the disease can be diagnosed on a single plasma glucose >7.0 mmol/l or a random plasma glucose >11.1 mmol/l is diagnostic. In an asymptomatic patient a second measurement should be made to confirm the diagnosis. An oral glucose tolerance test (OGTT) with a 75 g load is helpful in doubtful cases or in diagnosing gestational diabetes.

Management

The aims of treatment are to prevent acute metabolic problems, abolish hyperglycaemic symptoms (polyuria, polydipsia, weight loss, lethargy) and to reduce the risk of complications.

Type I diabetes

The results of the Diabetes Control and Complication Trial (DCCT) showed beyond doubt that patients with type I diabetes that had good long-term glycaemic control had significantly fewer complications. The trial found that if blood sugar is maintained near normal levels over a long period of time the risk of diabetic eye disease is reduced by 76%, and diabetic nephropathy by 35–56%. Mean glycated haemoglobin level was 7.2% in the intensively treated group, compared to 9% in the usual care group. In type I diabetes, insulin therapy is mandatory with supervision from a diabetes team (diabetologist, dietitian, diabetes specialist nurse, chiropodist). Patient education is a crucial part of management, with detailed advice on insulin technique, dietary intake and home blood glucose monitoring.

Exogenous insulin is now identical in amino acid composition to endogenous insulin, such that human insulin is normally used. Various insulin regimes are in use and the preferred combination will depend on the age, lifestyle and motivation of the patient. Traditional regimes involve twice daily injections with a combination of short- and intermediate-acting insulins. Standard pre-mixed formulas containing 10–50% short- and 90–50% intermediate-acting insulin are commonly employed. Four times daily injections (three short-acting injections and a long-acting injection at night) allow for more flexibility, and this may be important in relation to achieving tight glycaemic control in light of the DCCT trial results. The advent of new delivery devices, such as insulin pens has improved insulin acceptability for many patients. New insulin analogues have also been introduced which are rapid acting, given just prior to a meal (rather than the former advised 20 minute delay) and are associated with a reduction of hypoglycaemia in some patients. The price of tight glycaemic control in Type I diabetics is multiple attendance, regular home blood glucose monitoring, weight gain and increased risk of hypoglycaemia.

Urine testing for glucose is not an accurate way to monitor diabetic control but urinalysis is important in Type I diabetes to detect ketones. Home blood glucose monitoring is particularly important in Type I diabetes with glycosylated haemo-globin (HbA_1) or fructosamine estimations used to reflect longer-term glycaemic control. Type I diabetic patients are usually followed up in a diabetic clinic with a trained multidisciplinary team (usually secondary care) including the dietician and chiropodist. Close liaison between the diabetic physician and other specialists, e.g. ophthalmologist, vascular surgeon, is essential to ensure optimum management of the diabetic patient.

Type II diabetes

The first line of treatment in Type II diabetics is dietary control. The recommended energy requirements are very similar to a normal balanced diet, with 30–35% derived from fats, 10–15% from protein and 50% as complex carbohydrates. Many type II patients are overweight and appropriate advice on weight reduction is important. Alcohol consumption should be moderated and advice on smoking cessation stressed.

If type II diabetics cannot be controlled by diet alone, an oral hypoglycaemic drug should be added. There are two main groups: the sulphonylureas and biguanides. Sulphonylureas are generally well tolerated but may lead to hypoglycaemia and weight gain. Newer generation drugs are now preferred as there is less risk of hypoglycaemia than the first generations, e.g. gliclazide, glipizide, glimepiride. Other side effects include weight gain, hyponatraemia and facial flushing with alcohol (chlorpropamide). Biguanides require the presence of some endogenous insulin to be effective, and metformin is the only biguanide currently available. Metformin does not induce hypoglycaemia, but may rarely lead to life threatening lactic acidosis especially in patients with renal impairment and liver dysfunction if these contra-indications are not respected. For the above reasons, some authorities also suggest that biguanides should not be used in patients over 70 years of age. Unfortunately, biguanides have a high incidence of gastro-intestinal side effects which may necessitate cessation of this therapy. The alpha glucosidase inhibitors (e.g. Acarbose) may be used in combination with sulphonylureas and/or metformin. These agents slow breakdown of long-chain sugars to glucose in the gut and their use is limited by a high incidence of gastro-intestinal side effects.

More recently, a new class of agents, the thiazolidinediones have appeared on the market. These drugs are thought to act by interacting with a nuclear receptor, peroxizome proliferator activated receptor (PPAR) gamma, thereby improving insulin sensitivity with reduction in glycaemia, and favourable effects on the lipid profile. Troglitazone, the first of the agents, was widely used in the USA and Japan, and rosiglitazone (and maybe pioglitazone) is now licensed for use in combination therapy, either with sulphonylurea or biguanide therapy.

Good glycaemic control has been the cornerstone of management in type II diabetes. The United Kingdom Prospective Diabetes Study (UKPDS) reported the results of 5102 newly diagnosed type II diabetic patients who participated in a prospective randomized intervention trial since 1977. Over a mean of 10 years, follow-up of those patients in the intensive treatment group (treated with sulphonylurea, metformin, or insulin) achieved an 11% reduction in glycated haemoglobin (−0.9%) compared to conventional treatment. This resulted in a reduction of risk in the intensive group of any diabetes related endpoint by 12% and a 25% risk reduction in microvascular endpoints. These included significant reduction of diabetic retinopathy two-step progression, the need for photocoagulation and reduction in cataract extraction. There was a reduction in macrovascular disease endpoints, but this did not quite reach statistical significance. There was an increased risk of hypoglycaemia and weight gain. Intensive blood glucose control by either sulphonylurea or insulin therapy had the same efficacy, whereas metformin in obese subjects was particularly efficacious, with less adverse effects of weight gain and fewer hypoglycaemia attacks. The UKPDS reports have therefore confirmed that hyperglycaemia plays an important role in the development of diabetic microvascular complications. However, to prevent and ameliorate macrovascular endpoints, management needs to be focused also on hypertension, cholesterol metabolism and overall cardiovascular risk assessment, and suggested targets to be achieved are shown in Table 1.

Table 1. Targets of diabetic treatment

- Maintain 'normal life'
- Avoidance of macro- and micro-vascular complications
- Glycated haemoglobin (HbA$_1$) <7%
- BP ≤ 140/80
- Existing macrovascular disease (secondary prevention)
  Serum cholesterol <4.8 mmol/l (STATINS)
  Aspirin therapy
- Primary prevention: CHD risk (and total cardiovascular disease risk)
  Identified 10 year risk (primary prevention)
  and
  Action if: UK advice >30% (SMAC)
                  More reasonable >20%
                  Eventually target >15%
  BP lowering, statins, aspirin, smoking cessation

BP, blood pressure; CHD, coronary heart disease; SMAC, Standing Medical Advisory Committee (UK).

Complications and annual review

The long term vascular complications account for 80% of the costs of care and 80% of diabetic patients will die prematurely from cardiovascular disease. They can be subdivided into:

- Large vessel (macrovascular) disease (MI, PVD, stroke);
- Small vessel (microvascular) or microangiopathic disease;
- Neuropathy (which has a microvascular component).

Diabetes, hypertension, dyslipidaemia and obesity commonly co-exist in the same patient (comprising Syndrome X or chronic cardiovascular risk syndrome) and are amongst major independent risk factors for macrovascular disease, which are:

- Diabetes mellitus;
- Hypertension;
- Dysplipidaemia;
- Cigarette smoking;
- Family history;
- Presence of proteinuria.

Microvascular disease has specific features with basement membrane thickening of the capillary resulting in plasma protein leakage. These effects are clinically apparent in the eyes, kidneys, and vasa nervorum of peripheral nerves. The other non-ophthalmic complications are:

        1. *Long-term.* The long term complications of diabetes result largely from changes in the microvasculature, leading to retinopathy, nephropathy and neuropathy. Atherosclerotic changes in the arterial circulation are responsible for the high rate of cardiovascular death in diabetics.

2. *Nephropathy.* Approximately 25% of patients who have diabetes diagnosed before the age of 30 years progress to end-stage renal failure. Microalbuminuria, which is defined as an albumin excretion of 30–300 µg/min, is a good predictor of progression to diabetic nephropathy. Good glycaemic control and the use of ACE inhibitors in patients with microalbuminuria has been shown to slow progression and improve prognosis.

3. *Neuropathy.* A peripheral sensorimotor neuropathy is the commonest form of diabetic neuropathy and is thought to result partly due to microvascular changes to the blood supply of the nerves and partly from metabolic changes, particularly in the sorbital pathway. Mononeuropathies and autonomic neuropathy also occur as complications of diabetes, with up to 25% of male diabetics having some degree of sexual dysfunction, including impotence.

4. *Foot problems.* Diabetic foot problems are a major cause of morbidity in patients who have had diabetes for a long time. Peripheral neuropathy is the major aetiological factor but peripheral vascular disease plays a part in over 50% of cases leading to neuro-ischaemic ulcers. Chiropody advice on foot care, and avoidance of trauma is essential in the prevention of foot problems.

The risk factors for microvascular complications are as follows:

- Type I > Type II diabetes mellitus;
- Increasing duration of diabetes mellitus;
- Increasing blood pressure;
- Increasing serum cholesterol;
- Micro- or macro-albuminuria;
- Pregnancy;
- Smoking (this is still debated).

Annual review

Screening for risk factors and vascular complications is a vital part of diabetes care as early diagnosis may prevent or retard vascular progression. This must form a major part of the regular review of diabetes for every diabetic patient and comprises check of metabolic control, cardiovascular risk factors and search for complications as part of diabetic annual review.

Cardiovascular risk assessment and management

Recent trials of lipid lowering (4'S', CARE, LIPID, WOSCOPS and AFCAPS) have proven the benefit of statin therapy with a serum cholesterol target of < 4.8 mmol in those with established cardiovascular disease (i.e. secondary prevention), whilst there is less benefit in those at low risk of a cardiovascular (CHD) endpoint (i.e. primary prevention). It is therefore important to calculate overall coronary heart disease risk (either by Joint British Society Guidelines normogram or the Framingham Equation) to guide therapeutic intervention. The standing medical advisory committee advises lipid lowering if there is a 10 year CHD of ≥ 30%, where as the joint

British Society guidelines suggest an aim of treating above a threshold of 15%. Approximately 40% of diabetics on annual review have a 10 year CHD risk of $\geq$ 20%. Whilst the statins are most widely prescribed, recent trial data has suggested the fibric acid derivatives also to be effective. Aspirin is widely advocated as therapy in patients with >15% 10 year CHD risk, diabetic patients, providing adequate blood pressure control is achieved. Smoking is strongly discouraged.

Hypertension identification deserves special mention, owing to its role in the pathogenesis of macro- and micro-vascular complications and the substantial benefit conferred by treatment. In addition the potential role of angiotensin converting enzyme inhibitors in retarding microvascular complication has been highlighted.

Hypertension and diabetes

The last few years has seen impressive confirmation of the benefit of treatment of hypertension in diabetic subjects in large, well conducted, randomized controlled trials. These include the SHEP, STOP, ABCD, FACET, SYST-EUR, HOT, UKPDS and the HOPE Studies. With regard to macrovascular disease (myocardial infarction, cardiovascular disease, death and stroke), unequivocal benefit of anti-hypertension treatment has been demonstrated such that blood pressure thresholds and targets of treatment are $\geq$ 140/90 and <140/85 for type II and $\geq$ 140/90 and <130/80 mmHg, respectively for type I diabetic patients. The important UKPDS hypertension trial demonstrated a 37% reduction in microvascular endpoints achieved by a mean difference of 10mmHg systolic and 5mmHg diastolic pressure over a 10 year period. No difference was observed in the outcome comparing ACE inhibitor to beta blacker therapy. The most recent HOPE study has confirmed the substantial benefit of ACE inhibition (Ramipril) to increased survival even in normotensive subjects. The EUCLID Study has also suggested the potential of specific treatment of ACE inhibition (Lisinopril) to diabetic retinopathy with 45% reduction of progression.

In type I diabetes, ACE inhibitors are a clear first choice, with substantial evidence of delay in progression of diabetic nephropathy from the earliest stage of microalbuminuria. There is proven benefit in diabetic patients with established chronic renal impairment and failure. In type II diabetics, ACE inhibitors are a usual initial therapy, but calcium channel blockers, thiazides and cardioselective beta-blockers are used as these agents have proven benefit and safety.

The following lessons for diabetics can also be made from the trials:

- Often two or three antihypertensive agents are required to reach target blood pressure.
- Diastolic blood pressure measurement is of limited value.
- The agents with an evidence base of benefit are: ACE inhibitors, calcium antagonists, beta-blocking agents, thiazide diuretics.

Conclusion

Modern diabetic care now has a sound evidence base to advise a patient to achieve good glycaemic control, excellent blood pressure control, and attention to lipid profile, cardiovascular risk and weight reduction. If the current targets for medical treatment for diabetics (see *Fig. 1*) can be achieved, many more people with diabetes will be alive and enjoy a better .quality of life in the future, including preservation of vision.

Further reading

DCCT Research Group. The effect of intensive treatment of diabetes on the development and progression of long-term complications in insulin dependent diabetes mellitus. *New England Journal of Medicine*, 1993; **329:** 977–1034.

DIABETIC MACULOPATHY

Jon M. Gibson

Diabetic maculopathy is the commonest cause of visual loss in diabetic patients, and occurs in both insulin- and non-insulin-dependent diabetics. Diabetic maculopathy comprises focal and diffuse macular oedema and ischaemic maculopathy caused by reduced perfusion of the peri-foveal capillary network.

Problem

In the Wisconsin Epidemiologic Study, an increased prevalence of macular oedema was associated with increasing severity of retinopathy. Macular oedema was found in 2–6% of patients previously regarded as having background retinopathy (see Diabetic Retinopathy Topic), in 20–63% of patients with preproliferative retinopathy and in 70–74% of patients with proliferative retinopathy. The prevalence of macular oedema also increased with duration of diabetes mellitus, higher glycosylated haemoglobin level and proteinuria.

Background

The simplest classification of diabetic retinopathy divides macular oedema into focal or diffuse.

Group 1. Focal areas of leakage, sometimes with circinate ring.
Group 2. Widespread leakage from microaneurysms.
Group 3. Widespread leakage from capillaries.
Group 4. Cystoid macular oedema.
Group 5. Scattered areas of capillary non-perfusion.
Group 6. Non-perfusion of the capillaries around the fovea.

Focal macular oedema is derived from microaneurysms, either individually or in clusters, which leak fluid into the extracellular spaces of the retina. Focal oedema is usually seen in association with streaks or circinate rings of hard exudate, which represent lipid and lipoprotein material that is precipitated at the edge of the oedematous retina.

Diffuse macular oedema by contrast arises from larger areas of extensively damaged capillaries, microaneurysms and arterioles which are in a capillary bed of generally dilated vessels with hyperpermeable vessel walls. Cystoid macular oedema may also occur in diffuse oedema, and probably represents an overloading of the outer plexiform and inner nuclear layers by large amounts of extracellular fluid.

It is also suspected that the retinal pigment epithelial cells, which comprise the outer blood–retina barrier, may be abnormal in diffuse macular oedema. In this case the retinal pigment epithelium is unable to maintain the normal pump functions for the extracellular and subretinal space, allowing fluid to diffusely accumulate in the retina.

Clinical features

The Early Treatment Diabetic Retinopathy Study (ETDRS), a large prospective multicentre clinical trial, has defined clinically significant macular oedema by the following:

- Retinal thickening at or within 500 μm of the centre of the macula.
- Hard exudates at or within 500 μm of the macula centre, if associated with thickening of the adjacent retina.
- Retinal thickening at least one disc area in extent, any part of which is within one disc diameter of the macular centre.

In practice, clinically significant macular oedema is best detected by slit lamp biomicroscopy or fundus photography with stereo pairs of photographs. For slit lamp biomicroscopy the use of a contact lens is the most effective means of detecting macular oedema and is very useful in difficult, borderline cases. Otherwise the use of a hand-held 60, 78 or 90 dioptre lens may be more convenient for the patient and doctor.

Fluorescein angiography is not usually necessary to diagnose clinically significant macular oedema, and is unnecessary in straightforward focal macular oedema with circinate rings. It is very useful once the diagnosis and decision to treat macular oedema have been made, as a guide to laser treatment. It is particularly important in those cases where there may be marked perifoveal capillary hypoperfusion, because in these situations laser treatment might compromise the remaining perifoveal vessels. Imaging of macular oedema can also be achieved with the scanning laser ophthalmoscope and with ocular coherence tomography.

The ETDRS has produced its results in a series of reports and states that prompt laser photocoagulation of clinically significant macular oedema reduces visual loss by one half. The treatment guidelines in the ETDRS were based on the following.

Focal oedema – all leaking points between 500 μm and two disc diameters were treated directly with 50 to 100 μm spots of argon green or blue/green laser, so that whitening of the microaneurysm was observed. Leaking spots closer in, between 300 and 500 μm of the centre of the macula, were treated with gentler burns.

Diffuse oedema or capillary non-perfusion was treated with a grid of laser treatment, using gentle burns of spot size 50 to 200 μm.

Follow-up examinations were carried out at 4 months and further treatment could be given at that stage. The ETDRS provides clinically proven basis for management of diabetic macular oedema, and has been widely adopted.

Concern has been expressed about recommending laser treatment for maculopathy in those patients with vision of 6/6 or better. Further analysis of the ETDRS data has not produced any clear-cut recommendations, but leaves it very much up to the treating ophthalmologist. However in general it is suggested that laser treatment is best deferred in patients with vision of 6/6 or better, if the macular oedema does not involve or imminently threaten the centre of the macula.

Concern has also been expressed about the deleterious effects of laser treatment, particularly for diabetic maculopathy, on the visual function of patients. Studies with scanning laser ophthalmoscopy and fine automated perimetry are helping to quantify the amount of damage to visual function inflicted by laser photocoagulation therapy. New lasers which can be used in a micropulse mode may prove to be less damaging to visual function.

Special cases

Hypertension is an important risk factor for diabetic retinopathy, and in particular for ischaemic maculopathy. The United Kingdom Prospective Diabetes Study (UKPDS) has demonstrated the value of tight hypertensive control in type 2 diabetic patients (see Diabetic Retinopathy topic).

Pregnant diabetics may develop severe macular oedema that may be associated with capillary non-perfusion and the development of pre-proliferative and proliferative retinopathy. The oedema usually resolves following delivery, but careful and frequent follow up is advisable until stability is achieved.

It has been reported that macular oedema and proliferative retinopathy in general can worsen following cataract surgery, even with an intact posterior capsule. When possible it is important to treat diabetic retinopathy and maculopathy prior to cataract surgery, if the fundus can be adequately visualized.

Panretinal laser photocoagulation can cause worsening of pre-existing macular oedema and is well documented. Focal treatment of maculopathy should be given prior to commencing panretinal photocoagulation if possible. If urgent treatment is required a combined treatment can be given. Failing that, fractionating the panretinal photocoagulation over a longer time course can be successful, as long as the patient still receives full treatment.

Further reading

Bloom SM, Brucker AJ. 1997. *Laser surgery of the posterior segment.* JB Lippincott, Philadelphia.

Ferris FL, Davis MD. Treating 20/20 eyes with macular edema. *Archives in Ophthalmology* 1999; **117:** 675–6.

Moorman CM, Hamilton AMP. Clinical applications of the Micropulse diode laser. *Eye* 1999; **13:** 145–50.

Olk RJ, Lee CM. 1993. *Diabetic Retinopathy – Practical Management.* JB Lippincott, Philadelphia.

Rohrschneider K, Bultmann S, Gluck R, Kruse FE, Fendrich T, Volcker HE. Scanning laser ophthalmoscope fundus perimetry before and after laser photocoagulation for clinically significant diabetic macular edema. *American Journal of Ophthalmology* 2000; **129:** 27–32.

Related topic of interest

Diabetic retinopathy (p. 100).

DIABETIC RETINOPATHY

Jon M. Gibson

Diabetes mellitus is a common, chronic condition associated with serious ocular complications. The incidence of diabetes mellitus continues to rise and it is predicted that by the year 2010, there will be an estimated 221 million diabetic persons in the world. Since 1997 there have been important changes in its diagnosis and classification. The revised diagnostic criteria include a fasting plasma glucose level of 7.0 mmol/l or greater. The oral glucose tolerance test is no longer recommended for routine purposes.

Type 2 diabetes is by far the commonest type, affects at least 500 000 people in the UK and is a disease of ageing. Overall, the prevalence of type 2 diabetes varies from about 1% in the Caucasian population of the UK to approximately 5% in the Indo-Asian community, and it is predicted that by the year 2011 approximately 1 in 10 diabetic persons in the UK will be of Indo-Asian origin. Prevalence of type 2 diabetes is also characteristically high in migrant populations in other countries. It is important to realize that non-insulin-dependent diabetes mellitus (NIDDM) is not 'mild' diabetes. Overall mortality is increased 2–3 fold and life expectancy reduced by 5–10 years.

Problem

Diabetic retinopathy is the most serious ocular complication of diabetes mellitus, and is the commonest cause of blindness and visual impairment in the working age population in the UK and other Western countries. In the UK it has been estimated that diabetic eye disease results in approximately 1000 new blind registrations annually, and that currently a diabetic person is 10–20 times more likely to go blind than someone who is non-diabetic.

Background

The retinal changes associated with diabetic retinopathy are a consequence of small vessel changes. Pericyte degeneration in the retinal capillary walls are early findings, along with thickening of the basement membrane of the capillaries and the formation of microaneurysms. As a consequence of these changes the small retinal vessels either become occluded, causing an ischaemic response in the retina, or allow leakage into the retina, an exudative response. This is the basis for the classification of diabetic retinopathy.

Risk factors for developing retinopathy

1. Duration of diabetes. This is the strongest factor effecting the development of retinopathy in types 1 and 2 diabetes. Virtually all persons with type 1 diabetes will eventually develop retinopathy, but it is unusual to find retinopathy in diabetics of less than 10 years duration. In type 2 diabetes, 20–40% of persons will have retinopathy at the time of diagnosis of the diabetes. This increases dramatically with increasing duration.

2. Control of diabetes. Recent evidence from large-scale, well-constructed studies, has shown the importance of glycaemic control in lessening the risk of retinopathy progression in both types 1 and 2 diabetes patients.

3. Hypertension. The United Kingdom Prospective Diabetes Study (UKPDS) has shown that tight control of blood pressure (< 150 mmHg systolic and < 85 mmHg diastolic) reduces the risk of any non-fatal or fatal diabetic complications and also of death related to diabetes. The UKPDS was the first major study to report that in type 2 diabetes, tight blood pressure control is effective in reducing the risk of diabetic retinopathy. It demonstrated that with tight blood pressure control there was 34% reduction in the progression of retinopathy, 47% reduction in deterioration in visual acuity and a 35% reduction in the need for retinal laser photocoagulation.

4. Hyperlipidaemia. This is a risk factor mainly in type 2 patients who are at increased risk of developing macular oedema. Several studies are underway looking at treating patients with raised serum lipids with lipid-lowering agents.

5. Nephropathy. Renal failure, in diabetics, is associated with worsening of retinopathy, particularly maculopathy. It is in part related to hypertensive and lipoprotein abnormalities.

6. Pregnancy. Pregnancy may accelerate the development and advancement of retinopathy.

7. Cataract. The development of cataract which is common in diabetics, may obscure or prevent treatment of retinopathy. Cataract extraction in diabetic patients has been associated with worsening of maculopathy and proliferative retinopathy.

8. Smoking.

9. Non-attendance and late presentation. Patients presenting late with diabetic retinopathy have a much worse prognosis visually, than if the retinopathy is caught early.

Clinical features

1. Background retinopathy. The earliest changes seen are dilated retinal veins and retinal capillary microaneurysms. Intraretinal haemorrhages, the so-called 'dot and blot' haemorrhages, are situated within the tightly packed outer plexiform and inner nuclear layers of the retina, and are most numerous at the posterior pole. Hard exudates are extracellular accumulations of lipid and protein from leakage of serum through abnormal vessel walls.

2. Maculopathy. Clinically significant macular oedema is defined as thickening of the retina at or within 500 μm of the centre of the macula. Prolonged leakage of fluid into the macula can give rise to exudative maculopathy. Ischaemic maculopathy occurs when the perifoveal capillary network becomes occluded. This is best detected on fluorescein angiography, as enlargement of the foveal avascular zone.

3. Pre-proliferative retinopathy. This is an intermediate stage between background and proliferative retinopathy, and is characterized by increasing signs of retinal ischaemia. These are cotton wool spots, beading and sausage-shaped dilatations of the retinal veins, venous loops and reduplication of the vessels and intraretinal microvascular abnormalities (IRMA), which appear as flat, intraretinal areas of dilated and abnormal-looking vessels.

4. *Proliferative retinopathy.* Proliferative diabetic retinopathy (PDR) is divided into new vessels arising from the optic disc (NVD) or from the retina and elsewhere (NVE). The primary stimulus for the neovascular response is retinal hypoxia. NVD is seen as very fine, stringy vessels on the surface and edge of the optic disc, which become more obvious and form larger networks of loops as they progress. The new vessels grow between the internal limiting membrane of the retina and the posterior hyaloid face, to which they eventually become attached. It is now accepted that the intact vitreous acts as a scaffold to allow the new vessels to grow. In cases where a complete posterior vitreous detachment has occurred the neovascularization becomes aborted.

NVE usually arise from large retinal veins and are commonly seen along the major arcades. They are thought to occur in areas of perfused retina adjacent to areas of retinal capillary non-perfusion. The NVE are attached to the posterior hyaloid face. Movement and shrinkage of the vitreous gel gives rise to haemorrhage. If haemorrhage breaks through into the vitreous, vision is usually profoundly reduced and it may take months for the haemorrhage to spontaneously clear.

5. *Tractional retinal detachment.* As NVD and NVE progress, fibrous proliferations occur between the new vessels and the posterio-hyaloid face. Contraction of the fibrovascular tissue parallel to the retina is called tangential traction. Progression of the contraction can cause either extra macular or macular retinal detachment. Visualization of these features is often difficult because of associated vitreous haemorrhage and retinal ultrasound examination is usually necessary. Whilst most detachments with PDR are tractional, retinal holes can also occur associated with the traction.

In time the natural history of diabetic retinopathy is one of gradual regression of the new vessels to a so-called 'end stage' or 'burnt out retinopathy', by which time vision has normally been lost. Present management is aimed at stopping this natural progression before the active fibrovascular stage has been reached.

Treatment

The Diabetic Retinopathy Study (DRS) was a prospective, multicentre clinical trial which showed that scatter laser photocoagulation reduced the risk of severe visual loss by at least 50%. It also confirmed that argon laser and xenon light coagulation were equally effective, but that harmful effects were more common with xenon. The DRS and the British Multicentre Trial established guidelines for laser photocoagulation.

- Immediate panretinal photocoagulation is indicated for eyes with NVD alone which is at least one fourth to one third disc area in extent, NVD associated with retinal or vitreous haemorrhage or NVE which is at least one-half disc area in extent and associated with preretinal or vitreous haemorrhage.
- Panretinal photocoagulation treatment should be divided into several treatment sessions close together, rather than applying all the treatment at one visit.
- Scatter laser treatment should be given to flat areas of NVE, but disc neovascularization and elevated NVE should not be treated directly.

The Early Treatment Diabetic Retinopathy Study (ETDRS) showed that laser photocoagulation should be applied to eyes with clinically significant macular oedema (see separate topic).

Laser photocoagulation is the most effective treatment available at present for preventing visual loss in patients with diabetic retinopathy. However, other measures can also be helpful.

The management of cataract in the presence of active proliferative diabetic retinopathy and/or maculopathy is a recognized problem. Ideally laser treatment should be given prior to cataract surgery, but limitations in visualization of the fundus may make this impossible. One option is to perform indirect laser treatment PRP in theatre immediately after cataract extraction and lens implantation, and this has been reported with promising results. Careful and early postoperative examination is necessary to detect diabetic maculopathy. Fluorescein angiography may be helpful in differentiating this from other causes of postoperative macular oedema.

Tightening up control of the diabetes has been shown in the Diabetic Control and Complications Trial (DCCT) to cause a transient worsening of retinopathy followed by a sustained long-term benefit in type 1 patients. In the DCCT, intensive treatment with insulin significantly reduced progression of retinopathy by 63%, macular oedema by 26% and need for laser treatment by 51%, compared to conventional treatment. However, the successful implementation of these guidelines has been difficult because of the association of tight control with hypoglycaemic episodes in many patients. The Wisconsin Epidemiologic Study of Diabetic Retinopathy (WESDR) showed that after adjusting for other risk factors in persons with type 2 diabetes, a 1% decrease in HbA1c levels over the first 4 years of the study was associated with a 22% decrease in the odds of developing proliferative retinopathy and a 15% decrease in the odds of developing macular oedema, at the 10-year follow up.

In type 2 diabetes, the UKPDS has shown that compared with 'conventional treatment' the intensively treated group had a risk reduction of 21% for progression of retinopathy over a 12-year period, and a 29% reduction in the need for laser treatment.

The UKPDS has also shown that beta-blockers and ACE inhibitors for hypertension were efficacious in reducing the complications of type 2 diabetes, suggesting that the key element is the level of blood pressure reduction rather than the agent used.

Raised lipids should be treated either by diet or by using cholesterol-lowering agents, as there is evidence that hyperlipidaemia is a risk factor for progression of retinopathy.

Currently clinical trials are being conducted to investigate the efficacy of new drugs such as protein kinase C inhibitors and vascular endothelial growth factor that may play a role in the pathogenesis of diabetic retinopathy. Aspirin, aldose reductase inhibitors, vitamin E and free radical scavenging agents have all been tried but seem to have limited value.

Screening

In the early stages, diabetic retinopathy is completely asymptomatic. It is common, can be detected by simple means and there is effective treatment available if detected early enough. It therefore fulfils the criteria for disease screening and this should be vigorously carried out.

All diabetic persons should have a dilated fundus examination performed every year, combined with a measurement of vision. The performance of screening programmes based solely on direct ophthalmoscopy has overall been poor in terms of sensitivity and specificity. Two options have emerged as the most successful: photographic schemes based on 35 mm film or digital imaging, and slit-lamp based biomicroscopy performed by trained optometrists or doctors. Community screening of diabetic persons in the population is the subject of some debate, and in the UK is currently being planned to run as a national programme.

Further reading

Gillow JT, Gibson JM, Dodson PM. Hypertension and diabetes – what's the story? *British Journal of Ophthalmology* 1999; **83:** 1083–7.

Klein R. Diabetic retinopathy: an end of year perspective. *Eye* 1999; **13:** 133–5.

Sivestri G. Management of retinopathy in type 2 diabetes. *Eye* 1999; **13:** 131–2.

The DCCT Research Group. The effect of intensive treatment of diabetes on the development and progression of long-term complications in insulin-dependent diabetes mellitus. *New England Journal of Medicine* 1993; **329:** 977–86.

UK Prospective Diabetes Study Group. Tight blood pressure control and risk of macrovascular and microvascular complications in type 2 diabetes. UKPDS 38. *British Medical Journal* 1998; **317:** 703–13.

Related topics of interest

Diabetic maculopathy (p. 97); Hypertension and the eye (p. 135).

DIPLOPIA WORK-UP

Robert H. Taylor

Binocular diplopia results from disparate images from each eye, the most common cause being when the visual axes are not aligned or if there is a prismatic effect from spectacle correction. Monocular diplopia results from unilateral ocular pathology. Diplopia is infrequently encountered in young children with strabismus due to suppression of the image from one eye.

Problem

The overriding problem with the patient presenting with diplopia is to identify the cause from the multitude of possible aetiologies. It is important to exclude intracranial pathology. The cause can often be identified by taking a careful history and examination. There are numerous examination techniques, including a neurological and orbital assessment, and these may lead to confusion if not applied appropriately. Combined assessment with an orthoptist may be useful.

Background

1. Binocular causes.

- Neurogenic: These entities can be divided into palsies (total loss of activity in the nerve) or paresis (partial loss). An acute cranial nerve weakness will cause an incomitant deviation. Patients with a congenital or long-standing weakness may develop a degree of comitance. The patient will usually complain of diplopia unless the vision is reduced unilaterally (e.g. from ptosis) or if there is co-existent suppression.

- Myogenic: Can be divided into disorders of the neuromusclar junction (e.g. myasthenia) and restrictive (e.g. thyroid related, orbital entrapment and myositis). Problems such as myasthenia gravis may give rise to intermittent diplopia.

- Mechanical: Interference to the movement of the globe may occur as a result of an orbital space-occupying lesion for example an inflammatory mass or tumour.

- Decompensation of a pre-existing phoria: Convergence insufficiency may give rise to diplopia for near fixation. Diplopia may also occur following occlusion therapy for amblyopia, particularly if commenced in the older child. Loss of effective suppression may occur spontaneously or following strabismus surgery.

- Refractive: An anisometropic error dispensed with bifocals can induce vertical diplopia for near vision due to induced prismatic effects. Surgically induced anisometropia can cause diplopia following unilateral cataract surgery in ametropic patients.

- Cortical: Rarely, diplopia can be due to cortical lesions.

2. Monocular diplopia.
Monocular diplopia may result from anterior segment opacities, such as cataract or corneal scars which fractionate the image entering the eye. Incorrect spectacle lenses for astigmatism and anisometropia give a monocular blur and may be interpreted as diplopia. Diplopia may also be caused by a macular disturbance, such as secondary to an orbital lesion or choroidal melanoma.

Clinical features

Diplopia is a difficult subject, and frequently much information can be gained from a carefully taken history. With experience, characteristic patterns will be recognized.

1. History. The first step is to establish if the diplopia is binocular or monocular. Monocular diplopia can be demonstrated by covering the unaffected eye and observing continuing diplopia or blur from the viewing affected eye. Monocular occlusion will eliminate binocular diplopia. Occasionally diplopia will only be elicited by moving the eyes into eccentric positions of gaze. Careful questioning is required to ascertain if monocular or binocular diplopia is present. If binocular diplopia is present, ask about the two images: In which direction of gaze are they further apart? Are the two images separated vertically, horizontally or obliquely? Is one twisted? The history may suggest an acute or chronic problem, or perhaps an episodic course (characteristically, worse at the end of the day) that may suggest myasthenia gravis. Diplopia may be related to close work, suggesting convergence insufficiency. Ask about associated pain (e.g. local orbital pain in myositis). Headache may be due to aesthenopia, but a headache characteristically worse on waking suggests raised intracranial pressure. A history of an abnormal head posture, trauma, amblyopia and strabismus may be present. Any recent change in spectacle prescription may be significant. Co-existent high blood pressure, diabetes mellitus, multiple sclerosis, known cranial neoplasms and vascular events need to be considered. It is particularly important to ask directly about neurological symptoms, (e.g. paraesthesia, weakness and tinnitus). Thyroid eye disease can present with double vision in the absence of overt thyroid abnormality. Questions pertaining to hyper- and hypothyroidism are relevant. A past medical history should be documented with a systems review.

2. Examination. Once the question of monocular or binocular diplopia has been resolved the examination can be tailored appropriately. If the patient has recently changed spectacles, check for a dispensing error. Document any abnormal head posture. This may require removing the glasses if a prism is incorporated. Where possible a measurement of the tilt or turn should be made by protractor or other means. Look for proptosis or enophthalmos. Diplopia may become manifest after dissociation of the eyes or by straightening a compensatory head posture.

The documentation of binocular diplopia can be divided into three parts:

- the subjective description of double vision, in primary position and eccentric gaze;
- the deviation of the eyes in the nine positions of gaze;
- the ocular excursions.

A cover/uncover test can be performed to a distance target to demonstrate latent or manifest deviation in the primary position and the nine positions of gaze, with and without any head posture. The 'three-step test' is carried out for vertical deviations (which includes the Bielschowsky head tilt test). This test is only applicable in the presence of a single vertical muscle paresis. A restrictive aetiology will give false results. A prism cover test in the nine positions of gaze quantifies the amount of deviation. A cover test to a near target is also documented.

Look for limitation of ocular excursions for both versions and ductions into the nine positions of gaze. These can be charted on a drawing. Remember to check convergence, saccades and pursuit movements where indicated. Reduced saccadic velocity may indicate a mild paresis.

The sensory side of the oculomotor system is also important. If the diplopia is intermittent, a fusion range should be measured. High-grade stereopsis suggests normal ocular alignment at an early age.

In all cases, it is important to examine the lids, the pupils and visual fields. The conjunctiva is examined for previous strabismus surgery. The optic discs should be examined to exclude swelling or atrophy. It may be relevant to fatigue the muscles, a clinical sign suggestive of myasthenia gravis. Look for any scars on the face (e.g. from previous orbital surgery or trauma). Examine for proptosis, enophthalmos or any masses. It is easy to miss a subtle proptosis.

Restrictive lesions are confirmed on forced duction tests. These can be performed in the clinic in selected patients. A forced generation test can confirm muscle activity.

Complementary tests such as Hess/Lees charts and fields of binocular single vision are important and useful for documenting status and monitoring progression. Investigations are guided by clinical findings, but may include blood investigations for diabetes mellitus, vascular conditions, thyroid status and acetylcholine receptor antibodies. An edrophonium test is indicated in cases of suspected myasthenia gravis.

Neuroimaging is helpful if intracranial or orbital pathology is suspected. Imaging the muscles with magnetic resonance or computer tomography may also be useful. In picking up early orbital pathology such as thyroid eye disease, B-scan ultrasound may also be of value.

Further reading

Berry SM, Carter JE. Isolated diplopia. In: van Heuven WAJ, Zwaan JT (eds) *Decision Making in Ophthalmology*. St Louis: Mosby Year Book, 1992; 12.

Leigh RJ, Zee DS. *The Neurology of Eye Movements*, 2nd edn. Philadelphia: FA Davies, 1999; 9.5: Clinical testing in diplopia.

Mein J, Trimble R. *Diagnosis and management of ocular motility disorders*, 2nd edn. Oxford: Blackwell Scientific Publications, 1991.

Related topics of interest

Child with strabismus: work-up (p. 45); Myasthenia gravis (p. 168); Sixth (abducens) cranial nerve (p. 289); Superior oblique weakness (p. 298); Third (oculomotor) cranial nerve palsy (p. 306); Thyroid eye disease (p. 315).

DRUGS (TOPICAL) IN GLAUCOMA: MODE OF ACTION

Shakti Thakur & Peter Shah

In recent years there has been an explosion in the number of topical medications available to treat glaucoma. Continuous patient education regarding drug therapy benefits both patient and clinician.

Problem

It is important to have a thorough understanding of the various modes of action of these agents so that they can be used to maximum effect in each individual patient. Several drugs are now also available as combination preparations. As with any medication, it is essential that patients comply with therapy in order to produce a clinical effect. Compliance depends on many factors, one of the most important of which is patient knowledge.

Drug	Mode of action	Effect
Beta blockers		
Non-selective		
Timolol	B2 >B1 antagonist	D
Carteolol		
Levobunolol		
	[Nad accumulation ≥ vasoconstriction of ciliary vessels also suggested]	
Selective		
Betaxolol	B1	D
Sympathomimetics		
Non-selective		
	A1	D, T
Epinephrine &	A2 inhibits Nad release	D, U
Dipevefrin	B1	I
	B2	I, T
Guanethidine	Adrenergic neurone blocker Potentiates effects of adrenaline allowing smaller dosage	D, TU
Selective		
Apraclonidine	A1	D, T
	A2	D, U
Brimonidine	A2	D, U
	(also effect via imidazoline receptor stimulation)	

Carbonic anhydrase inhibitor

Dorzolamide	inhibits carbonic anhydrase isoenzyme II	
Brinzolamide	in ciliary epithelium ≥ bicarbonate production decreased	D

Prostaglandin analogue

Latanoprost	Ciliary body muscle fibre – extracellular matrix resistance decreased	U

Parasympathomimetics

Pilocarpine	ciliary muscle contraction	
Carbachol	≥ opens trabecular meshwork	T

Topical medications and mode of action

A1 = Alpha 1 receptor
(Ciliary body arterioles)

A2 = Alpha 2 receptor
(Ciliary body)

B1 = Beta 1 receptor
B2 = Beta 2 receptor
(Ciliary process epithelium)

D = Decrease aqueous production
I = Increase aqueous production

T = Increase trabecular outflow
U = Increase uveoscleral outflow
Nad = Noradrenaline

Further reading

ABPI. *Compendium of Data Sheets and Summaries of Product Characteristics 1999–2000.*
Donoghue EK, Wilensky JT. Dorzolamide: A review. *Seminars in Ophthalmology* 1997; **12**(3): 119–26.
Greenfiels *et al.* Brimonidine: A Review. *Seminars in Ophthalmology* 1997; **12**(3): 127–33.
Wyse TB *et al.* Latanoprost: A Review. *Seminars in Ophthalmology* 1997; **12**(3): 134–42.

Related topics of interest

Normal tension glaucoma (p. 187); Ocular hypertension (p. 199); Toxicology: drugs for ocular disease (p. 325).

ELECTRORETINOGRAPHY IN CHILDREN

Carole M. Panton & Carol A. Westall

An electroretinogram (ERG) is an electrophysiological test that measures the mass response of the retina. Carefully chosen stimulus parameters and testing conditions allow the evaluation of the functional integrity of different retinal elements.

Problem

There is debate about the most suitable type of electrode. Whether to sedate or not will be determined by the age of the child and the type of electrode used. Two testers are required, one to collect the data and the other to encourage compliance from the child.

Background

The ERG provides objective information about various retinal elements and can help distinguish an abnormality of outer or inner retinal function. ERGs are used to identify photoreceptor (rod or cone), middle retina (bipolar and Müller cells) and inner retina (amacrine and interplexiform cells) defects. ERGs are the primary diagnostic test for inherited retinal degenerations and dystrophies such as retinitis pigmentosa (RP), its many variants and other night-blinding disorders. Two electrodes are required, an active electrode and a reference one. The active electrode needs to be as near to the cornea as possible. We prefer to use contact lens electrodes for paediatric testing. Responses are of good amplitude with good repeatability. In addition the electrodes may have a speculum that prevents closure of the eye. Some visual electrophysiology laboratories prefer the use of non-contact lens electrodes. The most common are 27/7X-static silver coated conductive nylon yarn (Saquoit Industries, Scranton, PA, USA), a gold foil electrode and skin electrodes. All these methods may be tolerated better than a contact lens electrode by young children. However, skin electrodes in particular are relatively insensitive and produce greater variability than the other mentioned electrode types. For such reasons the International Society for Clinical Electrophysiology of Vision (ISCEV) strongly recommends use of electrodes that contact the cornea or nearby bulbar conjunctiva. Whatever the electrode of choice, the tester must be vigilant for variable responses caused by movement artefact or electrical noise. An electrode of the appropriate size for the child must be used to minimize movement artefact. Contact lens electrodes should be sterilized after each use.

For clinical application, two component parts of the ERG, a negative a-wave and a positive b-wave are analysed. Measurements are made of the amplitude of these components and of the time taken from the onset of a flash of light to reach the peak of each component (implicit time). ISCEV standards for electroretinography recommend that ERGs be recorded for the following five response types:

- rod-response ERG to very dim light stimulating a dark adapted retina;
- maximal response to a bright flash which is the rod-cone response of a dark adapted eye;

- oscillatory potentials (series of wavelets mainly superimposed on the ascending arm of the b-wave, formed by both rod and cone systems);
- cone-response from a light adapted eye, in the presence of a rod-suppressing background light;
- 30 Hz flicker response recorded from a light adapted eye.

Variables affecting the ERG response

The ERG develops rapidly during the first six months of life. Different ERG components develop at different rates. Most reach adult levels by 3 to 5 years of age. Visually normal infant and toddler ERG amplitudes appear diminished and implicit times delayed compared with adult control data. Therefore, in order to prevent a misdiagnosis of retinal disease it is essential to have age-matched control data for correct interpretation of paediatric ERGs. Likewise, axial myopia greater than – 4.00D is known to reduce ERG amplitudes. A-scan biometry should be used to measure axial length. Software is available to derive normal ranges according to age and refractive error (The Hospital for Sick Children, Toronto, Canada).

Once a neurological cause for early onset nystagmus has been ruled out, an ERG is performed to determine the presence of retinal dysfunction. Most children with early onset nystagmus are referred at an age when sedation is required. Chloral hydrate has no effect on the ERG but minimizes movement artefact caused by the nystagmus. In older children with coarse amplitude nystagmus testing with both eyes open may minimize movement artefact.

If the ERG amplitude varies visibly during testing, pupil position should be checked to see if the pupil is centred centrally through the contact lens. In sleeping/sedated children the eye is often elevated. Rousing the child slightly will result in the eye and pupil being repositioned.

Clinical application

Before ERG testing, visual acuity should be assessed. Pupils are pharmacologically dilated. Fully dilated pupils are required to allow maximum light to reach the retina. Bilateral patches are placed over both eyes for 20–30 minutes to facilitate testing of scotopic rod-isolated responses first. The cornea is anaesthetized with a suitable topical agent. A bipolar Burian Allen contact lens electrode of appropriate size for the child is chosen with a reference electrode built into the speculum. A drop of viscous artificial tears is placed into the contact lens to protect the cornea and provide good electrical contact. A gold disc electrode attached to the forehead serves as a ground. Rod-isolated responses are recorded first using a dim white light (standard flash attenuated by 2.5 log units). A series of mixed rod-cone responses are then recorded to a stimulus intensity between 1.5–3 candela second/m^2 (standard flash). The eye is then light adapted for 10 minutes using a background light to suppress the rod response and allow for cone-isolated testing. Most babies under 7 months are swaddled and tested lying supine. Most children between 7 months and 5 years are tested after choral hydrate sedation (80–100 mg/kg to a maximum single dose of 1 g). Those over 5 years sit with a parent or alone. In a few specific cases (e.g. older children with behavioural disorders or severe developmental delay) ERGs may be performed under general anaesthetic in a surgical theatre. Stimulus conditions must still comply with ISCEV recommendations.

Blink artefact, eye movements and electrical noise can contaminate the ERG signal and contribute to false results. The ERG is observed online to determine repeatability and where possible three repeatable responses are obtained. Appropriate software allows for the rejection of contaminated waveforms. Artefact from extraneous electrical noise often can be eliminated with the addition of artificial teardrops. These are placed in the lower fornix and will then seep under the contact lens.

ERGs are also helpful in the diagnosis of retinal involvement in lipopigment storage diseases such as Batten disease, metabolic diseases (mucopolysaccharidoses), inflammatory conditions, toxic retinopathies and in syndromes associated with RP-like dystrophies such as Bardet, Biedl or Usher.

Further reading

Heckenlively JR, Arden GB (eds) (1991). *Principles and Practice of Clinical Electrophysiology of Vision.* St Louis, Mosby Year Book, Inc.

Marmor MF, Zrenner E (for the International Society for Clinical Electroretinography of Vision). Standard for clinical electroretinography. *Documenta Ophthalmologica* 1994; **89:** 115–24.

Westall CA, Panton CM, Levin AV. Time course for the maturation of the human electroretinogram from infancy to adulthood. *Documenta Ophthalmologica* 1999; **96:** 355–79.

Westall CA. Electrophysiological testing. In: Leat SJ, Shute RH, Westall CA (eds). *Assessing Children's Vision: A Handbook.* Oxford, Butterworth-Heinemann, 1999; 311–43.

ESOTROPIA, CONVERGENCE AND ACCOMMODATION

Robert H. Taylor

A significant proportion of esotropia is associated with hypermetropia, accommodation and convergence. It is the most common form of strabismus encountered in children.

Problem

Various classifications exist and different terms will be encountered. Some children will change their position in the classification, for example satisfying the criteria for a fully accommodative esotropia, then subsequently breaking down to become a partially accommodative esotropia. Some will occupy two positions at the same time. Accommodation is not measured in routine clinical practice. Why some individuals become binocular once hypermetropia is corrected and some remain esotropic is unclear.

Background

1. Convergence. There are five recognized types of convergence: accommodative, tonic, fusional, proximal and voluntary. The amount of convergence is the sum of these component parts. The amount required is equal to the inverse of the distance to the object in metres × interpupillary distance (IPD) in centimetres. For example 18 prism dioptres is required, assuming a target at a third of a metre and an IPD of 6 cm. In a normal subject, fixing an object at 33 cm would induce 3 dioptres of accommodation.

2. Accommodative convergence/accommodation ratio AC/A. This is the ratio of how much convergence (measured in prism dioptres) is induced per spherical dioptre accommodation. Accommodation is assumed to have taken place, so a measurement of accommodation per se is not undertaken.

3. Normal example. If the AC:A ratio is 3:1, observing a target at 33 cm (IPD of 6 cm), would demand 3 dioptres of accommodation and so generate 9 prism dioptres of convergence (3 × 3). To this would be added approximately 3 prism dioptres of proximal convergence and 6 dioptres of fusional convergence, to total the 18 prism dioptres required. If the AC:A ratio was 6:1, the accommodative convergence would be 18 prism dioptres. If 3 dioptres of proximal convergence were present, 3 dioptres of fusional divergence would be required to maintain bifoveal fixation.

4. Gradient method. This is a measurement of the AC/A ratio. A prism cover test is carried out for distance fixation (to exclude proximal convergence), through a minus dioptre lens. The subject should read at least 6/12 through the negative lens to ensure accommodation has taken place. For example, an orthotropic patient reads 6/12 through a minus 3 dioptre lens, and breaks down to a 9 prism dioptre esotropia. AC/A = New angle-original angle/3, (9–0)/3 = 3:1. A ratio ranging from 3:1 to 6:1 is normal if measured by this method.

5. Heterophoria method. This is an alternative to the gradient method and ignores several concepts such as proximal convergence. It is generally considered less accurate and not widely used. A high ratio can be defined as 8:1 or higher.

Clinical features

The esotropias can be divided into (i) infantile esotropia, (ii) primary acquired esotropia, (iii) secondary esotropia, (iv) incommitant esotropia e.g. secondary to sixth nerve palsy, Duane syndrome and (v) consecutive esotropia (i.e. following surgery for exotropia).

Infantile esotropia

See separate topic.

Primary acquired esotropia

These can be divided into those in whom accommodation is an aetiological factor and those in whom it is not. For the former group, hypermetropic glasses improve or eliminate the esotropia for distance fixation.

1. Accommodative esotropia. Accommodative esotropia develops because of uncorrected hypermetropia. Overcoming hypermetropia causes increased accommodation, therefore increased accommodative convergence. Fusional divergence is required to maintain alignment. When this fails esotropia develops.

The esotropia generally presents in patients older than 6 months and before 7 years of age. The commonest age is between 2 and 3 years old. Children may complain of blurred vision, but more commonly an esotropia is noted by the parents, or detected in screening programmes. The esotropia is characteristically intermittent at first, often when tired. An acute onset may also occur. If spectacle correction is delayed the esotropia may become manifest and even unresponsive to hypermetropic correction (non-accommodative). This would increase the probability of the strabismic eye developing suppression and amblyopia. There is often a family history of strabismus, amblyopia or hypermetropia. Patients are hypermetropic (usually more than +1.5 dioptres) and may have anisometropia and amblyopia on presentation. Patients often have co-existent inferior oblique overaction and may develop dissociated vertical divergence (DVD). Latent nystagmus may exist but is less common than in infantile esotropia. The presenting angle is usually between 20 and 30 prism dioptres. Cycloplegic refraction is mandatory. The full hypermetropia should be prescribed particularly in the first years of life.

- **Fully accommodative esotropia.** These patients have an eso-deviation for near and distance fixation, and hypermetropia. The deviation may only be apparent to an accommodative target (i.e. they may be orthotropic when fixing a light). Once spectacle correction is worn, the esotropia disappears for both near and distance fixation. Patients generally have good vision in both eyes and may have bifoveal fixation with normal stereopsis. In some instances, patients are controlled with spectacle correction to a microtropia with a small residual angle (less than 10 prism dioptres) and sub-normal stereopsis. Surgery is not indicated.

- **Partially accommodative esotropia.** Patients have an eso-deviation for both near and distance which is reduced once their hypermetropia is corrected. However, they still have a significant angle of esotropia which may require surgical correction. These patients often have co-existent amblyopia.
- **Accommodative esotropia with convergence excess.** Patients have an esotropia for near when fixating an accommodative target. They are orthotropic or esophoric for distance fixation. Hypermetropic correction may reduce both angles, but the difference remains. These patients have a high AC/A ratio. Patients who demonstrate fusion for distance fixation with their glasses (if indicated) may benefit from bifocal glasses. Split pupil executive bifocal glasses are preferred. If the split is too low, the near segment will be difficult for the child to locate. Variable focus glasses are possible, with the near segment raised as compared to an adult. The power of the near add is calculated depending on how much is required to control the near deviation. Failure to measure this may result in more near add being ordered than is necessary, although 3 dioptres is commonly required.

2. Non-accommodative esotropia. There are a group of patients with eso-deviations who are either emmetropic or in whom correcting any hypermetropia does not change the angle of strabismus. Patients are usually over 6 months of age at presentation. Amblyopia is common in younger patients. Inferior oblique overaction, DVD and latent nystagmus may be present. The index of suspicion should be raised for intracranial pathology or myasthenia, especially with acute onset.

Occasionally a non-accommodative esotropia can occur acutely with the patient complaining of double vision. Possible causes include patching for an eye injury or following a period of emotional or physical stress. An accommodative or paretic cause needs excluding. If binocularity was normal prior to the breakdown, prognosis is good. Re-establishment of binocular single vision can be achieved with prisms or surgery.

- **Basic (or constant) esotropia.** The esotropia is manifest and equal for near and distance fixation. Treatment is usually surgical. A prism adaptation period may be beneficial to elucidate the maximum surgical angle.
- **Non-accommodative convergence excess or near esotropia.** These patients are straight in the distance and esotropic for near fixation. The near esotropia is present whether accommodation is exerted or not. The AC/A is normal so bifocals are useless. The near angle is thought to derive from a large proximal convergence. If treatment is contemplated at all, medial rectus recession or posterior fixation sutures are suggested.
- **Cyclic esotropia.** An esotropia is present intermittently, for example every other day. It is rare. Constant esotropia may evolve. Treat any hypermetropia and consider surgery if this fails.

Secondary esotropia

1. ***Sensory deprivation in childhood.*** Monocular causes of poor vision can induce an esotropia. Full dilated ocular examination is mandatory to elucidate the cause for visual loss.

2. ***Divergence insufficiency or distance esotropia.*** The esotropia is larger for distance fixation. Fusional divergence is poor. The index of suspicion is high for a lateral rectus weakness due to a sixth cranial nerve paresis.

3. ***Divergence paralysis.*** Similar clinical features exist as divergence insufficiency. This may be due to a pontine tumour or head trauma.

4. ***Spasm of the near reflex.*** Sustained convergence spasm is unusual. Spasm is often present as part of a conversion or 'functional' problem. The key to diagnosis is the associated pupillary miosis. Pseudomyopia may occur and a small amplitude nystagmus seen due to the accommodative effort. There may be limited abduction on versions, but monocular abduction is usually normal. Occasionally correcting hypermetropia may help. Patients may present with headache so intracranial pathology should be excluded.

Incommitant esotropia

There are various esotropias that occur because of poor abduction. This leads to an incommitant deviation, with esotropia increasing in the direction of abduction. This is not an exhaustive list, but would include sixth nerve weakness, Duane syndrome, medial rectus fibrosis from thyroid eye disease, and esotropia in association with high myopia.

Consecutive esotropia

Surgery for exotropia may result in an esotropia with or without double vision. In younger children care must be exercised to follow such patients carefully to treat any emerging amblyopia. Patients with diplopia can be treated with prisms. The angle usually resolves, particularly if a medial rectus resection has been part of the operation. Further surgery may be indicated. Careful attention should be paid to a duction weakness in the field of previously recessed muscle (e.g. a slipped muscle) or a restriction of a previously resected muscle.

Treatment

Treatment is largely a function of diagnosis. In accommodative esotropia treatment starts with full cycloplegic spectacle correction. Treatment of any co-existing amblyopia with occlusion therapy or penalization follows. Patients with a high AC/A, orthophoria for distance with correction may benefit from executive bifocals. Prisms can be used in non-accommodative esotropia to re-establish fusion. Surgical intervention is indicated if the angle for distance fixation is significant. In younger patients some degree of binocularity may be restored by ocular alignment and so is also an indication for surgery. A prism adaption trial may be employed to elucidate the surgical angle. In general a unilateral or bilateral medial rectus muscle recession is undertaken. If one eye has poor vision and the age of the child makes reversing amblyopia unlikely a unilateral medial rectus recession and lateral rectus resection may be favoured, to avoid surgical complications in the good seeing eye.

Strabismus surgery cannot eliminate the accommodative angle caused by uncorrected hypermetropia. Parents need to be warned that in cases of accommodative esotropia, an esotropia will be present postoperatively if the glasses are not worn.

Conclusion

Childhood esotropia is common and most often associated with hypermetropia. The measurement of the cycloplegic refraction and institution of spectacle wear is central to the understanding and management. Amblyopia treatment and possible surgical correction come later. Maintaining an open mind as to the possibility of intracranial pathology cannot be overstated.

Further reading

Prism Adaptation Study Research Group. Efficacy of prism adaptation in the surgical management of acquired esotropia. *Archives in Ophthalmology* 1990; **108:** 1248–56.

Wilson ME, Buckley EG, Kivlin JD, Ruttum MS, Simon JW, Magoon EH. Pediatric Ophthalmology Section 6. *American Academy of Ophthalmology* 1999; 76–84.

Wright KW. In Wright KW (ed.) *Pediatric Ophthalmology and Strabismus.* Mosby-Year Book Inc, St Louis, MO. 1995, Chap 12, 179–94.

Related topics of interest

Congenital nystagmus (p. 69); Exotropia, divergence and accommodation (p. 127); Infantile esotropia (p. 143); Latent nystagmus (p. 151); Refraction in children (p. 248).

EXOTROPIA, DIVERGENCE AND ACCOMMODATION

Robert H. Taylor

The exotropias are a group of disorders that involve all aspects of ophthalmology. Four groups exist, infantile exotropia, intermittent exotropia, consecutive exotropia (following surgery for esotropia) and sensory exotropia (poor monocular vision). This topic concentrates on intermittent exotropia, mentioning the latter two groups and other related conditions only briefly. The term secondary exotropia is avoided, as 'secondary' could relate to a poorly sighted eye or previous surgery.

Problem

The aetiology of intermittent exotropia is debated. The combination of factors that hold better alignment for near fixation are not fully understood. Binocular sensorial function may play a role in the aetiology. Intermittent exotropia has recently been reclassified, so multiple terms are likely to be encountered. The terminology relating to convergence weakness exotropia and convergence insufficiency can easily become confused.

Background

1. Divergence. No divergence nucleus has been identified. Increased tonic divergence has been suggested as an aetiological factor in exotropia. This is disputed as proximal convergence factors were not eliminated. Some authors feel that exotropia (in intermittent exotropia) occurs as a result of an abnormal resting position, a passive divergence. Some feel a combination of active and passive divergence is responsible.

2. Tenacious proximal fusion (TPF). This is a recently introduced term to describe a slow to dissipate fusional mechanism that holds patients aligned for near fixation. Monocular occlusion is required for up to an hour in order to obtain a correct measurement for near fixation. This term is not universally accepted. Proximal fusional convergence and postocclusion vergence after-effect are also used.

3. Accommodative convergence/accommodation ratio has been traditionally measured using the gradient method at near with a convex lens to relax accommodation. AC/A = Adjusted angle at near minus original angle at near)/3, where the adjusted angle equals the near angle measured with + 3 lens to relax accommodation. A high ratio can be defined as more than 6:1 if measured by this method. A high AC/A may be false and termed a pseudo-high AC/A, if the AC/A reduces to normal after elimination of TPF. Measurement of the AC/A using distance fixation may therefore be more accurate.

An alternative is the heterophoria method. This also can be falsely high as TPF has not been eliminated.

Failure to eliminate a pseudo-high AC/A has important implications for management. Patients who have a true high AC/A may develop a near esotropia following a surgical dose correcting the distance angle.

Clinical features

A useful classification includes the following groups, infantile exotropia, intermittent exotropia, consecutive exotropia and sensory exotropia. Primary convergence insufficiency and dissociated horizontal divergence are included for comparison.

1. Infantile exotropia. This is defined as an exotropia presenting after 2 months and before 6 months of life. A constant and large angle is usual. Co-existent ocular or systemic abnormality is more common in infantile exotropia (67%) than infantile esotropia (49%). Early surgery is generally accepted as the preferred treatment, but the potential for bifoveal fixation is probably poor. Consecutive esotropia and recurrent exotropia are both relatively common.

2. Intermittent exotropia. This is the most common form of exotropia encountered in children. While it is accepted that this condition may become constant with time, the term intermittent exotropia is widely accepted.

Onset is usually before 5 years old, but can be seen as young as 2 years old. An exotropic deviation may be observed by the parents when the child is fixing on a distance object, often when tired. When asked, the patient may be able to control the deviation. Patients tend not to notice diplopia. Patients may close the exotropic eye when outside on sunny days. This may be related to photophobia (the threshold for photophobia is higher for monocular viewing) or a reduction of fusional convergence (in those with a tenuous attachment to fusion). There is usually good vision in each eye with normal stereopsis when aligned, although some patients control to a microtropia. Inferior oblique overaction, A and V patterns may be present. The angle of deviation may increase while fixing a far distance target, particularly when the object is non-accommodative and approximates infinity (e.g. looking out of the window).

Over time the exotropia may be present more frequently, and stay manifest for longer periods. Young children may develop sensory adaptation, hemiretinal suppression, loss of high-grade stereopsis, amblyopia and abnormal retinal correspondence.

Traditionally intermittent exotropia management is based on the following progression. Stage 1 consists of a manifest deviation seen only for distance fixation for short periods, usually when tired or not concentrating. Stage 2 is when the deviation is still only present for distance fixation but is present for up to half of the waking hours. Stage 3 is present when fusion is lost and there is manifest deviation for both near and distance.

Intermittent exotropia can be further classified as follows:

1. **True divergence excess.** True normal AC/A. Patients have a larger measurement for distance fixation, but the eyes are controlled for near fixation or the angle is less for near fixation. This difference is maintained after monocular patching for 60 minutes. The term distance exotropia is sometimes used.

2a. **Simulated divergence excess** with pseudo high AC/A (i.e. normal AC/A after elimination of TPF). Patients have a near distance disparity with a small angle measured for near. If the AC/A ratio is measured using a near target and +3 lenses, an increase in the near angle suggests a high AC/A. However, the near angle also increases after TPF is eliminated with a 60 minute patch test. The AC/A is now normal.

2b. Simulated divergence excess without a pseudo high AC/A. Near/distance disparity is present and the AC/A is normal when tested with +3 lenses. However, TPF is present. After elimination of TPF, the near angle increases to within 10 prism dioptres of the distance angle.

3. (True) simulated divergence excess with a true high AC/A. Monocular occlusion does not increase the near deviation (i.e. TPF is absent), but +3 lenses do. A small esotropia may be seen if a cover test is performed at very close range (17 cm or 8 cm).

4. Basic exotropia. Patients have equal measurements (within 10 prism dioptres) for distance and near fixation. The AC/A ratio is normal.

5. Convergence weakness: (XT with low AC/A) (Burian's convergence insufficiency) (Near exotropia or IXT of the convergence weakness type). Patients control for distance fixation but have a exotropia for near. Older patients present with aesthenopic symptoms associated with near tasks. X(T) at distance is 10 pd less than near. Patients have a low AC/A ratio or good fusional convergence. Monocular occlusion does not change any angle.

6. Exotropia with simulated low AC/A (Kushner's pseudo convergence insufficiency) X(T) at distance is 10 pd less than near. TPF (or a distance variant) is present, so after monocular occlusion the distance angle increases to approximately the near. AC/A is normal after monocular occlusion.

Table of the intermittent exotropias

		AC/A	Pseudo AC/A	TPF	? Treatment
1	True DXs	Normal	Absent	Absent	BLR or Rc Rs
2a	Sim DXs (Sim H AC/A)	Normal	Pseudo high	Present	Rc Rs or BLR
2b	Sim DXs (Sim True)	Normal	Absent	Present	Rc Rs or BLR
3	Sim DXs	High	Absent	Absent	Myopic Bifocals
4	Basic	Normal	Absent	Absent	Rc Rs or BLR
5	Conv W	Low	Absent	Absent	BMResection
6a	Sim ConvW	Normal	Pseudo low	Present for D	Rc Rs or BLR

DXs = divergence excess; Sim = simulated; Conv W = convergence weakness; BLR = bilateral lateral rectus muscle recession; Rc Rs = unilateral lateral rectus muscle recession and medial rectus muscle resection; BMResection = bi-medial medial rectus muscle resection.

Treatment of intermittent exotropia. Refraction and amblyopia treatment are important. Small amounts of hypermetropia are often left untreated (assuming the vision is satisfactory) as full correction may increase the exotropia. However, hypermetropia over 4 dioptres or more, or anisotropia of more than 1.5 dioptres should be treated as exotropia control may improve with increased visual acuity.

Alternate patching or part time patching the non-deviating eye can be tried. The mechanism of improved control is not understood. Any improvement may be temporary but may delay the need for surgery.

Timing of surgical intervention can be difficult. It can be considered for stage 2 intermittent exotropia. Assessing this control, particularly if based on parental observation, has obvious inaccuracies. Control can be divided into excellent (only occasionally seen), good (manifest less than 5 times a day), fair (more than 5 times and only at distance) and poor (manifest frequently, near and distance viewing). Such control can be confirmed by clinical testing – assessing how easy it is to break down a phoria to a tropia (happens spontaneously or needs disruption of fusion), whether control is re-established spontaneously or by using a blink or re-fixation manoeuver. Decreasing distance stereo-acuity also suggests deteriorating fusion.

Age is an important consideration in surgical planning. Re-operations, amblyopia and loss of fusion are associated with early surgery.

In general the surgical dose is based on the maximum angle measured. This is often the angle measured for far distance or after one hour of occlusion. Patients with a true high AC/A ratio need to be treated more conservatively, with consideration given to myopic glasses with a bifocal for near.

The type of surgical intervention may be based on the diagnosis. Distance exotropia is treated with a bilateral lateral rectus recession and basic exotropia with unilateral surgery (either lateral rectus recession alone or a recess/resect) although this is disputed. There is some evidence that simulated divergence excess does well with bilateral lateral rectus surgery.

Slight over correction following surgery for exotropia is possibly desirable and spontaneous improvement common. If amblyopia is a risk, careful follow up is advised, with repeat cycloplegic refraction, correction of any hypermetropia, temporary prisms and meticulous attention to amblyopia detection and management.

3. Consecutive exotropia. This describes an exotropia that happens as a consequence of previous surgery for an esotropia. It is a common problem in clinical practice. Documentation of the previous surgery is informative if available. Examination needs to identify any under action of the previously recessed medial rectus or restriction in the field of the previously resected lateral rectus muscle. A forced traction test may be useful to differentiate these two entities. Sensory assessment is important to identify any diplopia that may be created by surgical alignment. The use of botulinum toxin may be useful to this regard. Treatment is usually surgical. Dissection of the medial rectus muscle can be challenging as a thin tennuous muscle may be present (sometimes termed stretched scar). Re-advancement of the previously recessed medial rectus muscle coupled with a recession of the lateral rectus muscle using an adjustable suture technique is commonly required.

4. Sensory exotropia. As a general rule a poorly sighted eye tends to become exotropic except in young children when sensory esotropia is equally common. Sensory assessment preoperatively is important to try and identify any diplopia. Use of botulinum toxin may be helpful to simulate the effects of surgical alignment. Treatment is surgical. In order to confine surgical risk to the lesser seeing eye, large recess/resect procedures may be needed. Patients should be warned preoperatively about reduced abduction postoperatively.

Primary convergence insufficiency

Primary convergence insufficiency is often included in a discussion on the exotropias. These patients have an inability to obtain and maintain adequate convergence without undue effort. In the early stage of the condition, an exotropia is absent. The near point convergence is increased from 10 to 30 cm from the nose. Repeated testing may be required to demonstrate poor convergence.

Symptoms often appear in the teenage years as demands increase for close work. Aesthenopia, diplopia for near work, blurred vision and reading problems are common. Patients may discover that monocular occlusion alleviates symptoms. There is no manifest tropia for near or distance, although some patients have an exophoria for near fixation.

Treatment with convergence exercises is often successful. Rarely prisms or surgery is required.

Dissociated vertical divergence (DVD)

Occasionally the horizontal component of dissociated vertical divergence or dissociated strabismus complex can mimic a true exotropia. DVD does not obey Herring's law. On occlusion of the fixing eye, the deviating eye will resume fixation without deviation of the occluded eye. DVD may be accompanied by vertical and excyclorotatory movements. If the movement is only horizontal, an ipsilateral lateral rectus recession can be considered.

Conclusion

Exotropia is common and intermittent exotropia the commonest exotropia entity encountered in childhood. The management and in particular the timing of surgical intervention is far from clear.

Further reading

Hunter DG, Ellis FJ. Prevalence of systemic and ocular disease in infantile exotropia: comparison with infantile esotropia. *Ophthalmology* 1999; **106**(10): 1951–6.

Kushner BJ. Exotropic deviations: A functional classification and approach to treatment. *American Orthopic Journal* 1988; **38**: 81.

Kushner BJ. Selective surgery for intermittent exotropia based on distance /near differences. *Archives in Ophthalmology* 1998; **116**: 324–8.

Kushner BJ. The distance angle to target in surgery for intermittent exotropia. *Archives in Ophthalmology* 1998; **116**: 189–94.

Kushner BJ. Diagnosis and treatment of exotropia with a high accommodation convergence-accommodation ratio. *Archives in Ophthalmology* 1999; **117**(2): 221–4.

Santiago AP, Ing MR, Kushner BJ, Rosenbaum AL. In: Rosenbaum and Santiago (eds) *Clinical Strabismus Management: Principles and Surgical Techniques.* WB Saunders Company, Pennsylvania, 1999, Ch. 12, 163–75.

Walsh LA, LaRoche GR, Tremblay F. The use of binocular visual acuity in the assessment of intermittent exotropia. *Journal of AAPOS* 2000; **4**: 154–7.

Wright KW. In: Wright KW (ed.) *Pediatric Ophthalmology and Strabismus*. 1995 Mosby-Year Book Inc, St Louis, Ch. 12, 195–201.

Yuksel D, Spiritus M, Vandelannoittee S. Symmetric or asymmetric surgery for basic intermittent exotropia. *Bulletin de la Societie Belge D'ophthalmologie* 1998; **268:** 195–9.

Related topics of interest

Esotropia, convergence and accommodation (p. 113); Refraction in children (p. 248).

GIANT CELL ARTERITIS

Mike Burdon, Robert H. Taylor & Peter Shah

Giant cell arteritis (GCA) is characterized by a necrotizing vasculitis affecting primarily the cranial branches of the arteries of the aortic arch. It occurs mainly in those over 50 years of age and becomes increasingly common with increasing age. The annual incidence in those in their sixth decade is quoted as 2.3 per 100 000, increasing to 44 per 100 000 in those in their ninth decade.

Problem

It is difficult to establish a diagnosis of GCA in some patients: ophthalmologists may be asked to see a wide spectrum of patients, varying from those with classical symptoms of GCA with an established anterior ischaemic optic neuropathy (AION), to those patients with few symptoms or temporal headaches with no or transient visual symptoms. Diagnosis must be prompt to avoid severe visual loss.

Background

GCA is an enigmatic condition in which visual loss can be sudden, devastating and bilateral. Systemic steroid therapy reduces the chances of visual loss, particularly in the second eye if the first is affected. Diagnostic confirmation can be made from a positive temporal artery biopsy (TAB), but a negative biopsy does not exclude the condition. Patients should be treated on the basis of clinical findings.

Clinical features

At presentation patients may have systemic symptoms including general malaise, fatigue, weight loss and headache, which is characteristically temporal and lancing in quality. These symptoms may predate acute visual loss by several months. Tongue and jaw claudication are said to be pathognomonic. Patients may have pain on brushing their hair. There is an association with polymyalgia rheumatica: a history of stiffness and pain around the shoulder girdle may be present. The temporal artery may feel normal or it may be tender, nodular and pulseless.

The most common ophthalmic presentation is sudden unilateral visual loss due to anterior ischaemic optic neuropathy caused by occlusive inflammation in the posterior ciliary arteries. Fifty per cent of affected eyes have hand movement vision or worse, with an obvious relative afferent pupil defect. The optic disc is pale and swollen, and peripapillary splinter haemorrhages may be seen. Cotton wool spots occur in approximately 8% of cases indicating concurrent retinal ischaemia. Occasionally, segmental optic disc infarction occurs causing altitudinal field loss. Up to 10% of patients present with central or branch retinal artery occlusions, and AION associated with a cilioretinal artery occlusion has been reported. Rarely a posterior ION occurs, presenting with acute visual loss, a relative afferent pupil defect and a normal appearing disc.

Patients may present with transient visual loss, offering the opportunity to prevent blindness if an early diagnosis is made. The visual loss may take the form of brief obscurations lasting seconds, or longer episodes of 30 seconds or more that resemble amaurosis fugax. Rarely, visual loss may be caused by cerebral infarction. Approximately 10% of patients present with transient or permanent diplopia. This may be due to either a third, fourth or sixth cranial nerve palsy, or by ischaemia of the extraocular muscles. Untreated, half of the patients who present with diplopia will go on to develop an anterior ischaemic optic neuropathy.

Investigations

ESR is markedly elevated in 95% of biopsy-proven GCA. However, a normal or moderately raised ESR does not exclude the diagnosis. A slightly raised ESR in the elderly may be normal. A useful guide to the age-induced elevation of the ESR is to divide the age by a factor of 2 in males, and for females divide the age plus 10 by a factor of 2. A normochromic normocytic anaemia may be present. IgG anticardiolipin antibodies are present in 50–100% of biopsy-proven patients with GCA. Unfortunately IgG anticardiolipin antibodies are found in non-arteritic patients, and the test is not in widespread clinical use. Serum levels of von Willebrand factor and C reactive protein can be raised but the tests are not specific. Fundus fluorescein angiography shows massive choroidal non-perfusion if there is AION.

Temporal artery biopsy (TAB) examines for giant cells in the artery wall and breaks in the internal elastic lamina. A positive biopsy establishes the diagnosis. The test is extremely specific, but is only 80–98% sensitive, as it is well described that histological findings may be focal and segmental ('skip lesions'). A 2 cm long specimen and multiple histological sections will increase the sensitivity. If the initial result is negative, the contralateral artery should also be biopsied. If both these are negative, GCA may still exist although alternative diagnoses, such as neoplasia, infection or systemic autoimmune disease, must be excluded.

Scalp necrosis and significant haemorrhage are rare complications of temporal artery biopsy. Cerebrovascular ischaemia is a very rare complication that arises because, on occasion, the superficial temporal artery provides a vital collateral blood supply to the internal carotid circulation. Care needs to be exercised if a bilateral biopsy is to be undertaken.

Treatment

Clinical GCA is a medical emergency. Before corticosteroids were available, 40% of patients with a unilateral AION progressed to bilateral disease. Treatment should be implemented in advance of the biopsy procedure in order to reduce the likelihood of further visual loss. Intravenous hydrocortisone (200–300 mg) and oral prednisolone (1.5–2 mg/kg/day) are given. Alternatively, some authorities recommend 1 g of intravenous methylprednisolone for the first 3 days.

It is sometimes difficult to decide which patients should be treated. There is no doubt that those patients with classical symptoms and an AION should receive treatment. The treatment is not altered on the rare occasions that the biopsy is negative, but a confirmed diagnosis is helpful if therapeutic complications arise. Difficulty exists regarding those patients in whom the clinical diagnosis is equivocal: each must be treated on an individual basis. The likelihood of GCA must be assessed on the basis of clinical features, ESR and TAB. TAB should be performed in those patients in whom the diagnosis is equivocal, accepting that a negative result will not aid the clinical management. In equivocal cases if the probability of GCA is considered moderate to high, treatment is instigated. If the probability is low then one should consider observation and referral to a physician to exclude other diseases.

Patients' symptoms in GCA respond well to steroids. Following control of the symptoms and a reduction of the ESR, tapering of steroids should proceed with caution, monitoring symptoms and the ESR. In cases of a sudden rise in ESR, without clinical symptoms suggestive of GCA, care needs to be exercised in implicating the vasculitis. The disease process is usually self limiting to 2 years, and steroids can be terminated by this time in most patients, but recurrent symptoms indicate that continued therapy may be required.

Prognosis

Visual loss from arteritic AION has a poor prognosis. For the fellow eye, treatment reduces the likelihood of loss from AION to around 10%. Treatment of GCA also reduces the cardiovascular and cerebrovascular complications, and life outcome statistics are similar to an age- and sex-matched population. Failure to treat GCA may result in the devastating complication of bilateral visual loss from AION. Treatment of GCA has to be balanced against the complications of long-term steroid therapy in a population prone to their side effects. Osteoporosis prophylaxis is important.

Further reading

Buchbinder R, Detsky A. Management of suspected giant cell arteritis: a decision analysis. *Journal of Rheumatology* 1992; **19**: 1220–8.

Hayreh SS. Anterior ischaemic optic neuropathy. Differentiation of arteritic from non-arteritic type and its management. *Eye* 1990; **4**: 25–41.

Kupersmith MJ. Giant cell arteritis. In: *Neuro-vascular Neuro-ophthalmology*, Kupersmith MJ, Berenstein A (eds) 1st edition. Springer-Verlag, Berlin, 1993; 208–18.

Miller NR. *Walsh and Hoyt's Clinical Neuro-Ophthalmology*, 4th edn., Vol. 4. Baltimore, MD: Waverly Press, 1991; 2601–27.

Watts MT, Greaves M, Clearkin LG, Malia RG, Cooper SM. Anti-phospholipid antibodies and ischaemic optic neuropathy. *Lancet* 1990; **335**: 613–14.

Related topic of interest

Non-arteritic anterior ischaemic optic neuropathy (p. 185).

HIV AND THE EYE

Philip I. Murray

The human immunodeficiency virus (HIV) is the retrovirus responsible for AIDS. The HIV target cell is the CD4+ T lymphocyte. With increasing CD4+ depletion the patient becomes more susceptible to opportunistic infection.

Problem

The emergence and management of new forms of ocular disease in AIDS patients on highly active anti-retroviral therapy (HAART) with clinically inactive cytomegalovirus (CMV) retinitis.

Background

HIV is a chronic infection taking on average 8 to 10 years before an infected patient develops symptomatic AIDS. By this late stage severe damage has occurred to the cell-mediated arm of the immune system and recurrent opportunistic infections and tumours occur, prior to death within 1 to 2 years. This depressing scenario has been transformed over the past 5 years with the introduction of effective combination anti-retroviral therapy resulting in, if not cure, at least prolonged suppression of viral replication and its associated clinical benefits. To balance against this we have become increasingly aware of the potential for drug resistance, side effects and drug interactions, which may limit the appropriateness and effectiveness of these agents.

Throughout the course of HIV infection, even during the prolonged asymptomatic stage, a patient infected with HIV produces millions of new viral particles every day. It therefore follows that to prevent the body being overwhelmed, an equally large number of viral particles and many infected cells are destroyed each day, putting an enormous strain on the immune system. Two markers are of particular relevance in assessing and monitoring viral turnover and the response of the immune system – the viral load and the CD4 lymphocyte count.

The viral load is expressed as the number of copies of virus per ml of serum ranging between a few hundred copies and several million copies per ml. Interpretation of the level of viral load will depend upon the stage of HIV infection. After initial infection the viral load rises rapidly prior to the production of anti-HIV antibody, peaking at around 6 to 12 weeks. It is therefore at this early stage of infection that the patient is at their most infectious, but still has a negative HIV antibody test using conventional assays. Some patients undergo a sero-conversion illness, which is usually non-specific with fever, rash and lymphadenopathy, but if they are identified at this stage then therapy should probably be initiated. Following sero-conversion the viral load falls and levels off at a 'set point' where it remains fairly steady over a period of many years. It is the absolute level of this 'set point' which is the single most reliable prognostic marker for HIV. For example, a patient with a viral load of between 3 000 and 10 000 has a median survival greater than 10 years, compared to a patient with a viral load of greater than 30 000 whose median survival is $4\frac{1}{2}$ years.

The serum CD4 lymphocyte count gives an estimate of the total number of CD4 lymphocytes, most of which are sequestered in lymphatic tissue. After the initial infection a fall in the CD4 count recovers partially following sero-conversion, and thereafter a steady decline occurs. Since there is a degree of over compensation in the immune system the level can drop from normal (approximately 500 cells/cm^3 upwards) to around 200 cells/cm^3 whilst the patient remains well. Below this level, patients are at increasing risk of opportunistic infections.

CMV retinitis

CMV retinitis is the commonest AIDS-related opportunistic infection of the eye but retinitis may also result from herpes simplex virus (acute retinal necrosis) and varicella-zoster virus (acute retinal necrosis, progressive outer retinal necrosis). Kaposi's sarcoma (human herpesvirus 8) can occur on the lids and conjunctiva. Other infections include toxoplasmosis, *Pneumocystis carinii*, cryptococcus, *Mycobacterium avium* complex and syphilis. Non-Hodgkin's B-cell lymphoma is another complication. Although HIV microvasculopathy (cotton wool spots and small retinal haemorrhages) is a frequent fundal finding, no specific therapy is required.

CMV retinitis occurs in about 25% of AIDS patients and those with an absolute CD4+ level of < 50 cells/mm^3 are at greatest risk of developing the disease. The clinical appearance is of a slowly progressive, necrotizing retinitis. It can affect the posterior pole, the periphery or both and may be unilateral or bilateral. White intraretinal lesions and areas of infiltrate and necrosis occur along the vascular arcades of the posterior pole. These are associated with prominent retinal haemorrhages within the necrotic area or along its leading edge ('pizza pie' appearance). Peripherally, it has a less intense white appearance with areas of granular, white retinitis that may or may not have associated haemorrhage ('brush fire' appearance). As the retinitis progresses, an area of atrophic, avascular retina remains. Active lesions have opaque or white borders, indicating 'active' viral disease. Inactive lesions are those with no opacity of the border and appear as transparent retinal scars with faint pigment mottling. There are usually only 1–3 foci of disease, the spread is relatively slow with anterior > posterior rate of progression, it is relatively fovea sparing with new lesions rarely in the fovea, and posterior spread of disease tends to be circumferential around the fovea. Documentation of disease spread using retinal photographs is important. There is usually only minimal vitreous activity and occasionally a few anterior chamber cells are seen. Small keratic precipitates, scattered widely over the corneal endothelium, are often found. Complications include blindness from retinal detachment (occurs in 20–30% and normally requires vitrectomy and silicone oil tamponade), optic nerve disease by direct involvement and optic atrophy secondary to vascular occlusion.

Treatment of CMV retinitis involves the use of ganciclovir, foscarnet, cidofovir, and more recently fomivirsen. Therapeutic strategies have included administration by a variety of routes; intravenous (ganciclovir, foscarnet, cidofovir), oral (ganciclovir), intravitreal injection (ganciclovir, foscarnet, cidofovir, fomivirsen) or intravitreal (ganciclovir) device. All are effective in controlling retinitis, but are virostatic and therefore do not eradicate retinal CMV in severely immunosuppressed individuals. Prevention of recurrent CMV retinitis has been dependent on lifelong maintenance treatment as active retinitis recurs in almost all patients within 3–4 weeks of stopping treatment. Despite the availability of effective treatment to control the retinitis (about 90% response rate with i.v. anti-CMV therapy reducing the possibility of disease in the second eye from 60% to between 0–15%) a number of important problems have arisen. Drug-related adverse reactions were common and included neutropenia (ganciclovir), nephrotoxicity (foscarnet, cidofovir), intra-ocular inflammation and hypotony (cidofovir). Prolonged use resulted in the emergence of drug-resistant strains and relapses invariably occurred. The time period between relapses became progressively shorter and the reactivated retinitis appeared increasingly more aggressive and more difficult to treat. Treatment of frequent recurrences required switching from one agent to another or using combination therapy. Ophthalmologists were becoming increasingly pessimistic with regards to preserving vision in their patients.

Anti-retroviral therapy

There are currently over a dozen different anti-retroviral drugs available within the UK, but they mostly fit into three groups – the nucleoside reverse transcriptase inhibitors (nucleosides), the non-nucleoside reverse transcriptase inhibitors (NNRTI) and the protease inhibitors (PI). To understand how these drugs work and the rationale for combination therapy it is helpful to consider how HIV replicates. Although the virus can infect many different cell types it has a predilection for cells carrying the CD4 receptor to which it attaches in order to gain entry. Since HIV is a retrovirus, the first step in viral replication is conversion from RNA to DNA requiring the enzyme reverse transcriptase. Both the nucleosides and the NNRTI drugs act by inhibiting reverse transcriptase at this point, early in viral replication. The nucleosides, however, become integrated into the extending DNA chain and act as chain terminators whilst the NNRTI drugs act only as competitive inhibitors of the enzyme. Following integration of the viral DNA into the host cell genome, transcription leads to the production of a long protein molecule which needs to be cut up into smaller pieces before re-assembly as new viral particles. The protease enzyme performs this function and it is here, at the opposite end of the reproductive cycle, that the PIs act.

The first anti-retroviral agent that became available was zidovudine, which is a nucleoside analogue, used initially as monotherapy for patients with advanced disease. Using a single agent in this way leads to a transient drop in the viral load of about three-fold, which translates into a survival benefit of around 12 to 18 months. Over subsequent years new agents have become available and the benefits of combination therapy initially with two drugs and, since the mid 1990s, with three or four drugs has consistently been shown to be superior. A typical initial combination would be two nucleosides with either a NNRTI or a PI. Combining drugs in this way can reduce the viral load by 500- to 1000-fold aiming to bring it below the current level of detection (50 copies per ml). Associated with this virological response many patients also achieve a rise in the CD4 lymphocyte count reflecting improved immune function, and this represents not just an expansion of existing memory CD4 lymphocytes but also the production of new naive cells. The effect of anti-retroviral therapy can be assessed using the viral load and CD4 count – a change in therapy can then be initiated in those who fail to have an optimal response.

A recent large cohort study suggested that over 90% of patients starting therapy for the first time would have an undetectable viral load after 2 years. This is associated with a clinical progression rate of less than 5% over the same time period that compares to a progression rate of 40% in patients previously treated with zidovudine monotherapy. In the UK this has translated into a marked decline in the number of reported opportunistic infections, which are now a rarity in patients taking effective treatment. In 1995, for the first time, a drop in the death rate from HIV was reported in the UK but since the number of cases of HIV being diagnosed remains stable, a rapid increase in disease prevalence has resulted.

Like other medications these agents can be associated with side effects and they require regular monitoring and caution when co-administered with other drugs. The nucleosides, including zidovudine, are generally well tolerated particularly in those patients with well-preserved immune function, but the possibility of myositis, peripheral neuropathy and pancreatitis need to be borne in mind. The main problem with the NNRTIs is skin rash occurring within a few weeks of starting therapy. Often therapy can be continued and the rash will subside, but a small proportion of patients will progress to the Stevens–Johnson syndrome and close monitoring is therefore advisable. The protease inhibitors have both short-term and long-term problems. Initially GI symptoms with marked nausea and diarrhoea tend to occur, although this often settles, at least partially, within a few weeks. In the longer term a lipodystrophy syndrome has been described in which patients lose fat from the limbs and face with accumulation of fat around the abdomen and the breasts, sometimes with a 'buffalo hump' on the back of the neck. This appears to be quite common affecting virtually all patients given PIs to a greater or lesser extent, with around 10% of patients developing fairly marked changes. For this reason many clinicians tend to avoid PIs as first-line therapy although they remain extremely potent drugs which may be required later in the disease course. Although the pathogenesis of lipodystrophy has not been identified it may be linked to another side effect seen with PIs – elevated serum lipids. In some patients this is quite marked, with cholesterol levels of over 10 raising the possibility of future cardiovascular disease.

Although the anti-retroviral drugs are effective in suppressing the virus, they do not eradicate it and low level viral replication persists. Thus the potential for developing resistant mutations exists and it is likely that all patients will eventually fail therapy. This is manifested by a rise in the viral load and necessitates a change in the anti-retroviral regimen. It is usually possible to find a second-line combination which will be effective but there is considerable cross-resistance between agents, and third- or fourth-line therapy tends to be less effective. Resistance is particularly likely to occur in patients where drug levels remain sub-optimal due to poor compliance and considerable efforts have been made to educate and support patients to ensure that they are able to take their medication at the appropriate time.

Paradoxically, the restoration of immune function can itself cause problems. For diseases where the immune response to infection is the major pathological process, restoring immune function may lead to an exacerbation of symptoms (see below).

New manifestations of ophthalmic AIDS

Over the past few years there has been a dramatic downturn in the number of new cases of CMV retinitis. Recent studies have confirmed a significant increase in survival of AIDS patients with CMV retinitis who were treated with HAART. HAART is effective in suppressing the viral load and reconstituting CD4+ T lymphocytes with a resultant increase in the time interval between relapses of CMV retinitis. Evidence is mounting that as sufficient immune reactivity against opportunistic infections, such as CMV, is restored, discontinuation of anti-CMV maintenance therapy should now be considered. In one series where anti-CMV therapy was discontinued, no reactivation or progression of retinitis was seen during the mean follow-up period of 11.4 months and retinitis did not develop in previously unaffected contralateral eyes. Many patients now have their anti-CMV maintenance therapy withdrawn. The replenished CD4+ T lymphocyte count induced by HAART is partly responsible for the emergence of a new pattern of ophthalmic AIDS, which is characterized by a heightened inflammatory response and more frequent complications associated with this response. In some patients with inactive CMV retinitis, the T lymphocyte rejuvenation is thought to mount an immune response to ocular CMV proteins which is seen as a vitreous inflammatory reaction (whereas paucity of inflammation has been considered to be the hallmark of CMV retinitis), occasionally associated with papillitis or cystoid macular oedema (CMO). This response has been termed immune recovery vitritis and usually occurs shortly after the initiation of protease inhibitors. Yet many patients on combination anti-retroviral therapy with partial immune reconstitution and inactive CMV retinitis do not develop inflammatory signs. Factors giving rise to the inflammatory response are unclear, but there have been indications that these CD4+ T lymphocytes are only partially functional and may give limited protection. Despite HAART, the CD4+ count in some patients will remain low and recurrences will occur. CMO causing loss of central vision, previously an infrequent occurrence with active CMV retinitis, is now an increasing cause of visual loss in patients with AIDS and inactive CMV retinitis. The aetiology is poorly understood, but it is thought that as the immune function improves, choroidal inflammation may be a causal factor. Whereas CMO associated with active CMV retinitis may respond to systemic antivirals, CMO associated with inactive CMV is more problematic. Effective treatment is essential, particularly as patients may already have extensive peripheral (navigational) visual loss from previous (now inactive) CMV retinitis and are now at threat of losing their central vision. Oral acetazolamide and topical non-steroidal agents have limited efficacy and despite the possible risk of CMV reactivation, treatment strategies include corticosteroids, given as periocular injections or by mouth.

Further reading

Holland GN. Pieces of a puzzle: toward better understanding of intraocular inflammation associated with human immunodeficiency virus infection. *American Journal of Ophthalmology* 1998; **125:** 383–5.

Karavellas MP, Lowder KY, Macdonald C, Avila C, Freeman WR. Immune recovery vitritis in patients with inactive cytomegalovirus retinitis: a new syndrome. *Archives of Ophthalmology* 1998; **116:** 169–75.

MacDonald JC, Torriani FJ, Morse LS, Karavellas MP, Reed JB, Freeman WR. Lack of reactivation of cytomegalovirus (CMV) retinitis after stopping CMV maintenance therapy in AIDS patients with sustained elevations in CD4+ T cells in response to highly active antiretroviral therapy. *Journal of Infectious Diseases* 1998; **117:** 1182–7.

Nussenblatt RB, Lane HC. Human immunodeficiency virus disease: changing patterns of intraocular inflammation. *American Journal of Ophthalmology* 1998; **125:** 374–82.

Vrabec TR, Baldassano VF, Whitcup SM. Discontinuation of maintenance therapy in patients with quiescent cytomegalovirus retinitis and elevated CD4+ counts. *Ophthalmology* 1998; **105:** 1259–64.

Walsh JC, Jones CD, Barnes EA *et al.* Increasing survival in AIDS patients with cytomegalovirus retinitis treated with combination antiretroviral therapy including protease inhibitors. *AIDS* 1998; **12:** 613–18.

Whitcup SM, Fortin E, Nussenblatt RB *et al.* Therapeutic effect of combination anti-retroviral therapy on cytomegalovirus retinitis. *JAMA* 1997; **277:** 1519–20.

Zegans ME, Walton C, Holland GN, O'Donnell JJ, Jacobson MA, Margolis TP. Transient vitreous inflammatory reactions associated with combination antiretroviral therapy in patients with AIDS and cytomegalovirus retinitis. *American Journal of Ophthalmology* 1998; **125:** 292–300.

HORNER'S SYNDROME

Peter Shah

Horner's syndrome is caused by an interruption of the sympathetic pathway at any point between the hypothalamus and the eye. When confronted with a patient with a possible Horner's syndrome one must first confirm the diagnosis and then attempt to localize the site of the lesion. Finally, one must identify the pathological process causing the lesion.

Background

The sympathetic pathway traces the following route. First-order neurones originate in the posterolateral hypothalamus and then proceed in a caudal route through the brainstem. They synapse in the intermediolateral part of the spinal cord from C8 to T2 (ciliospinal centre of Budge). Second-order neurones then emerge from the spinal cord in the ventral roots. They then ascend, cross the apex of the lung and course through the stellate and inferior cervical ganglia. After passing through the middle cervical ganglion, they synapse in the superior cervical ganglion (SCG) at the level of the angle of the mandible. Third-order neurones ascend from the SCG along the internal carotid artery, which enters the skull, passes through the carotid syphon and then enters the cavernous sinus. From here, fibres ride with the nasociliary nerve (a branch of the ophthalmic division of the trigeminal nerve) into the orbit. The long ciliary nerves emerge from the nasociliary nerve and supply the dilator pupillae muscle to the iris.

Note: the sudomotor fibres to the face and neck travel with the external carotid artery when fibres emerge from the SCG.

Horner's syndrome may be classified into congenital and acquired subgroups, and then further divided on the basis of the site of the lesion: (i) central, first-order neurone, between the hypothalamus and ciliospinal centre of Budge, (ii) pre-ganglionic, second-order neurone, between the ventral root of T1 and the superior cervical ganglion, and (iii) post-ganglionic, third-order neurone, between the superior cervical ganglion and the eye. There are 10 main regions in which the sympathetic nerves may be damaged:

- hypothalamus;
- brainstem;
- spinal cord;
- ventral root of T1;
- apex of the lung;
- neck;
- internal carotid artery at the base of the skull;
- middle ear;
- cavernous sinus;
- orbit.

A thorough history and clinical examination are essential and can give valuable information regarding the site of the lesion. For example, anhydrosis of the face implies a lesion proximal to the superior cervical ganglion, (i.e. central or pre-ganglionic). The help of a neurologist may be valuable at this stage.

Pharmacological testing can be used both to confirm the diagnosis of Horner's syndrome and to localize the site of the lesion. The cocaine (4%) test is used to confirm or refute the diagnosis. Cocaine blocks re-uptake of noradrenaline at the synaptic cleft and, if sympathetic damage is present (at any level), then the pupil will dilate poorly to cocaine. The hydroxyamphetamine (Paredrine 1%) test is used to further localize the lesion. Hydroxyamphetamine releases noradrenaline (NA) from normal nerve terminals. When post-ganglionic neurones are damaged then there is no production of NA and no pupil dilation occurs with hydroxyamphetamine. If central or pre-ganglionic neurones are damaged then the third-order neurones can still produce NA, and pupil dilation will occur with hydroxyamphetamine. This test identifies a lesion damaging the third-order neurone.

The adrenaline (0.1%) test relies on denervation hypersensitivity to a dilute solution of adrenaline, but may not be present immediately after damage occurs.

With all these tests it is important that no other drops have been administered. These tests are sensitive and the result may be affected by previous drops and applanation tonometry or any contact with the ocular surface.

Despite the careful assessment and investigation of patients with acquired Horner's syndrome, a definite pathological diagnosis is not reached in every case. In cases where the underlying pathology is a neoplastic lesion, the prognosis will be generally worse than in patients with other lesions. It is important to remember that any pathological process, whether neoplastic, vascular, infective, inflammatory degenerative, demyelinative, traumatic, metabolic or iatrogenic can interfere with the sympathetic supply in the eye.

Clinical features

Typical features of Horner's syndrome include a moderate ptosis of 1–2 mm with a miosis of the pupil and dilation lag, both of which are more noticeable in dim illumination. There is an elevation of the lower lid by 1–2 mm, giving the impression of an enophthalmos. The globe position is unaltered. If the lesion is congenital or acquired early in infancy then heterochromia iridis may be present. Features such as reduction in sweating of ipsilateral face and neck may help with localization of the lesion. Ocular hypotony, conjunctival hyperaemia and increased amplitude of accommodation have all been described as early signs and may be transient.

Further reading

Bajandas FJ, Kline LB. *Neuro-Ophthalmology Review Manual*, 3rd edn. Thorofare, NJ: SLACK, 1988; 113–24.

Related topic of interest

Anisocoria (p. 16).

HYPERTENSION AND THE EYE

Amanda Butcher & Paul Dodson

Hypertension is 'that blood pressure above which the benefits of treatment outweigh the risk of treatment'. The blood pressure measurement at which this level is set is arbitrary and a number of groups have suggested various thresholds and targets for treatment based on observational and study data.

Problem

There is debate about who needs treatment continued. The rationale for the treatment of hypertension is the reduction of clinical events due to atherosclerosis, and in particular ischaemic heart disease and stroke. The assessment of hypertension should therefore be carried out in the context of other risk factors for cardiovascular disease.

Background

Ninety-five per cent of hypertensive patients have no underlying cause and it is described as essential hypertension, 65% of accelerated hypertension is essential in origin.

Secondary causes:

1. **Renal disease**
   - intrinsic, e.g. glomerulonephritis, pyelonephritis;
   - renal artery stenosis;
   - chronic renal failure (it may be difficult to establish whether this is cause or effect);
   - renal tumours;
   - polycystic renal disease.

2. **Endocrine**
   - diabetes;
   - phaeochromocytoma;
   - primary aldosteronism (Conn's syndrome);
   - primary hyperparathyroidism;
   - hyperthyroidism;
   - Cushing's syndrome;
   - Acromegaly.

3. **Drugs**
   - oral contraceptive pill;
   - steroids;
   - NSAIDs;
   - excess liquorice.

4. **Rarer causes**
   - coarctation of the aorta.

5. *Baseline investigation of all hypertensive patients should include:*
- full history;
- physical examination, including fundoscopy;
- urinalysis (glycosuria, proteinuria);
- blood glucose;
- biochemical profile;
- ECG;
- serum cholesterol and high-density lipoprotein cholesterol.

Clinical features

Direct consequences of hypertension on the eye include: hypertensive retinopathy, hypertensive choroidopathy and retinal detachment. Retinal vascular events associated with hypertension include: retinal macroaneurysm, central/branch retinal vein occlusion and non-arteritic anterior ischaemic optic neuropathy. The consequences of systemic atherosclerosis on the visual tract are: field defects due to posterior cerebral vascular accident, diplopia due to infarction of cranial nerves e.g. III, VI, central retinal artery/branch retinal arteriolar occlusion and amaurosis fugax.

Hypertensive retinopathy

The main role of fundoscopy in hypertension is to establish the presence of target organ damage. A simplified grading system, which highlights the current use of fundoscopy in hypertension is as follows:

1. *Grade A Non-accelerated hypertension.* Generalized arteriolar narrowing and focal constriction.

2. *Grade B Accelerated hypertension.* Haemorrhages, exudates, cotton wool spots, with or without optic disc swelling. Optic disc swelling may also occur alone. A lesion of retinovascular damage must be present in both eyes for the diagnosis of this grade.

Although hypertensive retinopathy can be florid, when it does not involve the disc or macula visual prognosis is good. If vision is impaired this may resolve with anti-hypertensive treatment. The presence of optic disc swelling places the patient at an increased risk of permanent visual impairment due to non-arteritic anterior ischaemic optic neuropathy and optic atrophy.

More detailed investigation for underlying cause is also indicated in patients presenting with:

- accelerated hypertension;
- BP resistant to two drugs;
- age < 45 years.

Further investigations should be guided by initial findings and may include random growth hormone, ultrasound scan of the kidneys, renal arteriogram, imaging the adrenal glands, renin and aldosterone measurement and 24 hour urinary collection for catecholamines and urinary free cortisol.

Treatment

Most national and international societies (including the British Hypertension Society) now agree on the following statements:

Treat all sustained hypertension > 160 mmHg systolic
> 100 mmHg diastolic.

In the following context of higher cardiovascular risk, blood pressures of > 140 systolic and > 90 diastolic should be treated:

(a) the presence of target organ damage: hypertensive retinopathy, left ventricular hypertrophy or proteinuria;
(b) established cardiovascular disease (secondary prevention) or diabetes;
(c) the risk of coronary heart disease (CHD) is calculated to be > 15% in 10 years.

There are a number of published methods for establishing the 10-year CHD risk for an individual patient such as the Joint British Societies Cardiac Risk Assessor computer program or their CHD risk chart. There is broad agreement that blood pressure should be reduced to <140/< 85 mmHg.

Those patients presenting with retinovascular disease, known to be associated with systemic atherosclerosis or hypertension, e.g. with retinal emboli, or retinal vein occlusion should be assessed with an appropriate cardiovascular risk calculator and managed according to their risk. There is some evidence that the recurrence rate of retinal vein occlusion is reduced with tight control of the risk factors, including hypertension. Strict hypertension control in Type II diabetes is established as being effective in reducing the incidence of diabetic retinopathy.

Accelerated hypertension is not defined by a level of measured BP and is diagnosed on the basis of a significant rise in the BP and fundoscopic changes as outlined above. Pathologically it corresponds to fibrinoid necrosis occurring in small arterioles hence the fundal changes and renal effects leading to proteinuria and haematuria. Patients presenting with accelerated hypertension have an increased prevalence of underlying causes and should be investigated. Untreated accelerated hypertension carries an increased mortality risk, with only 1–20% survival at 5 years, but with modern treatment regimes this increases to > 80% five-year survival.

1. Lifestyle measures apply to all groups of hypertensive patient – optimize weight, increase exercise, reduce dietary salt, moderate alcohol, increase intake of fruit and vegetables.
2. Adequate control of blood pressure may require one or more of the following drugs:

- low-dose thiazide diuretics;
- beta-blockers;
- calcium channel antagonists;
- angiotensin converting enzyme inhibitors (ACE-I);
- angiotensin II blockers;
- alpha receptor blockers;
- minoxidil (third-line only).

Recommended first-line therapy is either beta-blocker or thiazide diuretic. Where necessary there are two methods of introducing combination therapy. Increase each drug to the maximum dose acceptable in terms of side effects then add a further drug or go to half the maximum recommended dose and then add the next drug.

3. An important part of the management of hypertension is to lower the patient's overall cardiovascular risk.

- Aspirin should be used in hypertensive patients > 50 years old, with well controlled BP in the presence of target organ damage, diabetes or 10 year CHD risk > 30%
- Statins should be used in hypertensive patients up to age 70, when serum cholesterol > 5.0 mmol and 10 year CHD risk is > 30%. Statins are used in secondary prevention (i.e. in established cardiovascular disease) up to the age of 75 when serum cholesterol is > 5.0 mmol.

Treatment of accelerated hypertension should result in a very gradual reduction in the BP using oral agents. The patient should initially be managed as an inpatient for monitoring of BP and further investigation for underlying cause. A rapid fall in BP can lead to severe consequences including myocardial infarct, stroke and infarction of the optic nerve heads as a result of disturbances in autoregulatory mechanisms that occur during the accelerated phase of hypertension.

Further reading

Dodson PM, Gibson JM, Kritzinger EE. *Clinical Retinopathies.* London: Chapman and Hall Medical, 1995.
Ramsay LE, Williams, Johnston GD *et al.* for the British Hypertension Society. Guidelines for management of hypertension: report of the third working party of the British Hypertension Society. *Journal of Human Hypertension* 1999; **13:** 569–92.
UK Prospective Diabetes Study Group. Tight blood pressure control and risk of mascrovascular and microvascular complications in Type 2 diabetes: UKPDS 38. *British Medical Journal* **317:** 703–12.

Related topics of interest

Diabetes mellitus: medical aspects (p. 90); Diabetic retinopathy (p. 100); Non-arteritic anterior ischaemic optic neuropathy (p. 185); Retinal vein occlusion (p. 259).

IDIOPATHIC INTRACRANIAL HYPERTENSION

Oliver Backhouse

Idiopathic intracranial hypertension (IIH), previously called pseudotumour cerebri or benign intracranial hypertension, is the diagnostic term used in an awake and alert patient who has signs and symptoms of increased intracranial pressure, the absence of localizing findings on neurologic examination (except abducens palsy) and normal neurodiagnostic studies, except for increased cerebrospinal fluid (CSF) pressure (> 20 cmH$_2$O in the non-obese and > 25 cmH$_2$O in the obese patient), with no other cause of increased intracranial pressure present. These are known as the modified Dandy criteria which must be met to make the diagnosis of IIH. In children the CSF pressure is lower (< 7.5 cmH$_2$O aged < 2 years and < 13.5 cmH$_2$O aged < 5 years).

Problem

This condition can present to the ophthalmologist with headaches or visual symptoms. Catastrophic visual loss can occur with speed in ischaemic papilloedema.

Background

Over 90% of IIH patients are obese and more than 90% are female suggesting an endocrinological disturbance. The incidence of IIH is negligible in countries where obesity is uncommon. In Iowa the incidence is 0.9 per 100000 in the general population; 3.5 per 100000 in women aged 20–44 years; 13 per 100000 in women who are 10% over ideal weight; and 19 per 100000 in women who are 20% over ideal weight. The age range at the time of diagnosis is broad with the mean age at 30 years. About 10% have symptomatic recurrences but asymptomatic raised pressure can persist for years. Rarely IIH can be familial.

Aetiology

Raised intracranial pressure may occur from increased venous sinus pressure, increased arachnoid resistance, CSF hypersecretion or other blockage of free CSF flow. Many previous cases, which would have been diagnosed as idiopathic, are now identified by magnetic resonance venography (MRV) as having venous sinus thrombosis, which is associated with a prothrombotic state. Other authors have also suggested a link of thrombophilia, collagen vascular disorders and IIH.

The possible link with oestrogens may link oral contraceptive use, obesity and menstrual dysfunction with IIH. Extraovarian oestrogen is produced from adipocytes and it is also known that raised oestrogen levels are prothrombotic by an effect on blood coagulation, fibrinolysis and platelets. However, the correlation of oestrogen, menstrual irregularities and pregnancy in IIH is not supported by case–control studies. Other associations include antibiotics (e.g. tetracyclines), vitamin levels (e.g. vitamin A), corticosteroid use and endocrinological disturbance but, in many of these compelling cases, validity is in doubt due to the poor adherence to the modified Dandy criteria needed for diagnosis.

Obesity and recent weight gain have the strongest association with IIH. Raised intra-abdominal pressure, which is significantly higher in obese patients, can cause a functional obstruction to cerebral venous outflow via the jugular venous system producing resistance to CSF absorption. It is probably the acuteness of the increase in central venous pressure that is important in producing the clinically significant rise in intracranial pressure. Some authors feel that the increase in intracranial venous pressure is the universal mechanism in IIH of varying aetiologies. Weight loss, medical or surgical, may cause papilloedema to disappear. How much is not fully known, but a reduction in weight of 6% has caused resolution of marked papilloedema in one study. In children the sex ratio is equal and obesity a feature in about 30%, rising up to 90% in the 15–17 year age group. Infectious disease (especially otitis media), drugs and trauma are the most commonly associated conditions but, in these studies, there was no case–control group.

Clinical features

Most studies into IIH presentation have been retrospective without any control group. Giuseffi *et al.* performed a case–control study comparing symptoms of 50 IIH patients with 100 controls. Headache is present in 94% of patients with IIH. These are usually severe and are frequently pulsatile in nature. Often accompanied by nausea, the headache is different from any previous headache, lasts hours, becomes worse on lying down and may wake the patient. Retrobulbar pain can be accentuated by eye movements. Transient visual obscurations are less common, occurring in 68% of patients. They often last less than 30 seconds and can be monocular or binocular. They are probably due to transient ischaemia of the optic nerve or disc and are sometimes posture-induced. Some patients (60%) mention intracranial noises on direct questioning. They may be in the form of pulsatile tinnitus. Temporary disappearance occurs after diagnostic lumbar puncture. Diplopia can occur usually due to an abducens nerve palsy as part of a false localizing sign in raised intracranial pressure. Other symptoms may include shimmering lights, lethargy and dizziness.

Examination signs may include reduced visual acuity, central, nasal and peripheral scotomas, increased size of blind spot (refractive), lateral rectus weakness and papilloedema. Other neurological abnormalities have been reported but these are so rare that the diagnosis of IIH can only be made after an underlying intracranial mass, infection or inflammatory process has been excluded. Papilloedema is usually bilateral but often asymmetrical. Optic nerve head drusen or an anomalous disc in the presence of a headache can lead to a mistaken diagnosis. Ischaemic papilloedema is characterized by the presence of haemorrhages and cotton wool spots and should initiate urgent pressure lowering to try and protect the optic nerves from further permanent damage. Strong warning signs for permanent optic nerve damage are: ischaemic papilloedema, an afferent pupillary defect, reduced colour vision/visual acuity and enlarging visual field defects. It is not strongly related to duration of symptoms or presence of visual obscurations.

Treatment

After normal CT/MRI and MRV imaging, a lumbar puncture must be performed. If the CSF constitution is normal and the pressure raised, then the diagnosis of IIH can be made. Because the natural history and underlying pathophysiology is still not fully clear and there is a lack of randomized, controlled, double-blind prospective studies of treatment, it is not possible to make evidence-based management recommendations. The two main reasons to treat IIH are to relieve the headache and prevent visual loss, which may be permanent. Despite the resolution of papilloedema, the CSF pressure may still be raised, even for years.

Weight loss should be coordinated by a dietitian and exercise encouraged. Gastric bypass or stapling surgery is an option if the above fails. Unfortunately weight loss can be difficult to achieve so acetazolamide 250 mg four times a day is given to reduce CSF production. The dose can be increased to 4 g a day but levels above 2 g a day are seldom tolerated due to unacceptable side effects. The dose is then gradually lowered over months according to the clinical response. Frusemide seems to be less effective and, although steroids may help in IIH of presumed inflammatory association, they may make the problem worse by inducing weight gain.

Multiple lumbar punctures have little place in a chronic treatment plan. The pressure-lowering effect may last only a few hours and is poorly tolerated by the patient. Lumboperitoneal shunting (LPS) can relieve headaches and papilloedema but there are complications such as shunt obstruction and low-pressure headaches requiring surgical revision. The long-term outcome of visual function following LPS is not known. Optic nerve sheath fenestration (ONSF) is presently the favoured treatment for deteriorating visual function when medical treatment has failed. The key to the success of this operation is early intervention by a surgeon of appropriate expertise. Papilloedema can resolve on the contralateral side, but eyes that have more than one ONSF rarely stabilize or improve after surgery. Ischaemic papilloedema requires urgent lowering of intracranial pressure.

In pregnancy, treatment of IIH is generally the same. Caloric restriction is not advised due to the effect of ketosis on the fetus. Steroids and acetezolamide used after 20 weeks gestation appear safe but other diuretics are contraindicated in the second half of pregnancy due to the risk of decrease in placental blood flow.

Permanent visual loss is the only serious physical complication of IIH. Blind spot enlargement is ubiquitous in IIH and is often eliminated with hypermetropic correction so should not be classified as a true field defect. Goldmann perimetry or automated perimetry of the central 30° are sensitive measures for IIH visual field monitoring. Serial indirect ophthalmoscopy, photography and/or the scanning laser ophthalmoscope aids interpretation of the field regarding the need for surgical intervention. Frequent visual field monitoring is recommended together with visual acuity, colour plate and papillary defect measurements. When the condition is considered 'non-sight-threatening' this monitoring may be performed at 4–6 month intervals.

Conclusion

The cause of IIH is probably variable, though obesity, recent weight gain and the female sex have the greatest association, particularly in the adult population. Management should involve an ophthalmologist, neurologist and a dietitian in close coordination. Despite this, a few patients have rapid irreversible visual loss.

Further reading

Blacer L, Liu G, Forman S *et al.* Idiopathic intracranial hypertension. Relation of age and obesity in children. *Neurology* 1999; **52:** 870–2.

Bloomfield G, Ridings P, Blocher C *et al.* A proposed relationship between increased intra-abdominal, intrathoracic, and intracranial pressure. *Critical care medicine* 1997; **25**(3): 496–503.

Giuseffi V, Wall M, Siegel P *et al.* Symptoms and disease associations in idiopathic intracranial hypertension (pseudotumour cerebri) a case–control study. *Neurology* 1991; **41:** 239–44.

Soler D, Cox T, Bullock P *et al.* Diagnosis and management of benign intracranial hypertension. *Archive of Diseases of Childhood* 1998; **78:** 89–94.

Sugerman H, Felton W, Sismanis A *et al.* Gastric surgery for pseudotumour cerebri associated with severe obesity. *Annals of Surgery* 1999; **229**(5): 634–42.

Wall M, George D. Idiopathic intracranial hypertension. A prospective study of 50 patients. *Brain* 1991; **114:** 155–80.

INFANTILE ESOTROPIA

Robert H. Taylor

Infantile esotropia is probably not present at birth so the term congenital is strictly incorrect. However the term congenital esotropia is often used. The onset is probably at around 2 months of age in most patients. Most authorities classify esotropia as infantile esotropia if the onset is before 6 months of age.

Problem

The pathogenesis of infantile esotropia is not fully understood, although there are some interesting associations that may prove important.

Background

Pursuit movement of the eyes is controlled through the magnocellular pathways. At birth the temporal to nasal movement is already developed. The opposite movement, nasal to temporal, usually develops at 3 to 5 months of age. This is associated with symmetrical oculokinetic nystagmus, stereopsis and aligned eyes. In congenital esotropia there is a failure of this development. This leads to an asymmetric oculokinetic nystagmus, poor monocular smooth pursuit in the naso-temporal direction and esotropia. There is also an increased prevalence of visually evoked potential asymmetry. It is suggested that the abducting nystagmus seen in Ciancia syndrome is due to a misperception causing an adduction pursuit movement with a refixation saccade. Why the nasal to temporal movement fails to develop, or if this is the primary abnormality remains unknown.

Clinical features

In general, patients with infantile esotropia have an otherwise normal development. There may be a family history. It has a relatively higher prevalence in patients who have developmental delay, hydrocephalus and some syndromes (e.g. Williams syndrome).

Examination findings at presentation include equal vision with cross fixation (i.e. the adducted eye looks into the contralateral field). The esotropia is usually large (over 40 prism diopters) and abduction is usually normal but this is often difficult to elicit. Refraction is weakly hypermetropic (i.e. normal) and fundus examination normal. In general, amblyopia is not a feature in the early stages, but is up to 5 times more likely after surgical correction. In most patients further features become obvious after the first year of life. They may also become apparent following corrective surgery for the esotropia, a fact worth warning parents about. These include inferior oblique over-action, dissociated vertical divergence (DVD) and latent nystagmus. Approximately half of patients will require a second operation for these abnormalities or recurrent horizontal strabismus later in life.

There is a subgroup of early onset esotropia patients, originally described by Ciancia in 1962, in whom there is nystagmus in abduction. This is a jerk nystagmus, fast phase towards the fixing eye, which has a larger amplitude in attempted abduction, and disappears in adduction. There is often a latent component. The child will adopt a compensatory head posture, turning the face towards the fixing eye, to bring it into adduction. If the other eye fixes, the nystagmus will change in direction, and the head turn will reverse. There is often a tilt to the side of the fixing eye, thought to be a response to the DVD. This must be differentiated from nystagmus blockage syndrome (see Congenital nystagmus topic). The term Ciancia syndrome is used by some authors to differentiate these patients.

Differential diagnosis

This includes a Duane retraction syndrome, unilateral or bilateral palsy of the sixth cranial nerve, nystagmus blockage syndrome (a dampening manoeuvre for congenital nystagmus using fusional convergence), Moebius syndrome, early onset of an accommodative esotropia and early onset sensory esotropia.

Treatment

In general glasses are not indicated, but if cycloplegic refraction reveals more than 2 dioptres of untreated hypermetropia, it is worth considering a trial. Any significant myopia or astigmatism should be corrected. There is active debate about the timing of horizontal surgical intervention with some authors proposing surgery between 3 and 6 months of age. The aim of such early intervention is to achieve a better binocular status, even high-grade stereopsis. However, most authorities plan surgical correction sometime after 9 months of age, with a view to aligning the eyes by age 18 months. Occasionally, large angle infantile esotropia can resolve spontaneously in the first year. Meticulous attention must be applied to the visual performance of each eye before and following surgery as the prevalence of amblyopia is higher with earlier surgery. Surgical intervention is usually either a bi-medial medial rectus recession (which may need to be more than the usually accepted maximum) or '3 muscle surgery' which combines a bi-medial rectus recession with a lateral rectus resection.

Management of any inferior oblique over action can be tackled simultaneously with the horizontal muscles if appropriate. Care needs to be exercised in selecting which weakening procedure is utilized. Dissociated vertical divergence is common in ensuing years and inferior oblique anteriorization a possible surgical procedure. Thus an inferior oblique myectomy may reduce the surgical options for the DVD that presents later.

Ciancia's syndrome patients who have a cosmetically important head turn may benefit from a large medial rectus recession on the fixing eye.

Conclusion

Infantile esotropia is a distressing condition at first for parents, and there is no doubt that surgical straightening achieves more than just an improved appearance. Parents often remark on improved motor coordination and general happiness of the child. Exactly how this is brought about is not clear. Surgical intervention should aim for a slight under correction rather than over correction. Measurements of less than 8 prism diopters are more likely to achieve some form of fusion.

Further reading

Ciancia A. 7th Bielschowsky Lecture. ISA. Infantile esotropia with nystagmus in abduction. *Journal of Paediatric Ophthalmology and Strabismus* 1995; **32**(5): 280–8.

Ciancia A. La esotopia con limitacion bilateral de abduccion en el lactante. *Arch Oftalm Buenos Aires* 1962; **36**: 207–11.

Ing MR. Progressive increase in the angle of deviation in congenital esotropia. *Transactions of the American Orthoptic Society* 1994; **XCII**: 117.

Tychsen L. Binocular vision. In: Hart WM (ed.). *Adler's Physiology of the Eye.* Mosby Year Book; 1992; 773–858.

Tychsen L, Lisberger SG. Maldevelopment of visual motion processing in humans who had strabismus with onset in infancy. *Journal of Neuroscience* 1986; **6**: 2495–9.

Wilson ME, Buckley EG, Kivlin JD, Ruttum MS, Simon JW, Magoon EH. Pediatric Ophthalmology Section 6. *American Academy of Ophthalmology* 1999; 74–78.

Wright KW, Edelman P, Terry A, McVey S, Lin M. High degree stereo acuity after early surgery for congenital esotropia. *Investigative Ophthalmology and Visual Science* 1993; **34**(suppl): 710. (Abstract)

Related topics of interest

Congenital nystagmus (p. 69); Esotropia, convergence and accommodation (p. 113); Latent nystagmus (p. 151).

IRIDOCORNEAL ENDOTHELIAL SYNDROME

Graham A. Lee, Peter Shah & Robert H. Taylor

Iridocorneal endothelial (ICE) syndrome, also termed primary proliferative endotheliopathy, is a group of conditions which are difficult to classify and may be regarded as either a dystrophy or dysplasia of the corneal endothelium. A common feature is degeneration of endothelial cells, with an associated proliferation of the remaining endothelial cells (ICE-cells). This endothelial cell–basement membrane complex encroaches the drainage angle and the anterior surface of the iris resulting in angle obstruction, peripheral anterior synechiae (PAS), secondary glaucoma, iris distortion and corneal oedema.

Problem

The identification of the ICE syndrome is important, as follow-up is necessary to detect the development of secondary glaucoma. Treatment of the glaucoma is frequently refractory to standard therapy. Other causes of corneal oedema should be excluded.

Background

Chandler's syndrome, progressive (or essential) iris atrophy and the iris naevus syndrome (or Cogan–Reese syndrome) are variants of this single pathological process. The conditions have been separated on the basis of signs in the early stages of disease. In Chandler's syndrome, corneal changes are most prominent; in essential iris atrophy, the iris changes are the main abnormality, and in the iris naevus syndrome iris nodules are the most striking feature. In the later stages of disease the separate entities are indistinguishable. The herpes simplex virus has been implicated in the pathogenesis of ICE, using polmerase chain reaction methods on corneal specimens. ICE-cells have been found to be morphologically similar to epithelial cells. It is proposed the cells may have arisen from an embryological ectopia of ocular surface epithelium or secondary to a metaplastic stimulus.

Clinical features

ICE occurs mainly in Caucasians, aged between 20 and 50 years old. Women are affected more commonly than men. The condition is nearly always unilateral, although subclinical changes in the other eye are common (endothelial changes and iris transillumination defects). Most patients have normal vision in the early stages of the disease and the abnormality may be detected as an incidental finding. Patients may present with the complications of the ICE syndrome. Failure of the corneal endothelium results in reduced vision or ocular pain from corneal oedema or bullous keratopathy. Clinically the corneal endothelium has a fine-hammered silver appearance with 'guttate' changes similar to those in Fuchs' endothelial dystrophy, but there is a visible junction between normal and abnormal endothelium. Specular microscopy reveals a characteristic diffuse abnormality showing pleomorphism in size and shape, dark areas within cells and loss of clear hexagonal margins.

In Chandler's syndrome, corneal oedema is an early finding with few iris changes. Essential iris atrophy results in displacement of the pupil towards an area of PAS (corectopia). Iris stromal atrophy and pseudopolycoria are seen in the sector opposite to the PAS. In the 'iris naevus syndrome' the anterior surface of the iris is covered with a sheet of membrane-like material. The appearance of 'naevi' is caused by nodules of normal iris tissue protruding through the membrane. It is also difficult to see precise normal iris details. The aberrant tissue may be seen in the angle on gonioscopy. All the above variants may develop unilateral, secondary glaucoma, by direct obstruction of the angle by the endothelial cell–basement membrane or indirectly, by the formation of PAS.

Treatment

Glaucoma may be treated initially with conventional topical drugs. Argon laser trabeculoplasty is not recommended as it may increase PAS formation. As argon laser is absorbed by trabecular pigment and not by the pretrabecular membrane, it is unlikely to be successful. When considering filtration surgery, the filtration site should be positioned in an area free of membrane, aberrant tissue on gonioscopy or PAS. Antimetabolites to reduce post-trabeculectomy scarring are useful, particularly in young patients. It is unlikely that antimetabolites have an effect on the pretrabecular membrane. Surgical failure occurs as the advancing edge of the membrane grows over the sclerostomy as well as due to subconjunctival scarring of the bleb. Management of refractory glaucoma may require Seton implantation or ciliary ablation. Corneal oedema may improve with reduction of the intraocular pressure, but if persistent, may require penetrating keratoplasty. Postoperatively, the graft is at risk of rejection, recurrent endothelial failure and primary failure due to raised IOP.

Further reading

Alvarado JA, Underwood JL, Green WR, Wu S, Murphy CG, Hwang DG, Moore TE, O'Day D. Detection of herpes simplex viral DNA in the iridocorneal endothelial syndrome. *Archives of Ophthalmology* 1994; **112**: 1601–9.

DeBroff BM, Thoft RA. Surgical results of penetrating keratoplasty in essential iris atrophy. *Journal of Refractive and Corneal Surgery* 1994; **10**: 428–32.

Hirst LW, Quigley HA, Stark WJ, Shields NB. Specular microscopy of irido-corneal endothelial syndrome. *American Journal of Ophthalmology*, 1980; **8**: 139–46.

Lanzl IM, Wilson RP, Dudley D, Augsburger JJ, Aslanides IM, Spaeth GL. Outcome of trabeculectomy with mitomycin-C in the iridocorneal syndrome. *Ophthalmology* 2000; **107**: 295–7.

Levy SG, McCartney AC, Baghai MH, Barrett MC, Moss J. Pathology of the iridocorneal-endothelial syndrome. The ICE-cell. *Investigative Ophthalmology and Visual Science* 1995; **36**: 2592–601.

Related topic of interest

Secondary glaucoma (p. 283).

JUVENILE IDIOPATHIC ARTHRITIS

Saaeha Rauz

In 1977, members of the American College of Rheumatology (ACR) and the European League Against Rheumatism (EULAR) independently defined the terms juvenile rheumatoid arthritis (JRA) and juvenile chronic arthritis (JCA) respectively, to describe a clinically heterogeneous group of idiopathic arthritides occurring in children under the age of 16. Although these terms are often used interchangeably, they do not describe identical spectra of disease, leading to much confusion. Both groups of disorders have an age at onset before 16 years, and are subtyped according to the mode of onset: pauciarticular (four joints or less), polyarticular (more than four joints) and systemic (with other features of systemic disease such as fever, hepatosplenomegaly, lymphadenopathy or rash), after the exclusion of other causes. Whereas the EULAR criteria define JCA by degree of joint involvement after a minimal duration of 3 months, the ACR criteria define JRA at 6 weeks. Other differences occur in the exclusion of the spondyloarthropathies (juvenile ankylosing spondylitis, juvenile psoriatic arthritis, Reiter's syndrome or arthropathies of inflammatory bowel disease) from the ACR classification of JRA, and the presence of rheumatoid factor (RF), which alters the EULAR criteria by replacing the term JCA with JRA. In an effort to unify the language, the International League of Associations of Rheumatologists (ILAR) has proposed a new set of classification criteria of juvenile idiopathic arthritis (JIA), the term intended to replace both JCA and JRA. Seven potential groups have been identified: systemic, oligoarthritis (four joints or less), polyarthritis (more than four joints) RF negative, polyarthritis RF positive, psoriatic arthritis, enthesitis-related arthritis, and other arthritides which fall outside, or fit more than one of the six main categories. The oligoarthritis group is further subcategorized into persistent (affecting no more than four joints throughout the disease course) or extended (affecting a cumulative total of five joints or more after the 6 months of disease). All have an age of onset before the sixteenth birthday and are characterized predominantly by an idiopathic arthritis, defined as arthritis persistent for at least 6 weeks, in which there is no defined diagnosis such as sepsis or rheumatic fever, and classification is made on the basis of listed criteria 6 months after disease onset.

Problem

The management of the ocular complications of these patients is difficult. As certain risk factors exist, screening programmes need to be implemented. Even with optimal therapy, glaucoma, cataract, band keratopathy and visual loss can occur.

Background

Overall 20% of children with JIA will develop intraocular inflammation, which is bilateral in over 70% of cases. Of these, 25% will have mild disease, 50% moderate to severe disease and the remaining 25% may develop severe sight-threatening complications. Although there is no correlation between activity of joint and eye inflammation, an association exists between the mode of onset of juvenile arthritis and subsequent risk of uveitis: systemic onset having the lowest and the pauciarticular the highest. Within the ILAR categories, uveitis forms part of the definition, or one of the disease descriptors, for four of the seven categories: oligoarthritis, polyarthritis

RF negative, psoriatic arthritis and enthesitis-related arthritis. Other accepted risk factors include young age of onset of arthritis (less than 6 years), female sex, the presence of circulating antinuclear antibodies (ANA) and HLA DR5.

As the onset of uveitis is usually asymptomatic, and the diagnosis relies on slit-lamp biomicroscopy, it is vital that these children are given continued screening ocular examinations. Several screening programmes have been suggested, with the most widely accepted categorizing children into high risk (onset less than 6 years, pauci-articular, ANA positive), medium risk (polyarticular and ANA-positive, or pauci-articular and ANA-negative), and low risk (systemic onset, HLA-B27 positive, or disease starting after age of 11 years). Screening recommendations require all children to be examined by an ophthalmologist as soon as possible after the diagnosis of JIA. If the eyes are found to be healthy, then children in:

- the high-risk group should be examined at 3 monthly intervals for the first year, then 6 monthly intervals for 5 years, and then annually;
- the medium-risk group should be examined at 6 monthly intervals for 5 years, then annually;
- the low-risk group should be examined annually.

The duration of screening should be for 10 years after the onset of JIA, or until the age of 12 years, whichever is shorter. However, some authorities recommend more intense screening regimens of longer duration.

Clinical features

In the majority of patients, JIA antedates the diagnosis of uveitis. The onset is usually insidious, often asymptomatic and chronic, with a non-granulomatous anterior uveitis frequently being detected on routine slit-lamp examination. In addition to the recognized risk factors, the severity of visual loss correlates with the degree of inflammation found on initial examination, the presence of posterior synechia at first eye examination, a delay in presentation to the ophthalmologist and duration of uveitis. The outcome of uveitis has been measured either by determining the visual acuity at follow up or by enumerating the ocular complications. Visual loss has been reported in up to 66% of patients and ocular complications, such as posterior synechiae, band keratopathy, secondary inflammatory glaucoma, complicated cataract, maculopathy and phthisis bulbi, in 75%.

Mild to moderate degrees of uveitis are treated with topical corticosteroids, usually in conjunction with a short-acting mydriatic at night. In more severe cases, periocular or systemic corticosteroids are needed especially if there is posterior pole oedema or serous elevation of the retina. Periocular injections may require the child having a general anaesthetic. Long-term systemic corticosteroids may have serious consequences on the child's growth. The use of systemic immunosuppressives (other than high-dose corticosteroids) is controversial, and the impact of drugs, such as methotrexate, on the activity and severity of uveitis has not been clarified, as many children already take these drugs to control joint inflammation. Yet, methotrexate (even at low dose orally) or other immunosuppressives, may allow for reduction or discontinuation of oral steroids. Cataract surgery is problematic due to posterior synechiae and poor view. Pars plana lensectomy combined with vitrectomy appears to be the technique of choice, but intraocular lens implantation is considered to be potentially hazardous. The control of postoperative inflammation is essential. Visual rehabilitation is usually facilitated by contact lens wear, although the risk of amblyopia in the younger child should not be underestimated. Secondary glaucoma tends to occur when the chronic anterior uveitis is relatively quiescent and will persist long after uveitis is no longer a primary concern. Topical treatment regimens (beta-blockers, α_2-agonists, carbonic anhydrase inhibitors) and oral carbonic anhydrase inhibitors are the mainstay, before augmented filtration surgery is considered. Pilocarpine and latanaprost should be avoided as they may aggravate the uveitis. Success of surgical intervention is often low, with hypotony being the most common postoperative complication. This may be reduced by maintaining a controlled intraoperative intraocular pressure environment, removal of cyclitic membranes, and a secure scleral flap and careful conjunctival wound closure. Band keratopathy occasionally threatens the visual axis, and may be removed by either a combined surgical and chemical approach, or by excimer laser.

Further reading

Kanski JJ. Uveitis in juvenile chronic arthritis: incidence, clinical features and prognosis. *Eye* 1988; **2**: 641–5.

Petty RE, Southwood TR, Baum J of *et al*. Revision of the proposed criteria for juvenile idiopathic arthritis: Durban 1997. *Journal of Rheumatology* 1998, **25**: 1991–4.

Report of a joint working party: The Royal College of Ophthalmologists and The British Paediatric Association. *Ophthalmic Services for Children*. December, 1994.

Southwood TR, Ryder CAJ. Ophthalmological screening in juvenile chronic arthritis: should the frequency of screening be based on the risk of developing chronic iridocyclitis? *British Journal of Rheumatology* 1992; **31**: 633–4.

Woo P, Wedderburn LR. Juvenile chronic arthritis [Seminar]. *Lancet* 1998; **351**: 969–73.

LATENT NYSTAGMUS

Robert H. Taylor

Latent nystagmus (LN) is commonly seen in patients with essential infantile esotropia although is also seen in patients with monocular vision or other disorders of binocular development. It can co-exist with congenital nystagmus.

Problem

The terminology is confusing. Some authors classify LN as a congenital nystagmus. It can have a profound effect on visual acuity.

Background

Latent nystagmus is defined as a nystagmus present when one eye is occluded. Manifest-latent nystagmus has a similar waveform and exists when both eyes are open. In some patients, both eyes are open but the individual is suppressing one eye. When this is present, the amplitude may increase further with occlusion of the suppressed eye. With sensitive recording, nearly all latent nystagmus has a manifest component.

The pathogenesis of latent nystagmus is essentially unknown but in experimental animals monocular deprivation affects the cortical areas that are responsible for seeing motion (area V5), and its projections to the nucleus of the optic tract (NOT). The NOT usually has bilateral innervation. If there has been monocular viewing during development, the contralateral NOT will be activated preferentially, which will produce a contralateral slow drift. Latent nystagmus can be reproduced in experimental animals.

Clinical features

The waveform in latent nystagmus is always a horizontal jerk nystagmus with the fast phase away from the occluded eye. The slow phase demonstrates a decreasing velocity. This reduces foveation time and explains the profound loss of vision when the nystagmus is provoked. This contrasts with the increasing velocity of the slow wave commonly seen in congenital idiopathic nystagmus. While a decreasing velocity is predominant, there are many variations – with some patients showing different patterns on sequential recordings.

Latent nystagmus may be asymmetrical in that the waveform differs with respect to which eye is occluded. The amplitude of the nystagmus is usually larger when the better seeing eye is covered. However, once elicited, the nystagmus is symmetric (i.e. both eyes move synchronously). This can be demonstrated by using a semilucent occluder. The nystagmus obeys Alexander's law, and is worse in abduction. The amplitude is usually less in adduction. Patients may prefer to fixate in adduction, particularly if there is a manifest component. In doing so they will adopt a compensatory head posture with a face turn towards the fixing eye. Latent nystagmus can also be unilateral if one eye is normal and the other very poorly sighted. Congenital nystagmus may co-exist and may be horizontal, rotatory or pendular. Dissociated vertical divergence often co-exists with latent nystagmus as may congenital esotropia, or any condition of disordered binocular development.

The examiner can elicit latent nystagmus in a variety of ways. Total occlusion is not necessary. Nystagmus can often be seen with just the visual axis occluded with a small occluder (e.g. a pen top), or even dazzled with a pen torch. The amplitude of the nystagmus is less if the degree of occlusion or blur is less.

Visual acuity can be profoundly affected by the nystagmus. This causes a problem in measuring individual visual acuities. The vision is better in adduction, and if a head posture is used to bring the eye into adduction. This should be allowed in order to maximize the measured visual acuity. It may be better to avoid occlusion and to optically blur the non-fixing eye with positive lenses to reduce the amplitude of the nystagmus to allow the maximum visual acuity recording.

Reduced abduction is invariably present in small children. However, in older children abduction can be seen to be full. This often induces a large amplitude nystagmus which seems to be unpleasant and avoided by these subjects.

Differential diagnosis should include gaze-evoked nystagmus (no latent component), and the abducting nystagmus in association with internuclear ophthalmoplegia (associated weakness of adduction or reduced adducting saccade). Infantile esotropia with nystagmus on abduction is closely related.

Treatment

The goal of treatment is the restoration of equal vision and binocularity. Use of a cycloplegic refraction is to be recommended. Any astigmatism is difficult to elicit in the presence of nystagmus and cycloplegia is therefore helpful. Correction of the full hypermetropic error in the presence of esotropia is likely to reduce the esotropia and may reduce the amplitude of the nystagmus. Surgery for any superimposed strabismus will reduce the amplitude of the nystagmus and may convert a manifest-latent nystagmus to a (clinical) latent nystagmus. Surgery for the head posture if fixation in adduction is preferred involves a large medial rectus recession on the fixing eye.

In the presence of latent nystagmus, occlusion therapy will reduce the vision by provoking latent nystagmus. It has been suggested to occlude for 48 hours continuously. An alternative is to use optical penalization. Results for amblyopia treatment are poorer in the presence of latent nystagmus.

Further reading

Dell'osso LF, Schmidt D, Daroff RB. Latent, manifest latent and congenital nystagmus. *Archives in Ophthalmology* 1979; **97:** 1877–85.

Harris C. Nystagmus and eye movement disorders. In Taylor D: *Paediatric Ophthalmology*, 2nd edn. Blackwell Science Ltd., 1997; 869–924.

Reinecke RD. Idiopathic infantile nystagmus: Diagnosis and treatment. *Journal of AAPOS* 1997; **1**(2): 67.

Simonsz HJ. The effect of prolonged occlusion on latent nystagmus in the treatment of amblyopia. *Doc Ophthalmol* 1989; **72:** 375–84.

Zubcov AA, Reiecke RD, Gottlob I, Manley DR, Calhoun JH. Treatment of manifest latent nystagmus. *American Journal of Ophthalmology* 1990; **110:** 160.

Related topics of interest

Congenital nystagmus (p. 69); Infantile esotropia (p. 143); Nystagmus 1: nystagmus (p. 190); Nystagmus 2: saccadic intrusions and other oscillations (p. 195).

MACULAR HOLE

Paul Jacobs

In 1991, Kelly and Wendel made a major contribution to the management of ophthalmic disease by demonstrating that macular holes could be closed by surgery and that closure was accompanied by improvement in vision.

Problem

Without treatment macular hole leads to loss of central vision but peripheral vision is generally maintained indefinitely. Surgery adds a small but definite risk of loss of vision, in particular from retinal detachment.

Over the past decade of macular hole surgery the reported success with one surgical procedure has risen to a level well above 90%. The incidence of retinal detachment is relatively high in some series and low in others. High rates of successful closure and a low incidence of retinal detachment are possible and it is the surgeons who can deliver these who should be undertaking this surgery.

Background

A macular hole is a full thickness absence of neural retinal tissue in the centre of the macula. The majority of macular holes are idiopathic, occurring in the absence of other ocular pathology usually after the age of 55 years. About 70% of macular holes occur in females. Macular holes are associated with other eye conditions including blunt trauma, cystoid macular oedema and rhegmatogenous retinal detachment. Epiretinal membrane formation may be associated with macular hole or a hole in the membrane may give the appearance of a macular hole (a pseudohole). This chapter is concerned with idiopathic macular holes, although surgical treatment for other types of macular hole is possible.

Clinical features

Idiopathic macular holes present with painless loss or distortion of central vision. Unilateral macular holes are often asymptomatic and may be detected during routine examination or may become symptomatic only when the fellow eye loses vision through macular hole or other eye disease (between 10 and 18% of fellow eyes will develop a macular hole).

Diagnosis is made by biomicroscopic examination of the macula at the slit lamp with a contact or non-contact fundus lens. The patient's perception of the slit lamp beam can be helpful. A thinning or break in the beam, seen by the patient, supports the presence of a full thickness retinal defect (Watzke–Allen sign). Optical coherence tomography has helped to clarify vitreoretinal anatomy in the diagnosis and staging of macular holes.

Gass classified the biomicroscopic appearances of macular holes into stages: stage 1A – foveolar detachment, small round yellow spot at fovea; stage 1B – further foveolar detachment, round yellow ring at fovea; stage 2 – early hole with full thickness defect in neural retina, either eccentric or central; stage 3 – fully developed hole but posterior hyaloid face of vitreous still immediately in front of hole; stage 4 – hole with posterior vitreous detachment.

Stage 1 holes are compatible with good visual acuity (6/7.5–6/24) approximately 50% of stage 1 holes will resolve spontaneously with good recovery of vision. Once a stage 2 hole occurs progression to stage 3 and decline in vision (without treatment) to between 6/60 and 6/120 usually occurs over the course of a few weeks or months.

Treatment

The success rate for surgical closure of stage 2 and recent-onset stage 3 holes is high (90% or more). Successful closure is accompanied by an early improvement in vision and a gradual further improvement in subsequent weeks. An average improvement of about three lines of Snellen acuity follows closure of the hole. Patients with a preoperative acuity between 6/24 and 6/36 or better can expect to recover vision to the standard required for driving a motor vehicle. Patients for who the recovery is less than this are often grateful for the reduction in central scotoma or distortion.

The success rate for closure of long-standing (more than one year duration) macular holes is less good (about 70%) and the visual recovery less certain but surgery for long-standing macular holes is still worthwhile.

The standard operation for macular hole involves three port pars plana vitrectomy. The posterior cortical vitreous is engaged by suction and elevated from the posterior retina and removed. A perifoveal epiretinal layer is removed if possible and the posterior segment is filled with gas (e.g. dilute SF_6 or C_3F_8). Patients are required to maintain a strict-face-down position for a minimum of 7 days following surgery. Variations include the use of silicone oil instead of gas. This permits air travel after surgery (which must be avoided for gas-filled eyes) and prone positioning may be less crucial. Reasonable success with gas without prone positioning has been reported. Various adjunctive agents (including growth factors and autologous serum or platelets) have been applied to the macular hole prior to the injection of internal tamponade but excellent success rates can be achieved without these.

Complications

Cataract is a common complication of vitrectomy and the majority of eyes undergoing vitrectomy for macular hole will require cataract surgery within a year of the macular hole operation. Simultaneous cataract surgery and vitrectomy is possible for eyes with pre-existing nuclear sclerosis.

Reported rates of retinal detachment following surgery for macular hole vary from 1% to 14%. The intraoperative creation of a posterior vitreous detachment is associated with the creation of retinal tears. The rate of detachment can be kept low by careful intraoperative identification and treatment of these tears.

Late re-opening of successfully closed macular holes may occur a year or more following surgery in up to 5% of cases. Some of these can be closed by further surgery.

Temporal visual field defects can occur following macular hole surgery. These may or may not cause symptoms. Trauma to the optic nerve head during vitreous elevation or gas exchange have been suggested as causes.

Conclusion

Idiopathic macular holes evolve through a number of stages. Stage 1 holes may resolve spontaneously with recovery of vision. Stage 2, 3 and 4 holes rarely recover without treatment and lead to significant loss of central vision.

Surgical treatment of macular holes has a high success rate. It can be performed using local anaesthesia but requires the ability and commitment of the patient to co-operate with maintaining a face-down position for several days following surgery. Factors which should be discussed with the patient prior to surgery include the prognosis with no treatment, the chance of developing a macular hole in the fellow eye, the possibility of failure to close the hole with surgery and surgical complications, such as cataract and retinal detachment.

Further reading

Desai VN, Hee MR, Puliafito CA. Optical coherence tomography of macular holes. In: SA Madreperla, BW McCuen II (eds), *Macular Hole*. Butterworth-Heinemann 1999; 37–47.

Duker JS. Macular hole. In: Yanoff M, Duker JS (eds) *Ophthalmology*. St Louis: Mosby, Inc. 1998.

Gass JDM. Reappraisal of biomicroscopic classification of stages of development of a macular hole. *American Journal of Ophthalmology*, 1995; **119:** 752–9.

Kelly NE, Wendel RT. Vitreous surgery for idiopathic macular holes. *Archives of Ophthalmology* 1991; **109:** 654–9.

Scott RAH, Ezra E, West JF, Gregor ZG. Visual and anatomical results of surgery for long standing macular holes. *British Journal of Ophthalmology* 2000; **84:** 150–3.

MICROBIAL KERATITIS

Raymond Loh, Andrew Morrell & Robert H. Taylor

Microbial keratitis is a sight-threatening disease and therefore represents an ophthalmic emergency. A delay in diagnosis and therapy has been estimated to reduce favourable visual outcome to 50% of affected eyes. Management protocols and guidelines for microbial keratitis have been published recently in an effort to rationalize treatment.

Problem

The aim is to identify a causative pathogen and match therapy appropriately to promote healing and maintain corneal clarity. This is influenced by the need to initiate therapy before the results of microbiological investigations are known. The success of microbial investigations is affected by culture techniques and previous antimicrobial therapy.

Background

Microbial keratitis is usually associated with predisposing factors identified from a clinical history. Examination will provide further clues to a diagnosis, which is confirmed by culture from sampling.

Any corneal epithelial defect may allow pathogen access and infection should be anticipated. Occupational and environmental factors should also be considered, for example fungal/amoebic infections if the patient is from a rural community, or certain fungi in tropical areas. Contact lens wear, especially extended wear, and poor cleaning methods are important risk factors. Culturing of contact lenses, lens cases and solutions can provide additional information. Ocular surface disorders including dry eyes, bullous keratopathy, herpes keratitis and corneal hypoaesthesia, exposure and lid dysfunction should be identified. Immune suppression predisposes to infections, especially fungal, and may inhibit the inflammatory response, altering presenting signs.

Clinical features

1. Viral. Herpes simplex classically causes a dendritic ulcer. Multiple punctate erosions with subepithelial infiltrates associated with follicular conjunctivitis are commonly caused by adenovirus. Other patterns of viral keratitis include disciform keratitis and acute stromal necrosis.

2. Bacterial. A central, paracentral or peripheral ulcer with purulent discharge, corneal stromal infiltration, circumcorneal injection, anterior chamber activity and often hypopyon with rapid onset of symptoms characterizes bacterial infection. These are usually due to Gram-positive bacteria including *Staphylococcus aureus, Staphylococcus epidermidis* and *Streptococcus pneumoniae*. Gram-negative bacteria are less common although *Pseudomonas aeruginosa* is the most common organism in soft contact lens users. Other less common causes are Neisseria, *Haemophilus influenzae* and mycrobacteria. Topical steroids, contact lens wear and corneal graft infection can predispose to infectious crystalline keratitis, the commonest bacterial cause being α-haemolytic Streptococcus.

3. _Fungal._ This is relatively uncommon accounting for 5–10% of corneal infections. Initially there are fewer signs and symptoms. Specific features include superficial or deep grey-white infiltrates with a feathery edge which may indicate a filamentous fungal infection. Satellite or multifocal lesions are possible. Hypopyon and endothelial plaque may occur if the lesion is deep or large. With progression the clinical picture may mimic a bacterial infection. Therefore, suspect fungal involvement if keratitis is unresponsive to antibiotics. Culture takes 48–72 h, sensitivities 7 days. Common pathogens are Fusarium, Aspergillus and Candida.

4. _Amoeba._ Acanthomoeba infections have increased incidence with widespread use of contact lens (see separate topic).

Ideally a corneal scrape to identify the pathogen is carried out prior to antimicrobial treatment. Samples should be obtained from the edges and base of the ulcer with a Kimura spatula or disposable hypodermic needle using preservative-free topical anaesthesia. Samples should be plated directly on blood agar, chocolate agar, thioglycollate and Sabouraud agar. Sufficient slide samples should be available for immediate staining with Gram and Giemsa stains as well as additional stains if indicated (eg. acid-fast, PAS, fluorescent and methenamine silver).

Repeated scrapes for unresponsive lesions may be carried out 24 h after stopping therapy. Consider culturing topical ocular medications, contact lens solutions/cases/lenses if corneal cultures are negative. Corneal biopsy in resistant cases is performed using a 2–3 mm trephine with the sample sent in liquid transport media. Liaison with the microbiologist is essential for immediate processing of samples. Diagnostic algorithms have been proposed in the management of such cases to rationalize further investigations/treatment.

In suspected viral keratitis, swabs may be taken. Adenovirus and herpes simplex virus are grown in tissue culture.

Treatment

Herpetic lesions are treated with the topical antiviral agent (Acyclovir) and local debridement. Alternatives include trifluorothymidine or idoxuridine. All are toxic to the cornea, although Acyclovir is less so.

Broad-spectrum intensive and fortified antibiotics drops are commenced for bacterial infections and modified, if necessary with the results of the Gram stain culture and clinical response. This usually constitutes combined aminoglycoside and cephalosporin (e.g. Gentamicin 1.5% and cefuroxime 5%). Penicillin 0.3% is the treatment of choice if streptococci infection is suspected. Common regimens consist of intensive administration hourly for the first 48 hours. This is then reduced depending on culture results and clinical course. Subconjunctival and systemic antibiotics are usually not required. Monotherapy with fluoroquinolones (e.g. ofloxacin) as primary treatment has been reported to be as successful as conventional treatment, with less toxicity. The use of fluoroquinolones as monotherapy may be most appropriate where pseudomonal infections are prevalent. Although fluoroquinolones provide good broad-spectrum cover, they are generally less effective against Streptococcal species. The use of monotherapy must also be tempered against emerging reports of increasing resistance by *Staphylococcus aureus* and *Pseudomonas aeruginosa* to ciprofloxacin in America and India. Single drug therapy is not advisable in children.

Topical natamycin 5% (a polyene) can be used for fungi. Flucytosine (a fluorinated pyrimadine) or amphotericin B (a polyene) is administered for yeasts. Topical imidazoles with broad-spectrum activity such as econazole 1% or micaonazole 1% are alternatives. Systemic treatment with itraconazole (a triazole) or ketoconazole (an imidazole) may be helpful though associated with systemic toxicity. Treatment should be continued for at least 6 weeks and combination with high-dose antibiotics avoided if possible. Treatment for acanthamoeba is discussed in a separate topic.

Complications

Failure to heal may result from inadequate therapy. Combined infection must be considered. If suspected, treatment should be stopped for 24 hours and corneal scrape repeated. Corneal biopsy is an alternative.

Drug toxicity is an important factor and may cause failure of epithelial healing, punctate staining and persistent conjunctival injection. It is more common with drops containing preservatives. It is important to use preservative-free drops when administration is more frequent than 2 hourly. Increased injection in the lower fornix may suggest the onset of conjunctival necrosis, which has been reported with fortified preparations.

The destruction of corneal stroma, scarring and vascularization can be reduced with topical steroids. In general, topical steroids have a role if the organism has been identified and appropriate antibiotics used. The exception is microbial keratitis in a corneal graft where topical steroid treatment should be initiated concurrently with antibiotic therapy, provided there is no evidence of fungal infection, to treat or prevent an induced concurrent rejection episode.

Thinning, descemetocele formation and perforation, are feared complications threatening globe integrity and survival. Infections may penetrate the cornea and cause an endophthalmitis. Medical cyanoacrylate glue can be used in the treatment of progressive corneal necrosis, thin descemetoceles or small perforated corneal ulcers. The glue has an inhibitory effect on bacteria but is toxic to lens and endothelium. A small perforation may also be treated with a patch graft. Penetrating keratoplasty is indicated for a large perforation, small perforation with continued active microbial growth or an oedematous necrotic cornea. Removed tissue should be divided and sent for pathological and microbiological assessment. An alternative therapy is to cover the defect using mobilized conjunctiva (Gunderson flap).

Further reading

Allan BDS, Dart JKG. Strategies for the management of microbial keratitis. *British Journal of Ophthalmology* 1995; **79:** 777–86.

Ficker L, Kirkness C, McCartney A, Seal D. Microbial keratitis – the false negative. *Eye* 1991; **5:** 549–59.

Garg P, Sharma S, Rao GN. Ciprofloxacin-resistant Pseudomonas keratitis. *Ophthalmology* 1999; **106**(7): 1319–23.

Goldstein MH, Kowalski RP, Gordon YJ. Emerging fluoroquinolone resistance in bacterial keratitis. *Ophthalmology* 1999; **106**(7): 1313–18.

Parsevio CE, Dart JKG. Microbial eye disease. *Current Medical Literature (Ophthalmology)* 1992; **2**: 63–7.

Portnoy S, Insler M, Kaufman H. Surgical management of corneal ulceration and perforation. *Survey of Ophthalmology* 1989; **34**: 47–58.

Related topics of interest

Acanthamoeba (p. 1); Postoperative endophthalmitis (p. 239).

MIGRAINOUS VISUAL DISTURBANCES

Mike Burdon

Migraine is a complex syndrome commonly encountered in clinical practice and defined by the World Federation of Neurology as:

"A familial disorder characterised by recurrent attacks of headache widely variable in intensity, frequency and duration. Attacks are commonly unilateral and are usually associated with anorexia, nausea and vomiting. In some cases they are preceded by, or associated with, neurological and mood disturbances. All the above characteristics are not necessarily present in each attack or in each patient."

Problem

Migraine symptoms may mimic a variety of other conditions and, conversely, patients with neurological disease may present with symptoms similar to migraine. Furthermore, individuals frequently experience a variety of migraine symptoms throughout life. For example, common migraine in early adulthood may disappear to be replaced in old age by acephalgic migraine. It is sometimes difficult, therefore, to make the correct diagnosis. Even when the correct diagnosis is made, treatment and control of symptoms is not always easy.

Background

The periodicity and variability of the attacks are of great diagnostic significance. Headache is not an integral part of the syndrome and the term 'migraine' can be used in its absence. The prevalence of migraine is estimated at 10% in the general population. It is more common in females and its prevalence peaks in the 15- to 30-year-old age group. Childhood migraine is less common, with a prevalence of 5%. The pathophysiology of migraine is poorly understood and a comprehensive review of this subject is outside the scope of this chapter. Most theories postulate that cerebral vasoconstriction followed by vasodilatation is the cause of symptoms. The 5-hydroxytryptamine (5-HT) receptors appear to be involved in this process. Platelets are the major source of 5-HT, and many patients with migraine are known to have platelet dysfunction, leading to the theory that migraine is a thrombocytopathy.

A careful history and examination are vital in making the diagnosis. A detailed description of the symptoms and their temporal sequence during an attack should be noted. Events that precipitate the attacks, such as stress, menstruation, smoking and dietary intake (e.g. chocolate, cheese, etc.) should be elicited. A previous history or family history of migraine is helpful but not always present. If the symptoms are atypical, or clinical signs suggest another underlying disease process, then further investigation is necessary. Guided by the age of the patient and the abnormal physical findings, these investigations may include: haematological evaluation (including erythrocyte sedimentation rate), cardiovascular assessment and cranial computerized tomography or magnetic resonance imaging. It is important to remember that migraine may manifest itself in many ways, and the classification below is a useful way of categorizing the various symptom complexes.

Clinical features

1. *Common migraine.* The patient presents with a throbbing headache that is often hemicranial and associated with nausea. If the pain is retro-orbital and severe it may be mistaken for ophthalmic disease. Apart from nausea, there is little other neurological dysfunction. Typically the headache is not preceded by visual or sensory phenomena, but non-specific prodromal symptoms, such as mood changes, may occur. The patient, who is often photophobic, seeks a quiet, dark environment for relief. Usually the attack lasts a few hours, but can last 1–2 days.

2. *Classic migraine.* This is similar to common migraine, but the patient experiences visual or sensory prodromal symptoms. Hemianopic positive scotomas are the most common visual symptoms. Classically these initially appear as a small central scotoma lined on one side by coloured zig-zag lines, oscillating in brightness (the 'scintillating fortification spectrum'). The fortification spectrum expands in the shape of a horseshoe with the open end pointing centrally. As it expands ('build-up'), drift to the temporal periphery may occur ('marching'). Usually the whole event lasts less than 1 hour. A headache similar to common migraine then follows.

3. *Ocular migraine.* Vasospasm of the ocular circulation may occur in isolation, leading to transient monocular loss of vision that may last for seconds or hours. During the attack the fundal examination may exhibit retinal venous or arteriolar narrowing. The attacks usually occur in patients with a history of common or classical migraine. Headache may or may not accompany the attack. Repeated episodes may result in permanent visual field loss and can be complicated by ischaemic optic neuropathy, cilio-retinal artery occlusion and, rarely, central retinal artery or vein occlusion.

4. *Ophthalmoplegic migraine.* This consists of severe ipsilateral hemicranial headache followed hours or days later by ophthalmoplegia, resulting in diplopia. The third nerve is most commonly affected, with or without pupil involvement. The ophthalmoplegia may be prolonged, lasting up to a month. Initial presentation is usually in the first decade and rare after the second decade. A high index of suspicion should always be maintained, and the diagnosis of subarachnoid haemorrhage, which may present in a similar way, must be excluded.

5. *Acephalic migraine.* Episodic neurological dysfunction, most commonly scintillating scotomas, may occur in the absence of headache. Usually patients over the age of 40 are affected. Children may experience 'abdominal migraine', characterized by episodic abdominal cramps, thought to be the result of mesenteric vasospasm.

6. *Cluster headaches/migraine.* This is a sudden-onset severe pain in the oculotemporal region, lasting 1–2 hours and ending abruptly. Horner's syndrome, lacrimation and rhinorrhea may accompany the attack. Males in their fourth decade are most commonly affected. In contrast to classical migraine, the patient is restless and finds comfort in moving around the room.

Many other forms of migraine exist (e.g. hemiplegic migraine and Raeder's syndrome [painful Horner's syndrome]). It is vital that all patients with migraine symptoms have a full clinical examination and neurological assessment. Scintillating scotomas may result from an occipital arterio-venous malformation or tumour, but such patients should have permanent visual field loss which will be missed unless specifically looked for. Patients presenting with an atypical history, particularly if neurological dysfunction such as ophthalmoplegia is present, should be managed with caution, referred for an early neurological opinion and considered for neuro-imaging. Although the neurological dysfunction associated with migrainous episodes are characteristically transient, migraine may rarely be complicated by permanent visual loss and hemiplegia.

Treatment

The treatment of migraine can be broadly divided into two categories: the treatment of the acute attack and the prevention of recurrence. The acute attack may be alleviated by simple analgesics (aspirin, paracetamol) in combination with an anti-emetic, particularly if taken during the early stages of the attack. Metoclopramide is the anti-emetic of choice since it increases gastric emptying and improves analgesic absorption. If the patient fails to respond to analgesic therapy then ergotamine (an alpha-receptor blocker) may be used. Ergotamine, however, is only effective if administered during the very early stages of the attack, and the profound vasoconstriction it can produce can lead to side effects such as abdominal pain and hypertension. It is contraindicated in patients with ischaemic heart disease or Raynaud syndrome. Sumatriptan is a new agent for the treatment of migraine. It is a 5-HT$_1$ agonist producing selective constriction of the carotid circulation. It is equally effective at whatever stage of the attack it is administered and, although it has a lower incidence of side effects, it is also contraindicated in patients with ischaemic heart disease.

Prevention of recurrence may be achieved by general measures, such as avoidance of precipitating environmental factors or the use of prophylactic treatment. Beta-blockers and calcium channel blockers are effective agents in a number of patients. The serotonin antagonist pizotifen and tricyclic antidepressants are also effective in reducing the frequency of attacks, but their long-term use is limited by their side effects.

Further reading

Hupp SL, Kline LB, Corbett JJ. Visual disturbances of migraine. *Survey of Ophthalmology* 1989; **33**: 221–36.

Related topics of interest

Giant cell arteritis (p. 124); Horner's syndrome (p. 133).

MULTIPLE SCLEROSIS AND THE VISUAL SYSTEM

Mike Burdon & Farida Shah

Multiple sclerosis (MS) is a demyelinating condition characterized by acute episodes of neurological deficit, which appear irregularly in time and place throughout the central nervous system (CNS), with spontaneous, but often partial, remissions.

Problem

The symptoms, signs and progression of MS are highly variable and there is no typical clinical picture. The sites most commonly affected are the optic nerves, brainstem, cerebellar peduncles, and the dorsal and pyramidal tracts.

Background

The prevalence of MS varies considerably around the world and varies from approximately 4–31 per 100 000 people. Prevalence is highest in temperate zones and the disease occurs more frequently in women than in men. The peak age of onset is 30 years. The cause(s) is (are) still unknown but evidence suggests it to be an 'immune mediated disorder in genetically susceptible individuals exposed to undetermined environmental factors'. There is a link with HLA-DR2 allele (high frequency of this allele in Scotland). The disease is the most common cause of neurological deficit in young adults in the UK.

Clinical features

1. Motor symptoms. Upper motor neurone deficit with weakness as a paraparesis, hemiparesis or monoparesis. Motor weakness is more common in the legs than the arms. The combination of bilateral visual loss from retrobulbar neuritis and transverse myelitis has been termed 'Devic's' disease, but this may actually be a separate entity from MS.

2. Sensory symptoms. Paraesthesia or loss of proprioception in a limb may occur. Lhermitte's sign is the sensation of an 'electric shock' in the back and legs on flexing the neck and is due to a lesion in the cervical spinal cord. Uhthoff's phenomenon is the worsening of sensory symptoms on exercise or in situations of raised external temperature.

3. Optic neuritis. See separate topic. This may be the presenting symptom in 20% of patients who go on to develop MS.

4. Ocular muscle palsies. Demyelinating plaques involving fibres of the III, IV or VI cranial nerves may cause isolated cranial nerve palsies and lead to diplopia. Internuclear ophthalmoplegia (INO) results from involvement of the fibres in the medial longitudinal fasciculus (MLF). Bilateral INO (especially in a young adult) is highly suggestive of a diagnosis of MS. If the demyelinating lesion involves the ipsilateral para-pontine reticular formation as well as the MLF, then the patient may have the combination of an ipsilateral horizontal gaze palsy and an INO on gaze to the opposite side (the one-and-a-half syndrome). Plaques affecting the cerebellum may cause gaze-evoked nystagmus or other features of cerebellar disease. Superior oblique myokymia is occasionally seen in MS.

5. Other ophthalmic features.   Chiasmal visual field defects are not commonly seen in MS, despite the fact that chiasmal plaques are seen in many patients with MS at autopsy. Similarly, it is unusual to clinically identify an optic tract lesion. Both congruous and incongruous homonymous hemianopic visual field defects have been described in association with retrochiasmal visual pathway disease, although again these defects are not often seen. It is very rare for the occipital cortex to be involved in primary demyelinating disease, although there have been isolated case reports. Ocular signs that may be seen in patients with MS include: anterior uveitis, intermediate uveitis and sheathing of retinal venules. The association of MS with neuroretinitis and optic disc oedema with macular star (ODEMS) is unlikely and a treatable infective cause should be ruled out in these cases.

6. Bladder symptoms.   Frequency, urgency, incontinence and difficulty in micturition are all common symptoms in MS.

7. Others.   Vertigo and vomiting are not uncommon. Psychiatric symptoms occur in about 10% of cases, with depression being the most common, although euphoria may occur in more severe disease. Chronic pain, cerebellar signs and sexual dysfunction may also occur. Prominent cortical signs (aphasia, apraxia, recurrent seizures, early dementia) and extrapyramidal phenomena of chorea and rigidity rarely dominate the clinical picture.

8. Investigations.   MS is a clinical diagnosis characterized by the demonstration of lesions, disseminated in time and place, which are not explicable by any other mechanism. Magnetic resonance imaging (MRI), visual evoked potentials (VEPs) and cerebrospinal fluid (CSF) abnormalities (oligoclonal IgG bands, pleocytosis and raised levels of myelin basic protein) can help support the clinical diagnosis but are not diagnostic in isolation. The Canadian Neurological Society now defines MS as having '... evidence of ongoing disease (clinical or radiological) rather than 2 documented relapses in 2 years'. Visual evoked potentials are useful as the visual pathway may be affected asymptomatically. Brainstem or somatosensory evoked potentials may also be abnormal.

MRI is the most useful investigation in supporting the diagnosis of MS. Areas of high signal on T2-weighted images are seen in over 95% of patients with a definite diagnosis of MS. A repeat MRI scan 3 months later in a patient 'at risk of developing MS' can increase specificity and sensitivity for future MS prediction. Gadolinium–enhanced MRI may be useful in detecting new lesions and their response to treatment. Currently, although MRI is good at predicting if an individual is going to get MS or not, there is poor correlation between the size and number of T2 MRI lesions and MS functional outcome. Other imaging techniques like magnetic resonance spectography may have better correlation between 'lesion load' and disability.

Treatment

1. *Demyelinating optic neuropathy.* See separate topic.

2. *Other neurological manifestations.* Corticosteroids are often used in the treatment of significant relapses, although it is thought that they do not alter the course of the disease. The steroids are best given as intravenous pulses of methyl-prednisolone (500 mg/day for 5 days or 1 g/day for 3 days) followed by an optional brief oral course. Oral prednisolone alone is now rarely used to treat acute optic neuritis as post hoc analysis of the ONTT trial suggested an increased recurrence rate of inflammation.

Many treatments for MS have been tried including azathioprine, cyclophosphamide, cyclosporin A, plasma exchange and hyperbaric oxygen. Several other immunomodulating drugs such as interferon β-1b (Betaseron), interferon β-1a (Avonex, Refib), glatiramer acetate (Copaxone) and mitoxantrone hydrochloride are still undergoing evaluation but some have shown encouraging results. All reduce MRI evidence of disease activity with variable effectiveness. In the UK the use of Avonex, Betaferon and Copaxone have been licensed for use mainly in relapsing-remitting forms of MS (see British National Formulary indications) and have strict criteria for their usage. The National Institute of Clinical Excellence is due to publish guidelines on all aspects of care for patients with MS late in 2002. Many MS support groups feel that these agents should be more widely available and used early on in the disease. They believe that these drugs are maximally effective at this point in time to limit irreversible axonal injury. It is unknown for how long or when to start interferon treatment and the clinical (not radiological) benefits of the patient need to be balanced against inconvenience, treatment related side-effects and cost effectiveness. The relation of axonal damage, inflammatory demyelination and clinical disability needs clarification. The current partially effective immunomodulatory drugs have a trend in delaying the disability of MS but statistical significance is poor. Other research treatment approaches are looking at ways of encouraging remyelination, delaying irreversible axonal loss and prevention of antibody-mediated demyelination.

Symptomatic treatment and support are essential in the management of patients with MS. This is usually via a combination of drugs, complementary medication, physiotherapy and occupational therapy. Making a diagnosis of MS may have many social and psychological implications for the patient, and these should not be underestimated. Patients should be informed that local and national self-help groups exist. They should be warned about some misinformation that may be available over the internet.

Prognosis

The disease has three typical clinical courses:

1. 85% Relapsing/Remitting, the most common form, with well delineated remissions of variable duration;

2. 50% of Relapsing/Remitting becomes Secondary Progressive after 10 years from onset (90% at 25 years). In the Secondary Progressive form there is steady worsening of neurological function with some superimposed acute events;

3.   10% have a progressive form from the outset leading to an accumulation of relevant disability.

Poor prognosis is more likely in the male sex, those who present after the age of 40 years, have permanent motor/cerebellar signs, a short interval between relapses or who have an early progressive course. In those diagnosed with 'probable MS' 84% have a clinical relapse in 7 years (58% of these occurring within the first year). In 10–20% there is no significant disability after 10 years and overall 75% are alive 35 years after the onset. Approximately 5% have a rapid progressive form and die within 5 years. Advanced MS is characterized by dementia, quadriplegia, blindness, incontinence and recurrent respiratory and urinary tract infections which is often the cause of death.

Further reading

Achiron A. MS – from probable to definite diagnosis. *Archives of Neurology* 2000; **57**: 974–9.
Brex P *et al.* Assessing the risk of early multiple sclerosis in patients with clinically isolated syndromes: the role of follow-up MRI. *Journal of Neurology, Neurosurgery and Psychiatry* 2001; **70**: 390–3.
De Stefano N *et al.* Evidence of axonal damage in the early stages of multiple sclerosis and its relevance to disability. *Archives of Neurology* 2001; **58**: 65–70.
Ebers G. Susceptibility to MS: Interplay between genes and environment. *Current Opinion in Neurology* 2000; **13**: 241–7.
Noseworthy J *et al.* Multiple sclerosis. *New England Journal of Medicine* 2000; **343**(13): 938–52.
Oger J. The use of disease modyfing agents in multiple sclerosis. *Canadian Journal of Neurological Science* 1999; **26**: 274–5.
WWW.NICE.ORG.UK

Related topics of interest

Nystagmus 1: nystagmus (p. 190); Nystagmus 2: saccadic intrusions and other ocular oscillations (p. 195); Optic atrophy (p. 208); Sixth (abducens) cranial nerve palsy (p. 289); Superior oblique weakness (p. 298); Third (oculomotor) cranial nerve palsy (p. 306).

MYASTHENIA GRAVIS

Mike Burdon

Myasthenia gravis is an acquired chronic autoimmune disease characterized by weakness and fatigability of skeletal muscles as a result of a defective neuromuscular transmission.

Problem

Between 50 and 75% of patients with myasthenia gravis present with ocular symptoms that may mimic a variety of other eye movement disorders. The correct management of myasthenia gravis is firstly to establish the diagnosis, secondly to look for associated conditions, and lastly to treat the patient while minimizing the side effects of treatment.

Background

Estimates of the prevalence of myasthenia gravis vary from 1/8000 to 1/20000. The disease may present at any age but is rare in childhood or after the age of 70 years. Women are more commonly affected (F:M 3:2). There is no racial or geographic predilection. The immune response is mediated by antibodies against post-synaptic acetylcholine receptors (AChRs). Pathological features include simplification of the post-synaptic membrane, widening of synaptic clefts, and a marked reduction in AChRs per neuromuscular junction.

Clinical features

Patients may present with either ocular or generalized muscle weakness, or a combination of the two. Variability is a key feature with symptoms tending to be worse at the end of the day or after exercise.

Ocular myasthenia gravis frequently presents with either diplopia or ptosis. Any combination of extraocular muscles may be affected. Therefore, myasthenia gravis must be considered in the differential diagnosis of all motility disorders. The direction as well as the degree of diplopia may change over time. Fatigue of either the levator muscles or the extraocular muscles can be demonstrated by sustained eccentric gaze (at least one minute) or by repeated saccades. Cogan's lid twitch sign may be present, but its absence does not exclude myasthenia gravis. Patients should be asked to look down for 15 seconds and then to rapidly refixate in the primary position. The sign is positive if an upward overshoot of the upper lid is observed before it falls to its normal or ptotic position. Weakness of the orbicularis oculi muscles, when present, differentiates myasthenia gravis from most other causes of ophthalmoparesis. The 'ice pack test' is a simple diagnostic procedure based on the observation that myasthenic ptosis may temporarily be improved by applying ice wrapped in a towel over the closed eye for 2 minutes.

Generalized myasthenia may cause proximal and distal limb weakness that worsens with exercise. Muscle tone and limb reflexes are normal. Muscle wasting may occur in advanced disease. Bulbar weakness may result in difficulty with speech, chewing and swallowing. Breathlessness suggests respiratory muscle involvement. Up to 80% of patients presenting with purely ocular disease will develop generalized myasthenia gravis, usually within 2 years. Ninety per cent of all myasthenics eventually develop eye movement abnormalities. The course of the disease is variable. In some patients it is progressive, and death occurs within a few years. In others long periods of remission occur. Intercurrent illness can exacerbate the condition. Patients with a thymic tumour have a poor prognosis. Certain drugs may cause an exacerbation of myasthenia, including suxamethonium, β-blockers, aminoglycosides and certain anticonvulsants.

Myasthenic crisis refers to a severe exacerbation of muscle weakness. It is treated with acetylcholine esterase inhibitors. Alternatively, severe weakness may be due to a cholinergic crisis precipitated by an overdose of acetylcholine esterase inhibitors for which anticholinergic agents such as atropine are required.

Associated diseases

Myasthenia gravis may coexist with other autoimmune diseases. Up to 5% of myasthenics also have autoimmune thyroid disease. Less strong associations have been reported with systemic lupus erythematosus, rheumatoid arthritis, polymyositis, pernicious anaemia, Sjögren's syndrome and pemphigus.

Hyperplasia of the thymus gland occurs in up to 70% of patients with myasthenia gravis. Thymomas occur in 12% of patents with generalized myasthenia gravis and 4% of ocular myasthenics. The incidence of thymomas increases with age. A patient with proven myasthenia gravis should have either a CT scan or an MRI scan of the chest to look for thymus hyperplasia or a thymoma.

Two per cent of patients given D-penicillamine for rheumatoid arthritis develop a myasthenic syndrome that is clinically indistinguishable from idiopathic myasthenia gravis. Onset varies from one month to several years after starting treatment. Affected individuals may have elevated anti-AchR antibodies, electrophysiological abnormalities, and thymic hyperplasia. Most remit within 9 months of stopping D-penicillamine.

Investigations

No single routinely available investigation has 100% sensitivity and specificity, but a combination of anti-AchR antibody assay, edrophonium test, and electromyographic studies allow a diagnosis to be made in up to 95% of cases. Quantification of AChRs on muscle biopsy is an extremely specific and sensitive test for MG, but the laboratory test is not routinely available. Occasionally, the diagnosis is only made after a prolonged trial of treatment.

Anti-AchR antibodies are detectable in 80 to 95% of patients with generalized myasthenia gravis and 50% of patients with purely ocular disease. Anti-skeletal muscle antibodies should also be requested because they are a marker for the presence of a thymoma, occurring in 85% of patients with thymoma but only between 5 and 45% of patients without. Antithyroid and antinuclear antibodies should also be requested.

The edrophonium (Tensilon©) test should only be performed where adequate support staff and resuscitation facilities are available. Secure intravenous access and cardiac monitoring are essential. Intravenous atropine (0.5 to 1 mg for adults, 20 micrograms/kg in children) must be available in case bradycardia develops. The adult dose of edrophonium is 10 mg. Two milligrams should be given as a test dose. If no adverse effects occur within 30 seconds the remaining dose should be administered slowly. (In children a test dose of 20 micrograms/kg is followed by 80 micrograms per kg.) A positive test results in clinical improvement within a minute or two. This is difficult to define particularly if the clinical problem is one of extraocular muscle weakness. The use of a pre- and post-injection Lees Screen may be of benefit. The false negative rate for edrophonium tests may be as high as 30%.

Repetitive supramaximal electromycography motor nerve stimulation studies show a characteristic decrement in muscle action potential amplitude. Single fibres studies show increased jitter. However, these responses are not observed in all muscles, and it is important to test clinically affected muscles. Overall 90% of myasthenic patients are reported to have abnormal electromyography.

Treatment

Acetylcholine esterase inhibitors act to improve muscle strength by increasing the amount of acetylcholine available to bind to the remaining AchRs. Pyridostigmine is the most commonly prescribed at a dose of around 30–120 mg a day in divided doses initially (in children up to 6 years 30 mg and 6–12 years 60 mg starting daily dose). Neostigmine is less often used because it has a shorter half-life. Side effects of treatment relate to increased acetylcholine at muscarinic receptors. They include increased gastro-intestinal motility, bradycardia, and increased sweating and saliva production. Side effects can be reduced with propantheline. Prisms and, rarely, surgery may benefit patients with stable ocular misalignment.

Oral corticosteroids are widely used in the management of myasthenia gravis in an attempt to modify the disease process. A typical maintenance dose is one of 10 to 20 milligrams of prednisolone per day. Patients with purely ocular disease may respond better to corticosteroids than to acetylcholinesterase inhibitors. Other immunosuppressive medications such as azathioprine may be used as 'steroid-sparing' agents. Plasmapheresis produces a short-lived improvement, and is very useful in a life-threatening myasthenic crisis. Thymectomy may be of use in patients with generalized muscle involvement. In non-thymoma patients, 80% remit following thymectomy, but only 10% of patients who have a thymoma remit following surgery. Thymectomy is not usually recommended for patients with purely ocular disease unless a thymoma is suspected.

Further reading

Blanton CL, Sawyer RA. Myasthenia gravis by another name: an elusive imposter. *Survey of Ophthalmology* 1993; **38**: 219–26.
Lee AG, Brazis PW. Ocular myasthenia gravis. In: *Clinical Pathways in Neuro-ophthalmology* 1998; 257–67. Thieme: New York.
Weinberg DA, Lesser RL, Vollmer TL. Ocular myasthenia: a protean disorder. *Survey of Ophthalmology* 1994; **39**: 169–210.

Related topics of interest

Diplopia work-up (p. 105); Sixth (abducens) cranial nerve palsy (p. 289); Superior oblique weakness (p. 298).

NANOPHTHALMOS

Maria Papadopoulos & Peter Shah

Nanophthalmos is a form of microphthalmos in which the eye is small, but of normal shape. The aetiology is believed to be due to arrested globe development after closure of the embryonic fissure. It is a rare, potentially blinding and usually bilateral condition which occurs with equal frequency in both sexes.

Problem

Nanophthalmos is a clinical entity that must not be missed, especially in any patient undergoing surgery. Recognition of the cardinal signs is of prime importance since angle-closure glaucoma and uveal effusion are common and potentially treatable if detected at an early stage. Complications following surgical intervention are very common and often sight-threatening. It is important to think of the possibility of nanophthalmos in any eye which is small and has a short axial length.

Background

Most cases occur sporadically but autosomal recessive and dominant patterns of inheritance have been reported. It is characterized by deeply set, small eyes (axial length less than 20 mm), high hyperopia (approximately +7.00 to +20.00 Dioptres), shallow anterior chambers with very narrow angles, small corneal diameters, thickened sclera and a tendency towards spontaneous and postoperative uveal effusion. Studies have shown that the thickened sclera in nanophthalmos is abnormal, with disordered collagen fibre structure and packing.

Clinical features

1. Angle-closure glaucoma. Angle-closure, and the associated elevated intraocular pressure, is a frequent complication of nanophthalmos, which may not present until the fourth to the sixth decade of life. The increase in lens volume and anteroposterior diameter which occurs with ageing leads to progressive angle crowding in the developmentally small anterior segment. Typically patients present with acute symptoms, but chronic angle closure is also common. Subjects with nanophthalmos who have open drainage angles and normal intraocular pressures should be closely observed every 3 to 6 months with sequential gonioscopy for signs of progressive angle closure.

2. Uveal effusion. Uveal effusion is a common complication of nanophthalmos and may occur spontaneously in the absence of any precipitating factor, but also commonly occurs following surgery. The effusions have an annular configuration and occur in the periphery. They are postulated to result from a combination of elevated ocular venous pressure from compression of vortex veins by thickened sclera, and reduced scleral protein permeability due to the abnormal sclera. Effusions can be associated with a non-rhegmatogenous retinal detachment which may be difficult to manage.

Treatment

For patients with elevated intraocular pressure, medical therapy with aqueous suppressants in the form of topical β-blockers is often effective. Miotics generally widen the angle, but the response is unpredictable as they can cause zonular relaxation and forward lens movement which aggravates pupil block and appositional closure. If miotics are used, they should be used cautiously, starting with low concentrations and the morphology of the drainage angle should be carefully assessed by sequential gonioscopy. Hyperosmotic agents are useful in providing short-term intraocular pressure control, especially during episodes of acute angle closure or before planned surgery.

The diagnosis and management of pupil block is central to the management of angle-closure in nanophthalmos. Laser peripheral iridotomy is indicated in the presence of pupil block, appositional closure and for angles that are graded as potentially occludable on gonioscopic assessment. Peripheral iridotomy may not always be successful in the management of angle-closure because of concomitant lens-induced appositional closure or peripheral iris apposition to the angle secondary to anterior ciliary body rotation related to uveal effusion. If a patent peripheral iridotomy cannot be achieved with laser therapy, then a surgical peripheral iridectomy should be considered. Laser gonioplasty should be considered after medical treatment and laser peripheral iridotomy if the angle progressively narrows or remains appositionally closed. In early angle-closure, a combination of medical and laser treatment are most effective in opening up the angle and relieving pupil block. Early diagnosis and intervention can retard or prevent appositional and synechial closure which otherwise progress to later complete and irreversible angle-closure and marked elevation of intraocular pressure. When medical and laser therapy fail, early lens extraction should be considered to relieve anterior chamber crowding. Phakoemulsification surgery can be performed with a closed, secure anterior chamber, and is probably safer than extracapsular surgery in these eyes.

Glaucoma filtration surgery is associated with very high risk of severe complications in nanophthalmos, and should only be considered after other treatment modalites have failed. In particular, one should always consider lens extraction before filtration surgery. Diode laser cycloablation should be considered for eyes with poor visual prognosis, however, even this treatment modality can be associated with marked postoperative uveal effusion and complications.

When the uveal effusions significantly contribute to anterior segment crowding or visual disturbance, then intervention should be considered. High-dose systemic steroids have been successful in treating uveal and retinal effusions, but relapses can occur. This may necessitate repeated courses and the effusions may eventually become refractory to treatment. Anterior and posterior lamellar sclerectomies with sclerostomies (+/– vortex vein compression) have been reported to be successful in the treatment and prevention of uveal effusion. An unsutured, V-shaped, full-thickness sclerostomy, anteriorly over the pars plana has been used with similar success. The anterior approach is technically easier and safer and may avoid the risks of posterior scleral weakness.

Any surgical intervention on a patient with nanophthalmos carries the risk of severe vision-threatening complications. Postoperative complications are frequent and include: malignant glaucoma, marked uveal effusion, suprachoroidal haemorrhage, vitreous haemorrhage and retinal detachment. It is considered wise to operate on patients with nanophthalmos only if there is no other course of management.

If surgery becomes inevitable with uncontrolled glaucoma or advanced cataract then precautions should be taken to minimize problems. Pre-operatively, the posterior segment should be carefully examined both clinically and with ultrasonography to look for pre-existing uveal and/or exudative retinal detachment and evidence of posterior scleral thickening. Prior to surgery, the intraocular pressure should be lowered as much as possible with medical therapy (including intravenous mannitol) to minimize the pressure differential when the eye is entered, and so reduce the extravasation of fluid from the choroidal vasculature into the suprachoroidal space. The risk of aqueous misdirection posteriorly and subsequent malignant glaucoma is very high, and care should be taken to prevent postoperative wound leaks and anterior chamber shallowing from aqueous over-drainage in glaucoma filtration surgery. It is essential to avoid both intraoperative and postoperative periods of hypotony in these eyes. Surgical intervention in nanophthalmic eyes is best performed under general anaesthesia. Some authorities recommend an unsutured, anterior, V-shaped sclerostomy whenever intraocular surgery is performed in a nanophthalmic eye to try and reduce complications.

Further reading

Calhoun FP Jr. The management of glaucoma in nanophthalmos. *Transactions of the American Ophthalmology Society* 1975; **73:** 97–122.

Jin JC, Anderson DR. Laser and unsutured sclerotomy in nanophthalmos. *American Journal of Ophthalmology* 1990; **109:** 575–80.

Kocak I *et al.* Treatment of glaucoma in young nanophthalmic patients. *Int Ophthalmol* 1997; **20:** 107–11.

Singh OS *et al.* Nanophthalmos – a perspective on identification and therapy. *Ophthalmology* 1982; **89:** 1006–12.

Wax MB *et al.* Anterior lamellar sclerectomy for nanophthalmos. *Journal of Glaucoma* 1992; **1:** 222–7.

NEOVASCULAR AGE-RELATED MACULAR DEGENERATION

Monique Hope-Ross

Age-related macular degeneration is the leading cause of blindness in people over the age of 50 in the Western world. There are two types of age-related macular degeneration: non-neovascular (dry) and neovascular (wet). Neovascular age-related macular degeneration is characterized by the presence of choroidal neovascularization. Choroidal neovascularization is the predominant cause of severe visual loss in age-related macular degeneration. Within 5 years of onset of choroidal neovascularization, 75% of eyes fulfil the criteria for blind registration.

Problem

The natural history of untreated choroidal neovascularization is poor with progressive loss of central vision. Laser photocoagulation is of benefit in only a small proportion of patients. The majority of patients have occult choroidal neovascularization or subfoveal disease and do not benefit from laser treatment. Laser photocoagulation results in destruction of retinal tissue. The recurrence rate, following successful treatment is high.

Background

The Macular Photocoagulation Study Group has established a classification of choroidal neovascularization based on the findings on fluorescein angiography.

1. Classic choroidal neovascularization. Characterized by a well-demarcated lacy area of hyperfluorescence that can be discerned in the early phase of the angiogram. Late leakage often obscures the boundaries.

2. Occult choroidal neovascularization, type I. Fibrovascular pigment epithelial detachment. Areas of irregular elevation of the pigment epithelium are seen on stereoscopic angiography and consist of an area of stippled hyperfluorescence noted within 1–2 minutes of fluorescein injection. Persistence of fluorescein leakage within this area occurs within 10 minutes of fluorescein injection.

3. Occult choroidal neovascularization, type II. Vascularized retinal pigment epithelial detachment. Areas of leakage at the level of the retinal pigment epithelium are noted in the late (but not the early) phase of the angiogram. There are no well demarcated areas of hyperfluorescence in the early phase to account for this leakage.

Treatment

1. Laser photocoagulation. The Macular Photocoagulation Study Group in well-designed, randomized, controlled trials has shown that laser photocoagulation is of benefit in the treatment of classic choroidal neovascularization. The degree of visual loss is reduced by limiting treatment to extrafoveal or juxtafoveal choroidal neovascularization. The group has also shown that patients with subfoveal classic choroidal neovascularization can also benefit from laser photocoagulation. In the long-term, the visual outlook is better with laser photocoagulation than without. An instant and irreversible loss of central vision occurs immediately following such treatment. Many surgeons do not perform subfoveal laser photocoagulation, for this reason.

The majority of patients with choroidal neovascularization do not have classic choroidal neovascularization but have occult choroidal neovascularization. This type of neovascular disease is not amenable to laser photocoagulation on the basis of fluorescein angiography. Indocyanine green angiography has been shown to delineate occult choroidal neovascularization. Indocyanine green angiography allows definition of occult choroidal neovascularization, permitting laser photo-coagulation of previously ill-defined or occult disease. A number of pilot studies have been published regarding the efficacy of indocyanine green guided laser photocoagulation of occult choroidal neovascularization, but no randomized controlled studies evaluating this technique have been conducted.

Following successful laser photocoagulation, the risk of recurrent disease is high and the risk increases with time. The majority of recurrences are subfoveal and not amenable to further laser photocoagulation.

2. **Photodynamic therapy.** This modality, originally used in tumour therapy, has been evaluated in the treatment of choroidal neovascularization. The endothelial cells within the choroidal neovascularization selectively take up verteporfin, a photosyn-thesizing dye. Photoactivation of the dye is accomplished by selectively irradiating the choroidal neovascularization by a low-power infrared laser (wavelength 689 nm). Focal damage to the vascular endothelial cells results. There is minimal effect on the photoreceptors and the retinal pigment epithelium. The treatment can be applied to those who have subfoveal disease. The TAP (Treatment of Age-related Macular Degeneration with Photodynamic Therapy) study has shown beneficial results, maintained at 2 years; 59.1% of patients treated lost less than three lines of vision compared to 31.3% of patients administered placebo. In a subgroup analysis, visual benefit was significantly greater when the leakage was wholly or mainly classic. Those with occult choroidal neovascularization do not seem to benefit. An average of 5.5 treatments were performed over a 24-month period. The drug is expensive.

3. **Submacular surgery.** Surgery can achieve removal of the neovascular com-ponent of the disease. However, the visual results are poor due to loss of the retinal pigment epithelium. The results of surgery are better in those patients with neovascularization not associated with age-related macular degeneration.

4. **Other.** Interferon, an antiangiogenic agent used in cancer therapy has not been shown to be of benefit in the management of neovascular age-related macular degeneration. Isolated reports have suggested that radiotherapy is of benefit in patients with subfoveal classic choroidal neovascularization. Radiotherapy is under evaluation with randomized controlled trials. It appears the visual results of teletherapy will however be disappointing.

Complications

Following successful laser photocoagulation, the risk of recurrent disease is high and the risk increases with time. The majority of recurrences are subfoveal and not amenable to further laser photocoagulation.

The risk of developing bilateral choroidal neovascularization is high. Once choroidal neovascularization has developed in the first eye, the risk of fellow eye involvement over 5 years varies from 7–87%. Risk factors for the development of choroidal neovascularization in the fellow eye are: the presence of five or more drusen, focal hyperpigmentation, one or more large drusen and systemic hypertension. The presence of all four risk factors confers an 11% chance of fellow eye involvement in the first year. There is no proven method of preventing the development of choroidal neovascularization. There is a suggestion from laboratory experiments and dietary analysis that vitamin and mineral supplements may play a role in prevention. The result of further research to evaluate the role of dietary supplements is awaited.

Further reading

Guyer DR, Yannuzzi LA, Slakter JA, Sorenson JA, Hope-Ross M, Orlock DA. Digital indocyanine green videoangiography of occult choroidal neovascularisation. *Ophthalmology* 1994; **101**: 1727–37.

Macular Photocoagulation Group. Risk factors for choroidal neovascularisation in the second eye of patients with juxtafoveal or subfoveal choroidal neovascularisation secondary to age-related macular degeneration. *Archives of Ophthalmology* 1997; **115**: 741–7.

Macular Photocoagulation Study Group. Argon laser for neovascular maculopathy: five year results from randomized trials. *Archives of Ophthalmology* 1991; **109**: 1109–14.

TAP Study Group. Photodynamic therapy of subfoveal CNV in AMD with verteporfin. *Archives of Ophthalmology* 1999; **117**: 1329–45.

Related topic of interest

Diabetic maculopathy (p. 97).

NEUROCRISTOPATHIES (ANTERIOR SEGMENT DYSGENESES)

Graham A. Lee, Robert H. Taylor & Peter Shah

The neurocristopathies are a group of embryological disorders in which there is dysgenesis of structures derived from the neural crest. Sequential waves of neural crest cells form the corneal endothelium and stroma, trabecular meshwork, iris, lens, most of the sclera, melanocytes, ciliary muscles, choroidal stroma and the ciliary ganglion. Defects in this process will lead to anterior segment dysgenesis.

Problem

Recognition of these conditions and the significance of the findings is important. Different interpretations of what may be included under the term of neurocristopathy will be encountered. The term 'anterior chamber cleavage syndrome' has been used to describe clinical problems resulting from anterior segment dysgenesis. Although this term is not strictly correct as no actual cleavage occurs during embryogenesis, its widespread use in clinical practice means that it is likely to be retained. Genetic linkage analysis will further sub-classify this group of diseases. Many of these conditions are associated with glaucoma.

Classification

1. **Cornea.**
- Endothelium: congenital hereditary endothelial dystrophy, Peters' anomaly.
- Stroma: congenital hereditary stromal dystrophy.

2. **Iris.**
- Aniridia: not a primary neurocristopathy, but as iris stroma is derived from neural crest it is included in some classifications.

3. **Trabecular meshwork.**
- Primary goniodysgenesis: trabecular dysgenesis (cause of primary infantile glaucoma), Axenfeld–Rieger syndrome.
- Secondary goniodysgenesis: Sturge–Weber syndrome, iris–lens membrane.

Axenfeld–Rieger syndrome (iridogoniodysgenesis)

1. **Posterior embryotoxon** is an abnormal thickening of Schwalbe's line and is present in up to 10% of the normal population, where it is not usually associated with glaucoma. It can be autosomal dominant.

2. **Axenfeld's anomaly** is a condition in which there are abnormal attachments from the peripheral iris to posterior embryotoxon. The view of the angle structures may be obscured on gonioscopy. The trabecular meshwork may be normal or abnormal, and consequently glaucoma is present in a small proportion of cases. Axenfeld's anomaly is sometimes classified under the term irido-trabecular dysgenesis.

3. Rieger's anomaly is an ocular condition where there are similar angle abnormalities to those found in Axenfeld's and in addition, the anterior iris stroma is involved in the dysgenesis. The hypoplastic iris stroma may lead to pseudopolycoria, corectopia and ectropion uveae. Glaucoma is present in about 50% of cases. There is an association with high myopia.

4. Rieger's syndrome is an autosomal dominant condition involving similar changes in the eye, with systemic involvement including maxillary hypoplasia, telecanthus with a broad, flat nasal root, microdontia and hypodontia and umbilical hernias. Less common associations include congenital heart defects, middle ear deafness, cerebellar vermis hypoplasia and mental retardation. As with Rieger's anomaly, glaucoma occurs only in about 50% of cases and may present anytime in childhood.

The *RIEG1* gene (chromosome 4) encodes part of the homeobox proteins known to be active as transcription factors. Mutations in this gene result in Axenfeld–Rieger syndrome.

Peter's anomaly

Peter's anomaly consists of a central corneal defect, which is variable in size. It is bilateral in 80% of cases. In its lesser form, there is a central posterior depression in the cornea. Central corneal opacity results from a defect of the corneal endothelium and Descemet's membrane and may have an attachment of the iris to the edge of the opacity. Lens involvement includes kerato-lenticular touch, displacement into the anterior chamber or central anterior opacity. Glaucoma occurs in about 50% of cases. Ocular associations include microphthalmos, aniridia, persistent primary hyperplastic vitreous and retinal dysplasia. Peter's anomaly is sometimes classified under the term irido-corneal dysgenesis. Peter's-plus consists of Peter's anomaly with additional features such as short stature, brachymorphia, mental retardation, cheilognathopalatoschisis and abnormal ears.

Management

The mainstay of management is close follow-up to detect secondary glaucoma. Antimitotic agents can be used as adjunctive therapy in trabeculectomy for glaucoma in Axenfeld–Rieger syndrome. Penetrating keratoplasty may be considered for significant corneal opacity, however this group carries a high complication rate due to associated glaucoma and poor vision due to amblyopia. Life-long follow-up is advised, as glaucoma has been known to present late. In those conditions associated with an autosomal dominant inheritance, examination of family members is essential.

Further reading

Butler L, Willshaw HE. Ocular and facial maldevelopment: the role of neural crest. *Eye* 1989; **3**: 64–8.

Kirkness CM, Ficker LA. Risk factors for the development of post-keratoplasty glaucoma. *Cornea* 1992; **11**: 427–32.

Kulak SC, Kozlowski K, Semina EV, Pearce WG, Walter MA. Mutation in the RIEG1 gene in patients with iridogoniodysgenesis syndrome. *Human Molecular Genetics* 1998; **7**: 1113–17.

Waring GO, Rodrigues MM, Laibson PR. Anterior chamber cleavage syndrome. A stepladder classification. *Survey of Ophthalmology* 1975; **20:** 3–10.

Williams DL. A comparative approach to anterior segment dysgenesis. *Eye* 1993; **7:** 607–16.

Related topic of interest

Secondary glaucoma (p. 283).

NEUROFIBROMATOSIS

Robert H. Taylor & Peter Shah

Neurofibromatosis is the most common of the phakomatoses. Type 1 (peripheral) is much the more common, having a prevalence of 1:2000 to 1:3000. Type 2 (central) is present in about 1:1 000 000.

Problem

The pattern of the disease is variable despite strict criteria that have been laid down to facilitate diagnosis. No therapeutic avenue has yet been found to prevent the occurrence of the tumours.

Background

1. Genetics. Type 1 neurofibromatosis (NF1, peripheral, von Recklinghausen's disease, VRNF) is inherited as an autosomal dominant disease with 100% penetrance and variable expressivity. The responsible gene is located at chromosome 17 q11.2. The gene product is neurofibromin, a GTPase activating protein (GAP), which normally acts as a tumour suppressor agent and interacts with the *ras* oncogene.

Type 2 neurofibromatosis (NF2, central, bilateral acoustic neurofibromatosis) also has an autosomal dominant inheritance with 95% penetrance and variable expressivity. The responsible gene is located at chromosome 22 q11.2. The gene product has been termed 'Merlin' or 'Schwannomin', and a defect of this protein is linked to the development of vestibular schwannomas and meningiomas.

Clinical features

For type 1, the diagnosis can be made with two or more of the following: six or more café-au-lait spots of approximate size greater than or equal to 5 mm before puberty or 15 mm or more after puberty; two neurofibromas or one plexiform neuroma; axillary or inguinal freckling; optic nerve glioma; two or more Lisch nodules; an osseous lesion or a first-degree relative with the disease. Patients are not uncommonly developmentally delayed. Other less common or specific associations include phaeochromocytoma, seizures, Wilms' tumour, rhabdomyosarcoma and leukaemia.

For type 2, there must be either bilateral VIII nerve neuromas, or an affected first-degree relative plus unilateral VIII nerve neuroma, or two of: neurofibromas, meningiomas, gliomas, schwannomas and juvenile posterior subcapsular cataract.

Ocular features in type 1 include: plexiform neuromas or neurofibromas of the lids; prominent corneal nerves; Lisch nodules (melanocytic hamartomas of the iris), which are present in 95% of cases; glaucoma and, rarely, retinal hamartomas. Optic nerve or chiasmal gliomas are present in up to 15% of patients. Optic nerve meningiomas occur uncommonly and may be multiple. Papilloedema may occasionally occur following aqueductal stenosis. Diplopia may occur following raised intracranial pressure affecting the IV or VI nerve or involvement of the cranial nerves with neurilemomas and schwannomas. Orbital asymmetry may occur due to sphenoid wing dysplasia with pulsatile proptosis. Proptosis may also occur from an orbital fibroma or plexiform neuroma. For Type 2 these include posterior subcapsular and capsular cataract, retinal membranes, hamartomas, retinal pigment epithelial abnormalities and optic nerve meningiomas.

Management

This involves genetic counselling and screening of the patient and close relatives to detect early lesions. Bilateral optic nerve gliomas are occasionally progressive. These may require chemotherapy. Surgery for acoustic neuromas is often followed by an ipsilateral facial nerve palsy leading to corneal exposure. Reconstructive surgery to prevent corneal infections may be required. Irradiation may also be used.

Further reading

Miller NR. Phakomatoses. In: *Walsh and Hoyt's Clinical Neuro-Ophthalmology*, 4th edn., Vol. 3. Baltimore: Waverly Press, 1988; 1747–827.

Ragge NK. Clinical and genetic patterns of neurofibromatosis 1 and 2. *British Journal of Ophthalmology* 1993; **77:** 662–71.

Rey JA, Pestana A, Bello MJ. Cytogenetics and molecular genetics of nervous system tumours. *Oncology Research* 1992; **4:** 321–31.

Truhan AP, Filipek PA. Magnetic resonance imaging. Its role in the neuroradiologic evaluation of neurofibromatosis, tuberous sclerosis and Sturge Weber syndromes. *Archives of Dermatology* 1993; **129:** 219–26.

Related topic of interest

Phakomatoses (p. 230).

NIGHT BLINDNESS (NYCTALOPIA)

Peter Shah & S.J. Talks

Night blindness is a feature of many diseases. On a worldwide scale it is seen commonly in association with vitamin A deficiency, but it is also a feature of many rare, inherited diseases of the choroid and retina.

Problem

The symptom of night blindness may be the primary visual complaint of a patient, but it is often only one element of the visual problem. Patients may not volunteer symptoms of night blindness and, unless the patient is asked directly about problems with night vision, the symptom may be missed. When confronted with a patient with night blindness, there are a large number of possible causes and a methodical approach is needed to reach a diagnosis. This diagnosis may have implications for other members of the family.

Background

Identification of the cause of night blindness requires a careful and detailed history, followed by a full ophthalmic examination with particular emphasis on examination of the posterior segment of the eye. In many patients the correct diagnosis will be apparent at this stage. However, further investigations, such as perimetry, dark adaptometry, electroretinogram (ERG) and electro-oculography (EOG), may provide additional useful information. Once a provisional diagnosis is made, it may be appropriate to perform a full neurological or systemic examination. It may be useful to examine the patient's relatives. In order to approach the problem of night blindness in a systematic manner, it is necessary to have a working classification of the possible aetiologies.

The main causes of night blindness may be divided into four main groups: general ocular disease, inherited diseases of the choroid and retina with progressive nyctalopia, inherited diseases of the choroid and retina with stationary nyctalopia, and acquired diseases of the choroid and retina.

1. General ocular disease. Many patients may experience difficulty in seeing at night as part of the overall visual disability from conditions such as cataract and advanced glaucoma.
2. Inherited diseases of the choroid and retina with progressive nyctalopia include the following:

   - choroideraemia;
   - gyrate atrophy;
   - degenerative myopia;
   - retinitis pigmentosa (RP);
   - RP variants (including: RP sine pigmentosa, sector RP, pericentric RP, retinitis punctata albescens, Leber's congenital amaurosis);
   - cone–rod dystrophy (advanced);
   - Goldman–Favre vitreoretinal dystrophy.

3. Inherited diseases of the choroid and retina with stationary nyctalopia include the following:

- congenital stationary night blindness (CSNB types I, II and CSNB plus myopia);
- fundus albipunctatus;
- Oguchi's disease.

4. Acquired diseases of the choroid and retina such as:

- Vitamin A deficiency (malnutrition, malabsorption, acute/chronic liver disease);
- drug-induced (toxicity: phenothiazines, isotretinoin, desferrioxamine);
- following panretinal laser photocoagulation.

Clinical features

Reduced vision at night may be due to glare, reduced visual field, reduced visual acuity, or true difficulty in adapting to conditions of reduced illumination.

One should attempt to identify the approximate age of onset of symptoms, and whether the night blindness is stationary or progressive. Initial difficulties with dim illumination which improve after several minutes may reflect a cone problem, as opposed to continued problems in dim illumination which are more characteristic of rod problems. An accurate family history should be obtained. A detailed previous and current drug history is necessary (e.g. previous use of retinoid drugs for dermatological disease). A full ophthalmic examination should be performed, including refraction, assessment of nystagmus and ocular motility, IOP and an anterior segment examination for media opacity.

Examination of the posterior segment is the key to diagnosis. Abnormal fundal appearances fall into six main groups: bone-spicule hyperpigmentation (e.g. classic RP); diffuse large areas of chorioretinal atrophy and associated hyperpigmentation (e.g. choroideraemia and gyrate atrophy); white retinal flecks (e.g. retinitis punctata albescens); retinoschisis, peripheral bone-spicule hyperpigmentation and vitreous liquefaction (e.g. Goldmann–Favre disease); diffuse chorioretinal degeneration (e.g. degenerative myopia); and mottled pigmentary retinopathy of the 'salt and pepper' type (e.g. Kearns–Sayre syndrome). In stationary nyctalopia, abnormal fundal appearances include: small white flecks (e.g. fundus albipunctatus); myopic changes (e.g. CSNB) and altered retinal colour (grey/green-yellow in light and slow change to normal in dark (Mizuo phenomenon; e.g. Oguchi's disease)). In both progressive and stationary nyctalopia the fundal appearance may be normal, but other ocular signs and information from electrodiagnostic testing may suggest the diagnosis.

A full examination is particularly important if one suspects that the patient has an RP-associated syndrome. Patients should be tested for signs of deafness (e.g. Usher's syndrome), and abnormal neurological signs (e.g. sensory loss and motor weakness in Refsum disease, cerebellar and long-tract signs in abetalipoproteinaemia, and myotonia in myotonic dystrophy). Cardiac conduction defects may be present in the Kearns–Sayre syndrome, which can be associated with fatal episodes of cardiac arrhythmia. In some conditions the patients have dysmorphic features (e.g. polydactyly, hypogonadism and obesity are found in patients with the Laurence–

Moon–Bardet–Biedl syndrome). Signs of malnutrition, vitamin A deficiency or chronic liver disease should alert one to the possibility of an acquired cause of the nyctalopia.

Dark adaptometry provides a quantitative measure of scotopic photoreceptor sensitivity. The test (using the Goldmann–Weeks dark adaptometer) is subjective and must be supervised by a trained technician. In an individual with normal retinal function, the dark adaptation curve has a characteristic shape with two components. The initial part of the curve (usual duration 5 minutes) is due to cone adaptation. The second part of the curve (usually measured for another 25–30 minutes) is due to a further increase in retinal sensitivity, because of rod adaptation. The point at which the curve levels off, between the cone and rod adaptation components, is called the rod/cone break. The site and type of the abnormality in the dark adaptation curve will reflect the type of underlying photoreceptor damage.

Examination of the visual fields may often provide striking evidence of field constriction, and may have implications for the patient's eligibility to drive a motor vehicle.

The ERG is an essential component of the work up to confirm or suggest a diagnosis, particularly when the fundus examination is normal (e.g. in Leber's congenital amaurosis). Testing should be performed under both scoptopic and photopic conditions according to ISCEV standards. Some diseases, including CSNB can be classified on the basis of ERG findings. An EOG can provide additional useful information. Electrodiagnostic findings should never be interpreted in isolation, but always in combination with the clinical findings.

If the patient has features of an inherited retinal disorder then it may be extremely helpful to examine other relatives. Retinal changes may be seen in female carriers of choroideraemia and X-linked retinitis pigmentosa. It is important to remember that affected relatives may be asymptomatic. Care should be taken to avoid causing unnecessary anxiety in family members. Ideally genetic counselling should only be undertaken in collaboration with a geneticist.

If clinically indicated one may consider further specific tests such as: serum vitamin A levels, serum phytanic acid (Refsum disease) or serum ornithine level (gyrate atrophy).

Further reading

Carr RE, Siegel IM. Unilateral retinitis pigmentosa. *Archives of Ophthalmology* 1973; **90:** 21–6.

Kaiser-Kupfer M, Kuwabara T, Askanas *et al.* Systemic manifestations of gyrate atrophy of the choroid and retina. *Ophthalmology* 1991; **88:** 302–6.

World Health Organization (WHO). *Control of Vitamin A Deficiency and Xerophthalmia* 1982. Technical Report Series No. 676 (2). WHO, Geneva.

Related topics of interest

Retinal dystrophies (p. 256); Retinitis pigmentosa (p. 265); Toxicology: drugs for non-ocular diseases (p. 319).

NON-ARTERITIC ANTERIOR ISCHAEMIC OPTIC NEUROPATHY

Mike Burdon, Peter Shah & Robert H. Taylor

Non-arteritic anterior ischaemic optic neuropathy (NAION) is a common cause of visual loss in the elderly.

Problem

Between 6 and 14% of patients with AION will have giant cell arteritis (arteritic AION), the remainder are termed non-arteritic (NAION). The first challenge is to recognize those patients with giant cell arteritis so that immediate steps can be taken to reduce the risk of further loss of vision. Having excluded GCA, patients should be screened for treatable risk factors for NAION.

Background

The average age at presentation is 66 years, but 10% are younger than 50 years. Apart from age, identified risk factors include a small crowded optic disc, smoking, hypertension, diabetes mellitus, hyperlipidaemia, vasculitis, massive/recurrent haemorrhage, cataract surgery and migraine. The strong association with cardiovascular risk factors supports the notion that NAION is due to occlusion or hypoperfusion of one or more branches of the short posterior ciliary vessels supplying the retrolaminar optic nerve. For unknown reasons NAION is only extremely rarely due to embolic occlusion of these blood vessels.

Clinical features

NAION usually presents with sudden painless visual loss (frequently overnight). Occasionally a stepwise deterioration of vision occurs over several weeks. Visual acuity is variably impaired ranging from 6/12 or better (18%) to 6/60 or worse (42%). Altitudinal field loss is most common (60%) with the inferior field being affected three times more commonly than the superior field. Other patterns of visual field loss include arcuate, quadrantic and central. A relative afferent pupil defect is usually observed, but may be subtle if visual loss is mild. Loss of colour vision indicates damage to the papillomacular bundle. In NAION there may be segmental or diffuse optic nerve head swelling, with segmental or diffuse pallor. Peripapillary splinter haemorrhages may be seen.

In general terms, visual loss due to giant cell arteritis is usually more severe and optic disc is likely to be very pale. However, for a given individual, it is not possible to distinguish between NAION and arteritic AION on these grounds alone.

Occasionally patients become aware of visual loss some months after the acute event. By then the optic disc is no longer swollen but shows diffuse or segmental pallor. In such circumstances other causes of optic atrophy have to be considered.

Investigations are directed at identifying underlying treatable risk factors for vascular occlusion. For patients over the age of 50 years urgent measures should be taken to diagnose or exclude giant cell arteritis by history, examination, haematological investigation (erythrocyte sedimentation rate, C reactive protein) and, if necessary, temporal artery biopsy. Patients over the age of 50 years should also be screened for smoking, hypertension, diabetes mellitus, hyperlipidaemia and anaemia. Patients less than 50 years old should additionally be screened for vasculitis (ESR, CRP, ANA, ANCA), clotting abnormalities (clotting factors, anti-phospholipid antibodies), and syphilis. As NAION is only extremely rarely due to emboli from the carotid artery or heart, investigations such as carotid duplex ultrasound are unnecessary unless there are specific indications on history or physical exam.

When patients have a delayed presentation with an uncertain history of visual loss and a pale disc, neuro-imaging is also required to exclude a compressive optic neuropathy.

Treatment and prognosis

There is no effective treatment for NAION. Anticoagulation, corticosteroids, iso-volaemic haemodilution, and optic nerve sheath fenestration have all been tried unsuccessfully. The 5 year mortality rate after an episode of NAION approaches 25% because of an appreciably increased incidence of cardiac and cerebrovascular events. Therefore, identified cardiovascular risk factors should be treated, in conjunction with a general physician.

At 6 months, 40% of affected eyes show a spontaneous improvement of at least two lines of Snellen visual acuity, and 20% deteriorate. It is rare for the same eye to experience a further episode of ischaemia, but one third of fellow eyes are affected within 5 years. Aspirin (75 to 150 mg/day) and treatment of underlying risk factors may reduce the incidence of second eye involvement.

Further reading

Acheson JF, Sanders MD. Coagulation abnormalities in ischaemic optic neuropathy. *Eye* 1994; **8**: 89–92.

Arnold AC, Helper RS. Natural history of non-arteritic anterior ischaemic optic neuropathy. *Journal of Neuro-Ophthalmology* 1994; **14**: 66–9.

Burde RM. Optic disc factors for non-arteritic anterior ischaemic optic neuropathy. *American Journal of Ophthalmology* 1993; **116**: 759–64.

Ischemic optic neuropathy decompression trial research group. Optic nerve sheath decompression for non-arteritic anterior ischaemic optic neuropathy is not effective and may be harmful: results of the Ischemic Optic Neuropathy Decompression Trial. *Journal of the American Medical Association* 1995; **273**: 625–32.

Johnson LN, Arnold AC. Incidence of nonarteritic and arteritic anterior ischaemic optic neuropathy. *Journal of Neuro-Ophthalmology* 1994; **14**: 38–44.

Kupersmith MJ. Vascular optic neuropathies. In: *Neuro-vascular Neuro-ophthalmology.* (Kupersmith MJ, Berenstein A, eds) 1st edition. Springer-Verlag, Berlin, 1993; 197–208.

NORMAL TENSION GLAUCOMA

Peter Shah & Karl Whittaker

Normal tension glaucoma (NTG) may be defined as a subcategory of primary open-angle glaucoma. However, disagreement exists as to whether it should be regarded as a separate disease entity from its higher tension counterpart. Although there is no consensus on a precise definition, the following criteria are in general use:

- IOP < 21 mmHg;
- open drainage angle;
- optic disc and visual field changes characteristic of glaucoma;
- the absence of a secondary cause of glaucoma.

One third of patients with open angle glaucoma can be classified as having NTG, and prevalence is estimated at 0.15% of the general population. NTG is more common in the elderly, although up to 30% are under 50 years of age. Females are probably more commonly affected than men. A genetic component is likely. There is a positive family history in 5–40%, and NTG and higher tension glaucoma have been reported in the same family.

Problem

NTG is a diagnosis of exclusion. Several diseases, some of which have systemic implications, may mimic the clinical picture of NTG. Careful consideration must be given to which patients require treatment, how aggressively to treat, and by what means. Different therapeutic options are being explored.

Background

There is clear evidence that IOP is a significant factor in the pathogenesis of NTG. However, non-pressure-dependent factors may also have an important role. In particular, attention has focused on the possibility of reduced blood flow to the optic nerve head or chronic ischaemia. A higher prevalence of vasospastic disease, such as migraine or Raynaud phenomenon, increased resistance of the ophthalmic and central retinal arteries and more severe dips in nocturnal systemic blood pressure have been demonstrated in NTG patients. Other factors have also been postulated to cause optic nerve damage, including autoimmunity, excitotoxicity and neurotrophic deprivation.

Differential diagnosis

1. POAG (primary open angle glaucoma). There is no doubt that many cases of apparent NTG are undetected POAG. Peaks of pressure and large diurnal variations in the IOP can be detected by phasing (which should include nocturnal pressure readings). Indeed, an estimated 40% of all patients diagnosed with POAG initially present with an IOP below 21 mmHg. Indentation tonometry may record IOPs which are falsely low in some patients, such as myopes with low scleral rigidity. A thorough drug history will identify patients who are taking systemic medications, such as beta-blocking agents or cardiac glycosides, which may mask raised IOP. In a small number of untreated cases of POAG, IOP has been reported to decrease to within the normal range, suggesting that NTG in these patients is 'burnt out' POAG.

2. *Secondary glaucomas.* Intraocular pressure may have been previously raised in patients with angle recession, pigmentary glaucoma, inflammatory uveitis or prior topical steroid use. Periods of normal IOP may also occur in patients with intermittent angle-closure glaucoma.

3. *Hereditary optic neuropathy.* A careful history and examination of both the patient and relatives may help to identify patients who have a hereditary optic neuropathy.

4. *Compressive lesions of the anterior visual pathways.* The disc cupping characteristic of glaucoma has also been reported with other optic neuropathies, including those associated with compressive lesions of the visual pathways. Therefore, a low threshold for requesting appropriate neuroradiological investigations is advised. In particular, one should be alert to poor correlation between field and disc changes, i.e. pale discs without cupping, a field defect which would not be predicted by the nature of disc cupping, or if there is a 'neurological' pattern to the field defect. If imaging techniques fail to demonstrate a compressive lesion, and the clinical picture is atypical or progressive, then consideration should be given to repeating the investigation.

5. *Other acquired optic neuropathies.* There are many causes of acquired optic neuropathy which may mimic NTG. A small group of patients give a prior history of a major haemodynamic crisis such as profound blood loss or a severe hypotensive episode. Differentiating NTG from ischaemic optic neuropathy can be difficult. The latter may produce nerve fibre bundle field defects typical of NTG and acquired glaucomatous discs. Excess disc pallor in these cases may help to identify that this is not a typical glaucomatous change. The possibility of a toxic optic neuropathy must be excluded. A history should be obtained of alcohol and tobacco intake, drugs which may damage the optic nerve (e.g. ethambutol), as well as abuse of methanol or illegal substances. Nutritional problems, including vitamin B12 and folate deficiency, may cause an optic neuropathy. Demyelinative and inflammatory diseases of the optic nerve, including neurosyphilis may occasionally produce changes suggestive of NTG. In addition, patients of West Indian descent sometimes develop an optic atrophy (Jamaican optic atrophy) that may be confused with NTG.

Clinical features

There are conflicting data as to whether there are genuine differences between NTG and POAG in terms of optic disc and visual field appearances. On balance, it appears that optic disc haemorrhages and acquired optic disc pits occur more often, the neuroretinal rim is thinner, and the optic cup is larger and shallower in NTG subjects compared to POAG. Monocular or asymmetrical visual field loss is also more common and field defects appear closer to fixation, denser, more localized and more often in the superior hemifield. Visual field loss appears to be linear, but can vary widely between patients. Progressive change has been demonstrated in 35–95% of patients after 6 years. A rise in IOP associated with topical steroid use occurs in 40%

of cases. Recent studies suggest that some patients with NTG have a significant reduction in corneal thickness compared with POAG and normal subjects. It has been suggested that this may result in an underestimation of IOP and erroneous diagnosis of NTG in these cases.

Treatment

Several factors should be taken into account when considering treatment, including severity of disease, rate of progression, prognosis, and the risks of medical or surgical intervention. It has been clearly shown that a 30% reduction in IOP leads to a slower rate of progressive visual field loss. This may be possible with topical medication and/or argon laser trabeculoplasty but often requires filtration surgery. It may be necessary to use adjuvant anti-scarring therapy to achieve these target pressures. Cataract formation and hypotonous maculopathy are potential complications of surgery.

Other treatment strategies may be employed to improve optic nerve blood flow, although their clinical benefit is controversial. Nocturnal dips in blood pressure can be detected by ambulatory monitoring and may be reduced in hypertensive patients by adjusting their systemic hypotensive medication. In such cases, one could also consider switching to a calcium-channel blocker (e.g. nifedipine); recent reports suggest these drugs may reverse vasospasm and could have a favourable effect upon visual fields. Some clinicians advocate the avoidance of non-cardioselective topical beta-blockers on the basis of their possible vasoactive effects in further lowering blood supply to the optic nerve head. Prostaglandin analogues (e.g. latanoprost) may be beneficial for NTG patients because of their greater IOP lowering effect at night, resulting in an increased pulsatile ocular blood flow. The neuroprotective action of recently introduced topical agents, such as brimonidine is not of proven benefit in NTG.

Further reading

Collaborative Normal Tension Glaucoma Study Group. Comparison of glaucomatous progression between untreated patients with normal tension glaucoma and patients with therapeutically reduced intraocular pressures. *American Journal of Ophthalmology* 1998; **126:** 487–97.

Collaborative Normal Tension Glaucoma Study Group. The effectiveness of intraocular pressure reduction in the treatment of normal tension glaucoma. *American Journal of Ophthalmology* 1998; **126:** 498–505.

Kamal D, Hitchings R. Normal tension glaucoma – a practical approach. *British Journal of Opththalmology* 1998; **82:** 835–40.

Related topics of interest

Drugs (topical) in glaucoma: mode of action (p. 108); Ocular hypertension (p. 199); Secondary glaucoma (p. 283).

NYSTAGMUS 1: NYSTAGMUS

Robert H. Taylor & Peter Shah

A practical classification is as follows: (i) physiological nystagmus; (ii) congenital nystagmus; (iii) manifest/latent nystagmus; (iv) peripheral vestibular nystagmus; (v) central nervous system causes of nystagmus; (vi) saccadic intrusions and (vii) other ocular oscillations.

Problem

When faced with a patient with nystagmus, one must try to identify an underlying cause. Correct identification of the type of nystagmus is fundamental for directing history, examination and further investigations. Patients with oscillopsia usually have an acquired oscillation, patients with congenital nystagmus usually do not. Appropriate neuroimaging studies should be performed in consultation with a neurologist or paediatrician where appropriate.

Background

Nystagmus may be defined as an involuntary, rhythmic, to-and-fro oscillation of the eyes. The initial slow phase may be followed by a refixation saccade (jerk), or there may be a constant sinusoidal pattern (pendular). The term saccadic intrusion can be used if the initial movement is a saccade. The direction of the nystagmus is described by the direction of the fast component, although it is the initial slow phase that is abnormal. Amplitude is arbitrarily described as fine, medium or coarse. Intensity is a product of both the amplitude and velocity of the nystagmus. The plane may be horizontal, vertical, rotatory or compound. When both eyes have a similar movement the nystagmus is described as conjugate. Dissociated nystagmus is when the two eyes have different movements. Asymmetry of ocular involvement is an important indicator of neurological abnormality. Null zone is the position of gaze in which the nystagmus is minimal. Alexander's law recognizes that jerk nystagmus increases in amplitude on gaze in the direction of the fast phase. Foveation time occurs when the eye is moving at less than 5° per second, usually as the nystagmus switches direction.

Recordings of the eye movements can be made to aid in interpretation. A variety of techniques are employed. The eye movements can be tracked by using corneal reflections or a contact lens with a coil, or an electromyographic recording can be made.

Clinical features

1. Physiological nystagmus.   There are many different types of physiological nystagmus, including end-point nystagmus, optokinetic nystagmus, caloric nystagmus and rotational (vestibular-induced) nystagmus. Their differentiation from pathological states is usually straightforward and no further investigation is necessary.

2. Congenital nystagmus.   See separate topic.

3. Latent nystagmus.   See separate topic.

4. *Peripheral vestibular nystagmus.* This is a primary position jerk nystagmus which is horizontal and often has a rotatory component. The nystagmus is characteristically unidirectional. The slow phase is linear and characteristically towards the diseased side. It is suppressed by fixation and lying down with the intact ear down. It is exacerbated by changes in head position, hyperventilation and the Valsalva manoeuvre.

Important associated symptoms include: vertigo, tinnitus and hearing loss. Peripheral causes of vestibular pathology include: inflammatory disease of the labyrinthine system, neuronitis, ischaemia and drug toxicity. If hearing is good then the diagnosis is probably labyrinthitis. If hearing is poor it is probably Meniere disease or other more major pathology.

5. *Central nervous system causes of nystagmus.* These causes may be divided into several distinct clinical entities. It should be remembered, however, that there may be considerable overlap between conditions. Localizing value varies.

- **Central vestibular nystagmus.** The jerk nystagmus of central vestibular disease may be vertical (upbeat or downbeat), horizontal or rotatory. In contrast to peripheral vestibular nystagmus, the nystagmus may be uni- or bi-directional.

  Associated symptoms of vertigo, tinnitus and hearing loss are less prominent. Romberg test may be helpful in differentiating central and peripheral types of nystagmus. In central vestibular disease, the direction in which the patient falls does not vary with head position, whereas in peripheral disease the direction alters with head position.

  (a) *Downbeat nystagmus*: Jerk nystagmus, fast phase down, may be worse after convergence and in lateral gaze. Fixation has little effect on amplitude. Alexander's law is usually obeyed.

  Downbeat nystagmus usually indicates disease affecting the cranio-cervical junction, degenerations in the vestibulocerebellum or drug toxicity. Oscillopsia may be present as well as postural instability. Causes include Arnold–Chiari malformation, spinocerebellar degenerations, tumours of the skull base, multiple sclerosis, brainstem cerebrovascular accident, lithium and anticonvulsant toxicity. A chin-down posture may be used to minimize oscillopsia. Bifocals are useless. Medical treatment has included baclofen and diazepam.

  (b) *Upbeat nystagmus:* Jerk nystagmus, fast phase up, usually obeys Alexander's law, but is often not accentuated on lateral gaze. Fixation has little effect on amplitude. Pathology is poorly localized but is often associated with intrinsic disease of the brainstem from medulla to midbrain.

  (c) *Horizontal central vestibular nystagmus:* The slow phase may have an increasing velocity, similar to congenital nystagmus. it may be caused by Arnold–Chiari malformation. The recent onset of oscillopsia will assist in differentiation.

- **Periodic alternating nystagmus (PAN).** This jerk nystagmus is always horizontal in the primary position with the fast phase to one side for about 90–120 seconds. After this period there is a short 5-second rest followed by a crescendo and decrescendo of the fast phase to the opposite side for another 90–120 seconds, then once again a period of about 5 seconds' rest. The cycle then repeats continuously. During the 'rest' period, there may be upbeat, downbeat or square-wave jerks. The congenital form can be much more irregular, and the disorder missed unless the examiner is careful to exclude it by observing the patient's spontaneous movements for 2–5 minutes. Vestibular stimuli can reset the mechanism and cause the nystagmus to stop for several minutes. Fixation has little effect on amplitude. Periodic alternating nystagmus may be congenital, secondary to vestibulocerebellar disease such as demyelination or associated with acquired bilateral visual loss. Baclofen abolishes acquired PAN in some patients. PAN is classified by some authors as a central vestibular nystagmus. In experimental animals PAN can be induced by lesions in the cerebellar nodulus and uvula and eliminated by Baclofen.

- **Gaze-evoked nystagmus.** These patients do not have nystagmus in the primary position, but demonstrate a specific nystagmus on eccentric gaze (e.g. right-jerk on right gaze, left-jerk on left gaze, up-jerk on up-gaze). The nystagmus is of low frequency and large amplitude. End-point nystagmus is a physiological gaze-evoked nystagmus which tends to have higher frequency and small amplitude. The amplitude of gaze-evoked nystagmus may decline with sustained eccentric gaze. There is often rebound nystagmus on returning to the primary position. There may be abnormalities in pursuit movement. A neurological examination may demonstrate other cerebellar signs. Gaze-evoked nystagmus may be found in association with cerebellar and brainstem posterior fossa disease. Gaze-evoked nystagmus can also be drug induced, particularly in states of drug toxicity (e.g. alcohol). Anti-epileptic drugs such as phenytoin and phenobarbitol, and members of the sedative/tranquilizer groups have been implicated. Gaze-evoked nystagmus may be seen in myasthenia or other causes of muscle paresis. This usually has an increasing amplitude with sustained eccentric gaze towards the weak muscle.

  (a) *Gaze-paretic nystagmus* is one form of gaze-evoked nystagmus seen in association with a gaze paresis. It is also seen in patients with cerebellar disease. It is thought to be due to a defect in the neural pathways responsible for gaze holding.
  (b) *Bruns' nystagmus*: A specific type of gaze-evoked nystagmus is seen with tumours of the cerebellopontine angle. Ipsilateral gaze evokes a large-amplitude, low-velocity nystagmus. In contralateral gaze there is a small-amplitude, high-frequency nystagmus, due to the vestibular imbalance.

- **See-saw nystagmus.** This pendular or jerk nystagmus has a conjugate rotatory component and a disconjugate vertical component. One eye supraducts and intorts, and the other infraducts and extorts. When a jerk nystagmus, it is sometimes known as a hemi-seesaw nystagmus, and the lesion is in the region of the interstitial nucleus of Cajal. There is a similarity in movement between the slow phase of a hemi-seesaw nystagmus and the ocular tilt reaction. Classic seesaw nystagmus is a slow pendular nystagmus. It is frequently associated with suprasellar compressive lesions with bitemporal field defects. The most common pathology is a craniopharyngioma. A congenital form exists in which usually one eye supraducts and extorts, and the other infraducts and intorts.

- **Internuclear ophthalmoplegia.** There is reduced adduction or reduced adducting saccade on the ipsilateral side, associated with a dissociated nystagmus, with postsaccadic drift on abduction in the eye contralateral to the lesion with increasing amplitude on abduction. Dissociated vertical nystagmus may be present, with down beat in the ipsilateral eye and torsional in the contralateral eye. Associated features include preserved convergence and sometimes a skew deviation. Asymmetry of ocular involvement often indicates pathology in the posterior cranial fossa.
- **Spasmus nutans.** This is a combination of a fine pendular nystagmus, anomalous head position (usually a tilt) and head nodding. The nystagmus is usually unilateral or asymmetrical, intermittent, small amplitude with a high frequency (3–11 Hz) which gives the appearance of a shimmering. There may be a variation over time, with conjugate, disconjugate, monocular movements seen in the same child. The plane is mainly horizontal with associated torsional or vertical components. Spasmus nutans starts between 3 and 15 months and usually resolves by 3 years old. The key point is that spasmus nutans must be regarded as a diagnosis of exclusion. Gliomas of the anterior visual pathway can cause such a constellation of signs and so need exclusion by neuroimaging.
- **Acquired pendular nystagmus.** This may show mixed horizontal, vertical or rotational components. The waveform may be suppressed or accentuated by lid closure, and may demonstrate postsaccadic suppression. The waveform may vary and appear monocular at times. Frequency is low, usually 2–8 Hz. Causes include demyelination, Pelizaeus–Merzbacher disease and toluene abuse.
- **Ocular myoclonus.** This is a rapid acquired vertical pendular nystagmus, but may be dysconjugate vertical-torsional. In addition to the nystagmus, there may be associated contractions of facial, palatal, pharyngeal, diaphragmatic and other musculature. These unusual eye movements are sometimes abolished by sleep, but the palatal movements are not. The nystagmus follows several months after brainstem or cerebellar infarction. Histological enlargement of the ipsilateral inferior olivary nucleus and destruction of the contralateral dentate nucleus have been described.

Further reading

Bajandas FJ, Kline LB. *Neuro-Ophthalmology Review Manual*, 3rd edn. Thorofare, NJ: SLACK, 1988; 67–76.

Harris C. Nystagmus and eye movement disorders. In Taylor D: *Paediatric Ophthalmology*, 2nd edn. Blackwell Science Ltd, 1997; 869–924.

Leigh RJ, Zee DS. Clinical features of ocular motor nerve palsies. In: *The Neurology of Eye Movements*, 3rd edn. New York, Oxford University Press, 1999; Section 10; 405–82.

Mein J, Trimble R. Nystagmus. In: *Diagnosis and Management of Ocular Motility Disorders*, 2nd edn. Oxford: Blackwell Scientific Publications, 1991; 375–405.

Wilson ME, Buckley EG, Kivlin JD, Ruttum MS, Simon JW, Magoon EH. Pediatric Ophthalmology Section 6. *American Academy of Ophthalmology* 1999; 125–32.

Related topics of interest

Child with strabismus: work-up (p. 45); Congenital nystagmus (p. 69); Latent nystagmus (p. 151); Nystagmus 2: saccadic intrusions and other ocular oscillations (p. 195).

NYSTAGMUS 2: SACCADIC INTRUSIONS AND OTHER OCULAR OSCILLATIONS

Robert H. Taylor

In addition to nystagmus, which strictly speaking has an initial slow movement, there are a number of other ocular oscillations. Some of these have important localizing value.

Problem

The terminology of some of these oscillations is confusing and classifications will vary. Yet, their importance in revealing underlying disease cannot be overestimated.

Background

Normal fixation is a complex neurological function. It is the direction of gaze that holds the visual image of the object of regard on the fovea. Some authors feel that the act of fixation represents a totally different system, an independent visual-fixation system, that has yet to be defined. Others feel that it is a form of smooth pursuit, an act that suppresses the image motion that would be present due to the natural drift of the eyes. There is also evidence that activity in the frontal eye fields and superior colliculus is responsible for suppressing saccades away from fixation when steady fixation is important, e.g. at times of concentration. This becomes important in certain disease states that interrupt fixation.

Clinical features

1. Saccadic intrusions. These are rapid movements of the eye that take it away from fixation. There is a spectrum that extends from a single saccade to a sustained oscillation.

- **Square wave jerks.** A square wave jerk is an involuntary break in fixation followed by a single re-fixation movement. They are usually of very small amplitude ($< 2°$ but up to $5°$) and return the eye after 200 msec. They can be a normal finding in elderly patients and often seen during ophthalmoscopy. They may be multiple. Cerebral hemisphere disease and cigarette smoking increase their occurrence.
- **Macrosquare wave jerks** are larger ($5–15°$) and return the eye after 70–150 msec. They are usually multiple and are seen most commonly in multiple sclerosis.
- **Macrosaccadic oscillations** occur in runs and increase in amplitude before declining. They can be intepreted as an extreme dysmetria, being stimulated by a refixation saccade and oscillating around the re-fixation point. Cerebellar disorders and pontine lesions have been identified as causes.
- **Saccadic pulses** consist of a saccade away from fixation and a rapid drift back. They can be seen in normals and with internuclear ophthalmoplegia.
- **Ocular flutter.** Saccadic oscillations without an intersaccadic interval are intermittent, with a small amplitude. Ocular flutter frequently co-exists with ocular dysmetria.

- **Opsoclonus** (saccadomania) is a repeated saccadic oscillation without an inter-saccadic interval. The plane is usually horizontal but can have vertical or torsional components. Frequency varies from six to 15 jerks per second. Opsoclonus usually persists during eyelid closure and sleep. It increases with light stimulation, attempted fixation, eye closure in response to sudden noxious stimuli (e.g. loud noise) and when upset. When acquired by an infant in the first weeks of life, opsoclonus may settle into ocular flutter by about 8 weeks of age, and disappears by 3 months. However, opsoclonus may also be a distant cerebellar effect of a neuroblastoma. Infants with opsoclonus secondary to an occult neuroblastoma may also have ataxia and myoclonus (dancing eyes and dancing feet). In both infant and adult, opsoclonus may be a relatively self-limiting disorder after viral encephalitis. When opsoclonus is acquired in adult life it can be a sign of remote malignant disease (lung, breast, ovary). There are metabolic and toxic causes. The presence of opsoclonus in adult or child mandates a full evaluation for systemic disease.

2. *Ocular dysmetria.* Sometimes termed saccadic dysmetria, describes the presence of an overshoot or undershoot in the saccade, followed by several oscillatory movements about the new direction of gaze, before coming to rest in the desired position. It corresponds in principle to cerebellar past pointing and is seen in cerebellar disease.

3. *Superior oblique myokymia.* Superior oblique myokymia consists of small rapid vertical and torsional oscillatory movements of one eye in the field of action of the superior oblique. Patients may present with either vertical diplopia or monocular visual blurring. They may also report odd tremulous sensations in the eye, with reduced vision. As the oscillations are very fine they are best detected by looking on a slit lamp or by observing the fundal details using a direct ophthalmoscope. Although often benign, with no underlying cause apparent, the condition is occasionally seen in multiple sclerosis.

4. *Convergence retraction nystagmus.* These unusual jerk convergence–retraction movements (due to co-contraction of extraocular muscles), seen especially on attempted up-gaze and convergence, should alert the clinician to the high probability of a lesion affecting the posterior midbrain, in particular the posterior commissure. It is not a true nystagmus as the first movement is a dysjunctive saccade. The oscillation is particularly well seen when a down-going optokinetic nystagmus drum is used to generate upward saccades. Look carefully at the upper sulcus, as the retraction may be subtle. A disinhibition of the third nerve nuclei occurs and all the muscles fire, giving the retraction. Convergence retraction nystagmus may be seen as part of the dorsal midbrain syndrome (Parinaud syndrome). The features of this include defective vertical up-gaze (first sign to occur), convergence retraction nystagmus, light near dissociation of the pupils (pupils are large), lid retraction (Collier sign), spasm/paresis of accommodation/convergence and occasionally skew deviation. Pathological lesions include aqueductal stenosis, pineal tumours, trauma, vascular anomalies and cerebrovascular events.

Pretectal pseudobobbing may be a variant, and seen in patients with obstructive hydrocephalus. The movement is fast-downward and medially followed by a slow return to the primary position.

5. _Voluntary nystagmus._ This is usually horizontal, high frequency, pendular and rarely circumrotatory. There may be a head tremor. There will be oscillopsia. There are no intersaccadic intervals. Fluttering of eyelids, concentrated facial expression and associated convergence usually make the diagnosis when patients present troubled with these signs.

6. _Monocular nystagmus._ Severe unilateral visual impairment (including profound amblyopia) can lead to a monocular pendular nystagmus, sometimes known as the Heimann–Bielschowsky phenomenon. The wave-form is usually vertical, low frequency, small amplitude and irregular. Monocular visual loss can also result in manifest latent nystagmus (see separate topic).

Eye movements in unconsciousness

1. _Ocular bobbing._ The oscillations consist of fast, conjugate movements downwards, followed by a slow drift back towards the primary position. The patient usually has no horizontal eye movements (either spontaneous or reflex). The causes include large pontine lesions, metabolic cerebral disturbances or obstructive hydrocephalus.

2. _Ocular dipping_ consists of a slow downward movement with a rapid return. It has poor localizing value.

Both the above can have a reverse picture with poor localizing value.

3. _Ping pong gaze_ consists of horizontal ocular deviations that reverse every few seconds. Patients usually have bilateral hemispheric damage.

4. _Periodic gaze deviation_ consist of alternating conjugate lateral gaze, alternating on average every 2 minutes. Can be seen in hepatic encephalopathy.

5. _Vertical myoclonus_ can be seen in the unconscious patient and suggests a pontine cerebrovascular accident.

6. _Monocular movements_ which are small and rapid, suggest pontine or midbrain damage.

- **Epileptiform nystagmus.** This is usually horizontal, conjugate, jerk nystagmus, but can be vertical, pendular or monocular. It is a form of epileptic seizure activity so there is no nystagmus when not active. One type has a large amplitude and crosses the midline. The slow phase is abnormal and may be due to stimulation of the parieto-occipital pursuit centre, causing ipsilateral slow phase with refixation. In the second type the fast phase is abnormal. The focus stimulates contralateral saccades with a slow decelerating phase that comes back to the midline without crossing it. Epileptiform nystagmus usually affects adults but can be seen in infants. There may be associated lid twitching. Conscious patients may report oscillopsia, blurred vision, blindness or hallucinations. Tonic eye deviation is more characteristic of other forms of seizure.

Lid nystagmus

This may be seen with horizontal nystagmus and has been described in a patient with lateral medullary infarction. Convergence inhibited the lid movement in this patient. Convergence can accentuate the nystagmus and be suggestive of medullary or cerebellar lesions.

Roving eye movements (searching)

Roving eye movements in a blind child are low frequency and large amplitude. There are often intermittent bouts of jerk nystagmus. The larger the amplitude the more anterior in the visual pathway the visual problem is likely to be. Cerebral visual impairment tends not to lead to nystagmus but roving eye movements may occur.

Further reading

Bajandas FJ, Kline LB. *Neuro-Ophthalmology Review Manual*, 3rd edn. Thorofare, NJ: SLACK, 1988; 67–76.

Harris C. Nystagmus and Eye movement disorders. In: Taylor D: *Paediatric Ophthalmology*, 2nd edn. Blackwell Science Ltd, 1997; 869–924.

Leigh RJ, Zee DS. Clinical features of ocular motor nerve palsies. In: *The Neurology of Eye Movements*, 3rd edn. New York, Oxford University Press, 1999; Section 10; 405–82.

Mein J, Trimble R. Nystagmus. In: *Diagnosis and Management of Ocular Motility Disorders*, 2nd edn. Oxford: Blackwell Scientific Publications, 1991; 375–405.

Wilson ME, Buckley EG, Kivlin JD, Ruttum MS, Simon JW, Magoon EH. Pediatric Ophthalmology Section 6. *American Academy of Ophthalmology* 1999; 125–32.

Related topics of interest

Congenital nystagmus (p. 69); Infantile esotropia (p. 143); Latent nystagmus (p. 151); Nystagmus 1: nystagmus (p. 190).

OCULAR HYPERTENSION

Karl Whittaker & Peter Shah

Ocular hypertension (OHT) is characterized by consistently raised IOP, anatomically open angles and no evidence of glaucomatous optic disc damage or visual field loss. A patient with this condition may be described as an 'ocular hypertensive' or 'glaucoma suspect'.

Problem

At present, there is no consensus as to which patients are likely to develop significant optic nerve damage and visual field loss. There are limited data on the efficacy of ocular hypotensive medication, although the clinical impression is that early initiation of treatment is more effective in preventing progressive field loss than treatment late in the course of glaucoma. OHT patients tend to be younger than those with glaucoma and, by definition, are asymptomatic. Therefore, careful consideration should be given to the potential risks of long-term treatment.

Background

Controversy exists as to what level of IOP is abnormally high. Population studies have shown that 97.5% of IOPs are < 20.5 mmHg, assuming a normal Gaussian distribution. However, IOP is, in fact, skewed to the right, suggesting the upper limit of 'normal' should be higher. Nonetheless, IOPs of > 22 mmHg are generally regarded as abnormal by clinicians in the UK. Some studies from the US have used an IOP cut-off of 24 mmHg. The prevalence of OHT increases with age. Of the population over 40, 4–10% have an IOP > 22 mmHg without any evidence of field loss. Long-term studies have shown that eyes with longstanding OHT will develop POAG at a rate of 0.5–1% per year, with 10% having converted after 10 years.

Clinical features

A thorough history and examination should focus on the following risk factors for the development of POAG.

1. Family history. There is a 1 in 8 chance of glaucoma developing if a first-degree relative has POAG. The hereditary tendency is strongest in siblings.

2. Age. The prevalence of glaucoma increases with age. This may relate to microvascular perfusion defects, changes in the supportive connective tissue of the optic nerve, or the length of time the optic nerve is exposed to raised IOP. Life expectancy of the patient should also be considered in relation to the likelihood of developing a visual field defect.

3. Optic disc and nerve fibre layer. By definition, the disc has a healthy appearance in OHT. Careful documentation is essential, and should include a disc drawing and estimation of cup:disc ratio. However, clinical evaluation is sometimes poorly reproducible and stereoscopic, or even single, colour disc photographs should be obtained if possible. Localized defects in the neuroretinal rim, and cup asymmetry are very suggestive of glaucoma. Disc splinter haemorrhages are suspicious but not pathognomonic. Other signs, such as peripapillary chorioretinal atrophy, circumlinear vessel baring and baring of the lamina cribrosa also occur in glaucoma but are less specific. Nerve fibre layer defects may be identified before optic disc changes. They are best seen with monochromatic high-contrast photography although an experienced examiner may observe changes using slit-lamp biomicroscopy or direct ophthalmoscopy with a red-free light.

4. **IOP.** Most clinicians will treat OHT patients whose IOP is > 30 mmHg as there is a high risk of developing glaucoma. There is good evidence that patients with an IOP > 28 mmHg and a vertical cup:disc ratio > 0.6 have an increased risk of developing field defects. In other patients with an IOP between 22–30 mmHg, the situation is less clear. Single IOP measurements may be misleading and phasing should be considered. Diurnal variation is normally 3–6 mmHg and this can be much higher in glaucoma patients. As a rule, IOP is highest in the morning and lowest in the evening, but it may be reversed or follow no particular pattern. IOP asymmetry is more common in patients with glaucoma. A difference of > 4 mmHg is seen in less than 4% of normals. Recent studies have shown that some OHT subjects have increased corneal thickness. It has been suggested that pachymetry should be performed to exclude an abnormally thick cornea as a reason for falsely high IOP measurements.

5. **Ethnic origin.** There is good evidence that POAG is more prevalent, is more severe and develops at an earlier age in black patients.

6. **Vascular disease.** Systemic hypertension, diabetes, angina and sleep apnoea syndrome are all associated with glaucoma, although a definite causal relationship has not been identified. Theories focus on reduced vascular supply to the optic nerve head. There are reports of lower blood flow velocities in the retrobulbar circulation of glaucoma patients compared with OHT and normal subjects.

7. **Thyroid-related immune orbitopathy.** IOP can be elevated due to tethering by fibrotic extraocular muscles or to orbital congestion and venous stasis limiting aqueous outflow. Prolonged persistence of active orbital involvement resulting in chronically elevated IOP may be associated with progression to glaucoma.

8. **Myopia.** Some studies indicate that myopes with OHT have a higher risk of developing visual field defects. This may be caused by structural alterations in the collagen and extracellular matrix of the optic nerve head.

Other considerations

1. **Retinal vein occlusions.** CRVOs and to a lesser extent, BRVOs occur more frequently in hypertensive eyes. Therefore, if there has been a vein occlusion in one eye it would seem reasonable to treat the fellow eye of an OHT patient.

2. **Only eye.** Some clinicians will consider early treatment if the patient has only one functioning eye.

Future developments

1. **Ocular hypertension treatment study.** This multicentre randomized clinical trial compares topical ocular hypotensive medication with close observation for OHT patients. It should provide useful information regarding: (i) the safety and efficacy of topical treatment in preventing or delaying the onset of POAG; (ii) the risk factors for development of field defects and optic disc damage.

2. *Earlier detection of glaucoma.* More sensitive diagnostic techniques are being developed, which may enable more effective prevention of disease progression.

3. *Visual field testing.* Conventional threshold perimetry of the central 30° only detects field loss after substantial numbers of retinal ganglion cells are lost. Several new methods are available, although their role in clinical practice is still being evaluated. Short-wave automated perimetry (SWAP) isolates the blue colour pathway by measuring the sensitivity of a blue Goldmann size V stimulus on a yellow background. High-pass resolution perimetry (HRP) measures peripheral visual acuity using a low-contrast target. Frequency-doubling perimetry (FDP) measures a function of a subset of specialized retinal ganglion cells by rapid reversal of black and white bars. Motion perimetry measures the ability to detect patches of spots or lines moving in one direction. Flicker perimetry measures temporal modulation (brightness threshold to detect flicker at different flicker rates) or critical fusion flicker frequency (flicker rate at which a bright flickering stimulus appears constant).

4. *Optic disc and nerve fibre layer (NFL) assessment.* Most ophthalmologists rely on clinical evaluation of the optic disc and NFL. Photographic assessment is more accurate but is a subjective and qualitative method. Various quantitative devices have been developed, although their usefulness in clinical practice is not proven. Confocal laser scanning gives a three-dimensional image of the optic disc and retina reconstructed from a series of scans of a thin 'slice' of tissue at sequential tissue depths. It can be used in subjects with small pupils and media opacities. Laser polarimetry can measure NFL thickness by measuring a change in the rotation of a polarized beam of laser light reflected from the retinal surface. Optical coherence tomography is analogous to B-scan ultrasonography except it measures the intensity of back-scattered infra-red light instead of sound to obtain a resolution of 10 microns. Laser polarimetry and OCT produce cross-sectional images.

Conclusion

One should not rely on a single IOP reading to guide management. There are a variety of factors that can lead to an artefactually high IOP.

Further reading

Copt R-P, Thomas R, Mermoud A. Corneal thickness in ocular hypertension, primary open angle glaucoma, and normal tension glaucoma. *Archives of Ophthalmology* 1999; **117:** 14–16.

Gordon MO, Kass MA. The ocular hypertension treatment study: design and baseline description of the participants. *Archives of Ophthalmology* 1999; **117:** 573–83.

Ritch R, Shields NB, Krupin T. *The glaucomas.* St Louis: CV Mosby, 2nd edn. 1996.

Related topics of interest

Drugs (topical) in glaucoma: mode of action (p. 108); Normal tension glaucoma (p. 187); Secondary glaucoma (p. 283).

OCULAR SURFACE SQUAMOUS NEOPLASIA

Graham A. Lee & Peter Shah

Ocular surface squamous neoplasia (OSSN) describes a spectrum of disease involving the cornea and/or conjunctiva ranging from dysplasia, carcinoma in situ to invasive squamous cell carcinoma. OSSN is an uncommon disease with an incidence of 2/100000 in Brisbane, Australia. It occurs most commonly in older Caucasian males around 60 years old, but has been reported in children as young as 4 years old.

Problem

The diagnosis and extent of the disease are difficult to assess from clinical examination. Various modalities of treatment are available, however all are associated with risk of recurrence. These patients require life-long follow-up.

Background

The limbus is an area of transition from conjunctival to corneal epithelium. It is akin to other areas such as the uterine cervix which are predisposed to dysplastic change. Cumulative exposure to excess ultraviolet-B light has been identified as a major aetiologic factor, with Caucasian populations living at latitudes closer to the equator than 30° at particular risk. Human papillomavirus-16 has also been associated with OSSN, but is thought to act in combination with other factors.

Clinical features

Patients present with a history of surface irritation, chronic red eye or a visible growth on the ocular surface. Most lesions straddle the limbus between the palpebral fissures, but may involve the cornea or conjunctiva alone. Appearance is quite variable ranging from flat to elevated; gelatinous, papilliform, nodular, leukoplakic or diffuse; pearly grey to reddish grey. The lesions may be accompanied by characteristic 'corkscrew' feeding blood vessels. Intraocular invasion can present as a low-grade inflammation with secondary glaucoma. Metastasis is rare, but spread may occur to preauricular, submandibular and cervical lymph nodes, as well as parotid gland, brain, lung and bone.

It is difficult to assess the severity of neoplasia by clinical appearance alone. It may mimic many other ocular surface conditions such as pterygium, pinguecula, papilloma, dyskeratosis, naevus, pyogenic granuloma, dermoid, keratoacanthoma, pseudo-epitheliomatous hyperplasia, amelanotic melanoma and chronic blepharoconjunctivitis. Rose bengal staining may be useful to delineate the extent of the lesion. This dye stains cells with an abnormal surface mucin layer. Impression cytology using cellulose acetate filter paper strips to sample superficial cells has recently been used to grade the lesions prior to treatment. Partial biopsy of more extensive lesions can be performed for grading, however the section may not be representative of the whole lesion.

Dysplasia can be graded as mild (<1/3 thickness atypical cells), moderate (1/3 to 3/4 thickness atypical cells) or severe (>3/4 to nearly full thickness atypical cells). Carcinoma in situ is full thickness dysplasia with loss of the normal surface layer. Squamous cell carcinoma is diagnosed when the basement membrane has been breached and the substantia propria/stroma has been invaded. Rare variants include muco-epidermoid, pigmented and spindle cell.

Treatment

Surgical excision is the most accepted form of treatment. A margin of 2–3 mm will generally suffice for the majority of lesions. As this can not always be achieved, in practice only as much normal surrounding tissue as possible is excised. Deep corneal or scleral involvement requires lamellar keratectomy or sclerectomy. Intraoperative frozen section has been advocated, however the technique is technically difficult to perform due to the small nature of the tissue fragments. In addition, poorer staining, compared with paraffin sections, make interpretation a problem. Cryotherapy to the conjunctival margins and/or the base of the lesion can provide adjuvant treatment, particularly in areas of inadequate excision margins. Beta-radiotherapy applied with a Strontium-90 cup-shaped applicator has also been proposed, however this is associated with significant complications including scleral necrosis. Recently, topical mitomycin C and 5-fluorouracil have been used in the treatment of OSSN. Long-term efficacy is not established as follow-up is short and the number of cases reported is small. Treatment of local invasion requires enucleation or if more extensive, exenteration.

Recurrence rate following treatment is approximately 20–40%. The major risk factor for recurrence is inadequacy of excision margin. Most lesions tend to recur in the first 2 years following treatment, but patients require life-long follow-up. Sequential drawings or, ideally, anterior segment photographs are useful to document any early sign of recurrence (e.g. re-growth of abnormal vessels, areas of rose bengal staining or re-growth of a mass). Local invasion and metastasis are rare, but when present can result in blindness or death.

Further reading

Lee GA, Hirst LW. Ocular surface squamous neoplasia. *Survey of Ophthalmology* 1995; **39**: 429–50.

Majmudar PA, Epstein RJ. Antimetabolites in ocular surface neoplasia. *Current Opinion in Ophthalmology* 1998; **9**: 35–9.

Shields JA, Shields CL, De Potter P. Surgical management of conjunctival tumors. The 1994 Lyn B. McMahan Lecture. *Archives of Ophthalmology* 1997; **115**: 808–15.

Tabin G, Levin S, Snibson G, Loughnan M, Taylor H. Late recurrences and the necessity for long-term follow-up in corneal and conjunctival intraepithelial neoplasia. *Ophthalmology* 1997; **104**: 485–92.

OCULAR ULTRASOUND

Ken K. Nischal

Ocular ultrasound can be classified as A-scan, B-scan, Doppler and high-frequency ultrasound (ultrasound biomicroscopy, UBM).

Problem

Like all examination techniques ophthalmic ultrasound requires an understanding of the basic principles of physics involved, a routine of examination and supervised practice before the clinician can reliably use this mode of examination.

Background

The basic physics of ultrasound involves the appropriate electrical stimulation of a piezoelectric crystal, which then emits ultrasound waves. As some of these are reflected back they re-stimulate the crystal which in turn produces an electric current. This electric current is converted to display either a single ultrasound amplitude display (A-scan) or a cumulative display of many ultrasounds as a grey scale (B-scan). In order for the same crystal to emit and then receive ultrasounds the electric current used to stimulate it must be switched off momentarily and then turned on again; this on/off cycle is continuously repeated. The component, which houses the crystal and the necessary electrical hardware, is called the transducer. This transducer is usually placed in appropriate casing, the ultrasound probe.

The higher the frequency of the ultrasound the less the tissue penetration. Therefore, for the best imaging of the orbit 4–5 MHz is used, for ocular ultrasound 8–10 MHz and for the anterior segment (5 mm tissue penetration) a high frequency of 50–60 MHz.

Most modern day ultrasonography is contact rather than immersion in nature i.e. the probe is in contact with the skin (if the eyelids are closed) or the sclera (if the eyelids are open) with a lubricating agent between the transducer head and the surface. Immersion techniques involve the use of a water bath or methylcellulose bath. This is only now used for some high-frequency ultrasound examinations.

Clinical features

Routine ocular ultrasound (B-scan, two-dimensional, 8–10 MHz transducer) is usually performed with eyelids closed. The probe has a marker which correlates with one side of the display screen (usually left side). There are various scanning protocols and the reader is referred elsewhere to decide which best suits the patient's needs. A simple protocol involves scanning with the probe marker pointing horizontally to the nose (horizontal scan) or vertically with the probe marker nearest the eyebrow (vertical scan). If the patient's left eye is stationary in the primary position and the probe is moved temporally, the nasal retina is being scanned (irrespective of whether the probe marker is horizontal or vertical). If the patient moves the left eye nasally while the probe is moved temporally, the nasal retina anterior to the equator is now being scanned. In this manner the posterior segment can be examined in 10 scan planes: 4 quadrants (supero-nasal, supero-temporal, infero-nasal, infero-temporal) each anterior and posterior to the equator and each horizontally and vertically, with an additional vertical and horizontal scan of the optic nerve head.

The scans described so far are static but if the probe is held still and the patient asked to move the eyes back and forth, dynamic scans can be taken. These are useful to examine the vitreoretinal interface (e.g. posterior vitreous detachment vs retinal detachment).

The advent of three-dimensional B-scan ultrasound has allowed reliable estimation of volumes especially for tumours.

Orbital ultrasound (B-scan, 3–5 MHz transducer) is usually performed with eyelids closed. Vertical scan planes are used to measure extraocular muscle thickness, while both horizontal and vertical scans are used to assess orbital masses.

High-frequency ultrasound (50 MHz transducer) is used to examine the eye with the eyelids open with methylcellulose as a coupling agent between the transducer head and the ocular surface. Scans are taken radial and parallel to the limbus at various clock hour positions, e.g. 4 o'clock. The view encompassing the pupil can be termed pupillary or axial scan.

Doppler ultrasound utilizes a B-scan grey scale display on which a specific area can be examined (usually with the use of a tracker ball and highlight box on the screen) for evidence of blood flow. Colour enhancement allows the examiner to distinguish between venous and arterial flow.

Diagnostic uses

1. *Ocular ultrasound (A-scan)*. Measurement of axial length (AL) is an integral part of biometry. An error of 0.1 mm in AL measurement will result in a 0.25 D error in postoperative predictive refractive error. Although the velocity of sound through the human lens varies with the amount of cataractous change, becoming higher as the lens becomes more cataractous, this does not appear to have a significant effect on IOL calculations. In post-vitrectomy eyes filled with silicone oil the AL may be artifactually longer because the speed of sound in silicone oil is slower than in vitreous. Artifactually low AL may be found in an eye with asteroid hyalosis as a result of confusingly strong echoes from the mid-vitreous. Most A-scans use an applanation technique but this may indent the eye and cause artifactually low AL.

A-scans are also used as part of standardized echography for tissue differentiation. However, it is used very uncommonly now with the advent of better resolution machines.

2. *Doppler ultrasound*. To assess the flow of blood in the central retinal artery, posterior ciliary arteries, ophthalmic artery and central retinal vein. The superior ophthalmic vein can be imaged to look for arterialized blood flow within it, in suspected cases of carotico-cavernous fistulas. An orbital lesion may be vascular in nature or not.

3. *Ocular and orbital ultrasound (B-scan)*. In the presence of opaque media (corneal opacification, cataract or vitreous haemorrhage) B-scan ultrasound can be very useful to exclude retinal detachment, tumour or retinal tear (dynamic ultrasound is essential for this) or structural anomaly e.g. coloboma. Malignant melanomas classically display four features on ultrasound namely smooth round elevation, relative hypoechogenicity (due to the homogeneous tumour absorbing ultrasounds and not reflecting them), choroidal excavation and an orbital shadow (due to ultrasounds not getting through the tumour but being absorbed by them). Retinoblastomas are hyperechogenic due to their intrinsic calcification. Posterior scleritis or orbital inflammation (orbital pseudotumour) both cause fluid in Tenon's space. Also severe flattening of the posterior pole curvature at the insertion of the optic nerve giving the so-called 'T-sign' (the vertical limb of the letter is represented by the optic nerve and the horizontal limb of the letter, by the flattened posterior pole) is seen, the 'T' being on its side.

4. _High-frequency ultrasound._ This can be used to confirm the presence of plateau iris syndrome. The ultrasound shows the classic plateau iris configuration with anteriorly rotated ciliary processes and body. In the pigment dispersion glaucoma, the iris can be seen to bow posteriorly with lens iris touch in the mid-periphery when the patient is asked to accommodate. Other anterior structures can be examined in detail such as iris tumours, the anterior segment if the cornea is opacified, e.g. Peter's anomaly and sclerocornea. Corneal thickness can be measured and the position of intraocular lens haptics assessed.

Therapeutic uses

Ocular ultrasound has been used to apply cryotherapy to retinal tears in the presence of a vitreous haemorrhage. Orbital ultrasound has been used to perform needle biopsy of orbital lesions

Table of uses of A and B scan ultrasound

Ultrasound scan	Uses	Structure	Diagnosis	Characteristics
A	Biometry	Axial length	Cataract	
A	Tissue differentiation	Varies	Most useful for differentiating retina from posterior vitreous face	
A: Doppler	Blood flow	Cen Ret artery Post ciliary art Ophthalmic art Cen Ret Vein	Occlusion	No flow seen
A Doppler	Blood flow	Sup Oph Vn	CC fistula	High flow
B Dynamic	Differentiation	Retina/viteous	PVD vv RD	RD attached at disc
B Scan	Diagnostic features	Post segment	Retinoblastoma	Hyperechogenic
B Scan	Diagnostic features	Sclera	Posterior scleritis	Fluid posterior to sclera

B Scan	Diagnostic features	Optic Disc	Optic disc Drusen	Hyperechogenic
B scan	Diagnostic features	Choroid	Malignant melanoma	Smooth round elevation Relative hypoechogenic Choroidal excavation Orbital shadow
B Scan	Diagnostic features	Choroid	Haemangioma	v. Hyperechogenic Smooth elevation
B Scan	Diagnostic features	Choroid	Metastasis	Irregular shaped Hyperechogenic Irregular internal structure
B Scan	Localization	Eye	IOFB	Hyperechogenic
B Scan	Delineate extent	Periorbital	Haemangioma	Varies
B scan	Size assessment	Eye Extraocular m	Thyroid eye dis./ myositis	

Further reading

Boldt HC, Byrne SF, DiBernardo C. Echographic evaluation of optic disc drusen. *Journal of Clinical Neuro-Ophthalmology* 1991; **11**(2): 85–91.

Byrne SF. Standardised echography in the differentiation of orbital lesions. *Surveys of Ophthalmology* 1984; **29**(3): 226–8.

Byrne SF, Green RL. *Ultrasound of the Eye and Orbit*. St Louis, Mosby-Year Book, Inc.

Cushmano A, Coleman DJ, Silverman RH *et al*. Three-dimensional ultrasound imaging. Clinical applications. *Ophthalmology* 1998; **105**(2): 300–6.

Flaharty DM, Lieb WE, Sergott RC *et al*. Color Doppler imaging. A new non-invasive technique to diagnose and monitor carotid cavernous sinus fistulas. *Archives of Ophthalmology* 1991; **109**(4): 522–6.

Fuller DG, Snyder WB, Hutton WI, Vaiser A. Ultrasonographic features of choroidal malignant melanomas. *Archives of Ophthalmology* 1979; **97**(8): 1465–72.

Lieb WE, Cohen SM, Merton DA *et al*. Color Doppler imaging of the eye and orbit: technique and normal vascular anatomy. *Archives of Ophthalmology* 1991; **109**(4): 527–31.

Ossoinig KC. Standardised echography: basic principles, clinical applications and results. *International Ophthalmology Clinics* 1979; **19**(4): 283–5.

Pavlin CJ, Harasiewicz K, Sherar MD, Foster FS. Clinical use of UBM. *Ophthalmology* 1991; **98**(3): 287–95.

Related topics of interest

OPTIC ATROPHY

Mike Burdon

Optic atrophy is a pathological term referring to optic nerve shrinkage caused by degeneration of retinal ganglion cell axons.

Problem

Optic atrophy is not a diagnosis, but rather a sign of disease affecting some part of the visual pathway. In adults this means the retinogeniculate section of the visual pathway. Glaucoma is the most common cause of optic atrophy. However, the changes to the optic disc caused by glaucoma differ from those caused by non-glaucomatous disease, and the diagnosis (of glaucoma) is not usually in doubt. Optic nerve disease in the presence of pre-existing amblyopia is particularly difficult to diagnose.

Background

Clinically, non-glaucomatous optic atrophy is recognized by diffuse or segmental pallor of the optic disc accompanied by evidence of optic nerve dysfunction (loss of visual acuity, field, colour vision, and a relative afferent pupil defect). Depending on the underlying aetiology, optic disc pallor may be accompanied by optic disc swelling, thinning of the neuroretinal rim, retinociliary collateral vessels, peripapillary nerve fibre defects and retinal arteriolar attenuation.

In contrast to other causes of optic atrophy, glaucoma does not cause pallor of the remaining neuroretinal rim. Furthermore, glaucomatous field defects tend to occur with glaucomatous cupping. Loss of visual acuity is a marker of very advanced disease. By comparison, the other causes of optic atrophy frequently cause loss of both visual acuity and visual field with only minimal, if any, optic disc cupping.

The pathological changes resulting in optic disc pallor (loss of nerve axons, reduced blood supply, and the formation of glial tissue) develop over a period of at least 4–6 weeks, and are permanent. By the time that optic atrophy is apparent, the underlying disease process may either have resolved (e.g. anterior ischaemic optic neuropathy) or still be active (e.g. compressive optic neuropathy).

The management of optic atrophy is firstly to try to establish the underlying aetiology. This may lead to treatment that either improves the vision in the affected eye, or minimizes the risk to the fellow eye. Where a diagnosis cannot be established, it is important to monitor visual function in order to determine whether there is evidence of progressive visual loss that would require further investigation.

Differential diagnosis

The differential diagnosis of non-glaucomatous optic atrophy encompasses a wide range of diseases affecting the eye, optic nerve chiasm or optic tract. A limited differential diagnosis is listed in the following table.

1. Congenital optic neuropathies
- Isolated: dominant, recessive, Leber's hereditary optic neuropathy
- Associated with other neurological or systemic disease

2. Extrinsic compression
- Pituitary adenoma
- Intracranial meningioma
- Craniopharyngioma
- Metastasis
- Aneurysm
- Mucocele
- Papilloma

3. Intrinsic optic nerve tumours
- Optic nerve glioma
- Optic nerve sheath meningioma
- Lymphoma

4. Vascular disease
- Anterior and non-arteritic anterior ischaemic optic neuropathy
- Central retinal artery occlusion

5. Inflammatory disease
- Demyelinating optic neuritis
- Sarcoidosis
- Systemic lupus erythematosus
- Polyarteritis nodosa
- Chrug–Strauss syndrome
- Sinusitis

6. Infection
- Syphilis
- Tuberculosis
- Lyme disease
- Aspergillosis
- Cryptococcus
- Chicken pox
- Measles
- Mumps

7. Toxic and nutritional optic neuropathies

8. Trauma
- To optic nerve
- Compression from haematoma
- Damage from orbital fracture

9. Swollen optic nerve
- Papilloedema
- Anterior ischaemic optic neuropathy

10. Retinal disease
- Retinitis pigmentosa
- Macular dystrophies

Clinical features

Symptoms consistent with optic nerve disease including blurring or loss of part or the whole of the visual field, reduced colour saturation and dimming of vision. Not all patients with optic atrophy are aware of when they lost vision. Unilateral visual loss may not be noticed unless the patient has occasion to compare the vision of one eye with the other. Bilateral loss may progress so slowly that the patient subconsciously adapts to the visual impairment. Where visual loss can be accurately dated, it is important to determine whether sight was lost acutely or over days or months.

Important points in the history include the patient's age, the presence or absence of symptoms such as headache, proptosis and diplopia, past medical history, current and past medications, occupation and family history. If a systemic inflammatory disease is suspected, specific inquiry should be made into past thrombotic episodes, respiratory disease, skin disease and joint disease.

All patients must have the visual acuities, colour vision and visual fields of both eyes assessed. This aids diagnosis and provides a baseline for repeat tests. When interpreting the visual field it is essential to remember that compressive optic neuropathies may produce any pattern of field loss. Field defects respecting the vertical midline in one or both eyes suggest a peri-chiasmal lesion. Bilateral central scotomas are characteristic of inherited optic neuropathies, toxic or nutritional optic neuropathies.

The optic disc should be carefully examined for clues to the underlying diagnosis. Optic disc swelling and retinociliary collateral vessels both suggest an optic nerve sheath meningioma, glioma or chronic papilloedema. Bowtie atrophy is seen with chiasmal compression. The list of possible causes of optic atrophy makes a complete ocular and systemic examination essential. Specific attention should be paid to the retina and retinal vessels, eye movements, the presence or absence of proptosis, and the cranial nerves. Sometimes, the diagnosis can only be made by examining the patient's relatives.

The number of investigations performed is determined by the clinical findings. Unless there is an obvious alternative, it is essential to exclude a compressive optic neuropathy by neuroimaging of the anterior visual pathways. Having excluded a compressive lesion, an older patient with cardiovascular risk factors who has an altitudinal field defect has almost certainly suffered an episode of anterior ischaemic optic neuropathy, and probably only requires an ESR measurement to exclude giant cell arteritis. By contrast, a young patient with unexplained optic atrophy may undergo extensive investigation similar to that described for atypical optic neuritis.

Treatment

This is based on whether an underlying diagnosis has been established. Treatment may be available to improve vision in the affected eye (e.g. surgery to remove a compressive lesion), or to reduce the risk to the fellow eye (e.g. treatment of vascular risk factors).

When initial investigations fail to identify an underlying cause, patients should be monitored for at least 6 months with repeated assessments of their visual function. Progressive visual loss suggests that the underlying disease process is still active, and the patient should be reinvestigated for compressive, infiltrative or inflammatory disease.

1. *Inherited optic neuropathies.* See separate topic.

2. *Toxic optic neuropathy.* A wide range of substances and vitamin deficiencies are known or suspected to cause optic neuropathy. They include amiodarone, chloramphenicol, ethambutol, isoniazid, lead, tobacco and vitamin B12 deficiency. Typically the neuropathy progresses slowly and symmetrically producing central scotomas with loss of visual acuity and colour vision. The optic discs may initially be normal or hyperaemic, but, if untreated, they will eventually develop temporal pallor. It is important to remember that compressive lesions may cause bilateral central scotomas. Therefore, neuroimaging of the anterior visual pathway is advisable before making a diagnosis of a toxic or nutritional optic neuropathy.

Ethambutol is one of the most clinically significant causes of toxic optic neuropathy because of its frequent and prolonged use in the treatment of tuberculosis. At present the British National Formulary advises that it should normally only be prescribed for the first 2 months of treatment. Screening of visual acuity, colour vision, central visual field is advisable before and during treatment. Cessation of ethambutol treatment usually, but not invariably leads to an improvement in vision.

Patients with so-called tobacco/alcohol amblyopia frequently neglect their nutrition and there is some debate as to whether toxicity or nutritional deficiency is responsible for the optic neuropathy. Treatment by abstinence and vitamin supplementation (B vitamins including B12, and folate) can lead to dramatic improvement in visual function.

Further reading

Bajandas FJ, Kline LLB. *Neuro-Ophthalmology Review Manual*, 3rd edn. Thorofare, NJ; SLACK, 1988; 135–40.

Dutton JJ. Optic nerve sheath meningioma. *Survey in Ophthalmology* 1992; **37**: 167–83.

Glaser J. Diseases of the optic nerve. In: Miller S (ed.) *Clinical Ophthalmology*. Bristol: IOP Publishing, 1987; 321–40.

Lessell S. Toxic and deficiency optic neuropathies. In: Miller NR, Newman NJ (Editors), *Walsh & Hoyt's Clinical Neuro-Ophthalmology*, Vol. one, 5th edn. William & Wilkins, Baltimore, 1998; 663–79.

Quigley HA, Anderson DR. The histologic basis of optic disc pallor. *American Journal of Ophthalmology* 1997; **83**: 709–17.

Riordan-Eva P, Sanders MMD, Govan GG, Sweeney MG, Da Costa J, Harding AE. The clinical features of Leber's hereditary optic neuropathy defined by the presence of a pathogenic mitochondrial DNA mutation. *Brain* 1995; **118**: 319–37.

Related topics of interest

Anisocoria (p. 16); Clinical colour-vision testing (p. 60); Giant cell arteritis (p. 124); Multiple sclerosis and the visual system (p. 164); Neurofibromatosis (p. 180); Non-arteritic anterior ischaemic optic neuropathy (p. 185); Optic atrophy in childhood (p. 213); Optic neuritis (p. 217); Toxicology: drugs for non-ocular diseases (p. 319); Visual-evoked potential testing in children (p. 344); Visual field testing (p. 348).

OPTIC ATROPHY IN CHILDHOOD

David E. Laws & Mike Burdon

Optic atrophy in childhood presents its own specific problems in diagnosis and management. The wide variety of pathological mechanisms and anatomical sites that result in optic atrophy mean that a systematic approach to management is particularly important.

Problem

The severity of optic atrophy in children may vary from an incidental finding that will not affect quality of life to a portent of blinding or life-threatening disease. The diagnosis may also be made difficult in children by confusion with disorders mimicking atrophy, such as Bergemeister's papilla, myopia and optic nerve hypoplasia.

Background

Optic atrophy in children may occur due to disease in the retina, optic nerve or caused by disorders elsewhere in the visual pathway. Damage to the visual pathway posterior to the lateral geniculate body can cause trans-synaptic optic atrophy if the timing of the injury occurs earlier enough in gestation (thought to be 30 weeks).

Differential diagnosis

The infant optic nerve may have a normal appearance that is slightly grey. Optic nerve hypoplasia may mimic atrophy if surrounded by a sclera ring. This can be differentiated by the presence of this double ring sign. Maturity of the healing response may determine the subsequent development of either hypoplasia or atrophy. If a glial response happens atrophy will result, but if an intrauterine insult occurs prior to the development of this healing mechanism hypoplasia will occur. This is thought to be after 30 days and before 10 weeks gestation. High myopia may give an appearance that can be mistaken for atrophy. Embryological remnants of hyaloid vessels on the disc (Bergemeister's papilla) leave white glial tissue over the cup. A disc coloboma will produce a white chorioretinal defect extending inferonasally from the disc margin. Morning glory discs have excavation of the fundus involving the disc, often with vessels entering the eye separately, but they are not usually pale. Myelinated fibres should not be mistaken for disc pallor. Infiltrative lesions such as from leukaemia or sarcoidosis may cause disc pallor in children.

Aetiology

1. CNS disease. Retrograde trans-synaptic degeneration is recognized more commonly in children than adults. Cerebral damage from meningitis, periventricular haemorrhage, cerebral tumours or porencephalic cyst may present as atrophy. Periventricular leucomalacia may be present in premature infants and cause retrograde optic atrophy. Disc pallor may be a sign of hydrocephalus, either new or as a result of a blocked shunt. Raised intracranial pressure leads to disorganization of the nerve fibres so that the disc appears grey and the degree of pallor underestimated. This is particularly difficult to assess when raised intracranial pressure occurs with craniosynostotic conditions which may have chronic swelling related to poor venous drainage. Neurometabolic diseases may have direct nerve toxicity or result in damage due to central effects. Storage diseases need to be considered, although the retinal signs predominate.

2. *Chiasmal compression.* Craniopharyngioma is the most common supratentorial tumour in childhood and causes band atrophy. The subtle appearance may delay diagnosis. The presence of dissociated vertical nystagmus is very suggestive of chiasmal lesion. Endocrine problems must be excluded in a child with chiasmal problems as pituitary dysfunction may coexist. Hypothalamic damage in association with chiasmal tumours can cause the diencephalic syndrome or be associated with clinical features similar to spasmus nutans.

3. *Optic nerve.* Optic nerve glioma associated with neurofibromatosis may extend to the chiasm causing variable visual loss and with variable rates of growth. Radiation or surgery for chiasmal tumours may damage the visual pathway. Post-infectious optic neuritis is uncommon and can result in atrophy. Possible causes include measles, mumps, chickenpox and other viral illnesses. Disc swelling can be prominent and associated with a macula star (Leber idiopathic stellate neuro-retinitis). The aetiology is unknown but an autoimmune process is suggested. Intravenous methylprednisolone can result in dramatic improvement of vision, and is to be considered in bilateral cases.

The association of noninfectious optic neuritis and multiple sclerosis is less clear.

4. *Orbit.* Contiguous inflammation from sinus disease may also damage the optic nerve. Compression from orbital tumours or abnormal bone growth (e.g. fibrous dysplasia) can also cause optic nerve damage. Assessment of orbital disease is therefore a part of optic atrophy assessment.

5. *Ocular.* Loss of ganglion cells in primary retinal disease will result in atrophy. If pigmentary retinal changes are not present arteriolar narrowing should be excluded. Many retinal dystrophies are associated with refractive errors. Irregularities in the internal limiting membrane may be an early sign of juvenile retinal dystrophy. An electroretinogram should be performed if a retinal problem is suspected. Glaucoma should be considered in a child with a pale disc with an enlarged cup.

6. *Hereditary.* Autosomal dominant atrophy is the most common pattern of inheritance (approximately 1:10000) with a high degree of penetrance but variable expressivity. The condition may be found on routine screening and families may only be aware of a vague history of poor vision amongst relatives. Onset is around 10 years of age and visual loss is usually stable but may be slowly progressive. Vision may be reduced to 6/24 but may be as good as 6/9 and as poor as 3/60. Blue yellow dyschromatopsia is characteristic. The disc appearance has typical sectoral temporal pallor with relative sparing of the nasal portion.

Leber hereditary optic atrophy is inherited via mitochondrial DNA from the maternal line and affects males more commonly. Three primary mutations are recognized, 11778, 33460 and 14484. There is a wide variety of age of presentation from the first to the sixth decade, but rapid onset sequential bilateral asymmetrical visual loss usually occurs in the second or third decade. Up to 25% of affected patients suffer simultaneous visual loss. Patients develop central scotomas that worsen over 4–6 weeks, resulting in visual acuities that range from 6/9 to vague perception of light. The disc may be noted to have telangiectatic vessels, but this is not a universal finding. No treatment is available but some patients experience spontaneous partial recovery, which may start several years after onset of visual loss. Younger patients and those with the 14484 mutation are the most likely to recover vision. Questions that remain unanswered include: what triggers the visual loss, not all patients with the mutation develop the disease, why are males more commonly affected and why the percentage of abnormal mDNA does not correlate with the risk of visual loss?

Autosomal recessive atrophy is severe and rare but more common in consanguineous relationships. Presentation is usually shortly after birth with poor vision and nystagmus. Visual acuity is usually 6/60 or worse. Before the diagnosis is made intracranial lesions must be excluded by neuroimaging and retinal diseases excluded by electroretinography. Wolfram syndrome is a constellation of diabetes insipidus, diabetes mellitus, optic atrophy and deafness (DIDMOAD) but renal disease and ptosis, amongst others, have been reported. Behr optic atrophy is found predominantly in males and is associated with severe cerebella ataxia hypotonia, external ophthalmoplegia and developmental problems.

7. Miscellaneous. Trauma can affect any part of the visual system and non-accidental injury should be considered in children with either unilateral or bilateral atrophy. Toxic drugs should be excluded particularly if anti-tuberculous treatment has been given. Vigabatrin is increasingly being recognized as a cause of optic nerve damage and is very difficult to monitor in children. Vigabatrin prevents GABA breakdown and clinically presents with optic atrophy and pseudo cupping presumably due to retinal toxicity. Heavy metal exposure or nutritional problems can rarely damage the optic nerve.

Clinical features

1. Presentation. This may be with reduced vision, nystagmus or disc pallor found on routine examination or screening. The presentation of reduced vision depends on the severity and age at which it occurs. Babies may not fix on the mother's face when feeding or react to bright toys. If the onset is rapid, toddlers may bump into things and older children might ask for the light to be turned on in the daytime. Nystagmus may be the presenting feature of more severe optic atrophy in infants, particularly if visual loss occurs before 2 years of age. Less severe forms may be detected at routine screening or by specific screening of patients at risk from an associated condition or family history.

2. History. A search for causes should included the following. Antenatal history of febrile illness may indicate transplacental spread of infection. Excess maternal alcohol consumption during pregnancy should also be excluded. Prematurity is associated with periventricular leukomalacia, intraventricular haemorrhage and hydrocephalus, all of which can cause optic atrophy. Specific enquiries should be made about birth trauma, meningitis and other neurological problems. A working knowledge of developmental milestones is invaluable. Nystagmus is associated with a disease onset before 2 years, but may be acquired later as well. It is essential to ask about family history and consanguinity; it only takes a few minutes to record a three generation family tree. If visual loss is a presenting feature the level of vision before the rate at which vision was lost and the current stability of vision should be assessed.

3. Examination.   Vision should be recorded using a method appropriate to the child's age but normal vision does not exclude atrophy. Eye movements are examined with particular attention to any nystagmus. A horizontal conjugate nystagmus is the most common pattern. Chiasmal compression can cause a vertical dissociated (seesaw) nystagmus. A relative afferent pupil defect will indicate asymmetrical disease and sluggish pupils are associated with severe anterior visual pathway pathology. Signs of orbital disease such as proptosis may indicate optic nerve compression. Colour vision tests can also help to confirm optic nerve disease with yellow/blue problems being more common. Fundoscopy should be undertaken so that the disc, macula and retinal periphery are clearly seen. The appearance of the disc is not usually helpful in identifying the site of the lesion but band atrophy can indicate damage to decussating fibres (NB – the temporal fibres between the fovea and disc serve the nasal field). Thinning of the nerve fibre layer causes the small vessels between the disc and the macula to become proud of the internal limiting reflex disturbing its reflection. Static or kinetic perimetry can be undertaken in older children giving information about the site of the lesion. Failing this the fields of smaller children can be grossly assessed using simple finger waggling which can be made into a game. Any previously well child who develops optic atrophy should have a thorough neurological examination.

Conclusion

The finding of optic atrophy in a child has a wide variety of visual, anatomic and systemic implications. The astute clinician can steer a course through this diagnostic maze reducing unnecessary investigation to a minimum but being alert to more serious possibilities. Electrodiagnostic tests are relatively non-invasive and if CNS or systemic disease cannot be excluded paediatric referral and neuroimaging are indicated.

Further reading

Brodsky MC, Baker RS, Hamed LM. In: *Pediatric Neuro-Ophthalmology.* New York: Springer Verlag, 1996.
Online Mendelian Inheritance in Man: *http://www.ncbi.nlm.nih.gov/Omim/searchomim.html*
Taylor D. Optic nerve: Congenital abnormalities. In: Taylor D (ed.). *Paediatric Ophthalmology.* 2nd edn. Blackwell Science Ltd, 1997; 660–718.
Wilson ME, Buckley EG, Kivlin JD, Ruttum MS, Simon JW, Magoon EH. Pediatric Ophthalmology Section 6. *American Academy of Ophthalmology* 1999; 300–2.

Related topics of interest

OPTIC NEURITIS

Mike Burdon & Oliver Backhouse

Optic neuritis is typically an acute demyelinating inflammation of the optic nerve. The inflammation may be idiopathic or associated with multiple sclerosis. The incidence of optic neuritis is between one and five per 100 000 per year. Women are affected three times more commonly than men. Approximately one third of patients with idiopathic optic neuritis will develop multiple sclerosis within 5 years. This risk increases with longer follow up, and is greater for women than men.

Problem

Patients with demyelinating optic neuritis usually present with characteristic features that allow a clinical diagnosis to be made. The diagnosis carries important management and prognostic implications, not least of which is the reassurance, both to the patient and the clinician, that the majority of affected eyes will recover vision over a period of several months. However, the differential diagnosis of demyelinating optic neuritis includes many conditions that require urgent treatment to prevent permanent visual loss. The ability to recognize an atypical presentation is essential to avoid misdiagnosis.

Background

The differential diagnosis of demyelinating optic neuritis includes local and systemic inflammatory disease (sinusitis, sarcoidosis, systemic lupus erythematosus; polyarteritis nodosa; Churg–Strauss), infection (syphilis, tuberculosis, Lyme disease, cryptococcus, aspergillus), vascular disease (arteritic and non-arteritic ischaemic optic neuropathy), tumours and compression (meningioma, glioma, pituitary adenoma, lymphoma, metastasis, aneurysm, mucocele), and miscellaneous causes (toxic, Leber's hereditary optic neuropathy).

Clinical features

Demyelinating optic neuritis is a clinical diagnosis. The Optic Neuritis Treatment Trial (ONTT) has confirmed that investigations are not required. This study recruited 457 patients between the ages of 18 and 45 years old who had an acute clinical syndrome consistent with unilateral optic neuritis, with visual symptoms of 8 days duration or less; a relative afferent pupil defect; and a visual field defect in the affected eye. All patients underwent a brain MRI scan, a chest X-ray, and haematological investigations for syphilis, antinuclear antibodies and diabetes. One patient was found to have a pituitary adenoma. Six had positive syphilis serology but no evidence of active disease. Fifteen had an antinuclear antibody titre greater than 1:320 of whom only one was later diagnosed as having a collagen tissue disease.

In order to be able to make a confident clinical diagnosis one must have a clear understanding of the features of a typical episode of optic neuritis.

1. Age. Demyelinating disease usually presents between the ages of 16 and 50. Patents outside this age range should be investigated, even if they have 'typical' symptoms.

2. *Visual loss.* Typical optic neuritis presents with unilateral loss of acuity, visual field and colour perception, and a relative afferent pupil defect. Symptomatic bilateral visual loss is atypical and requires investigation. Data from the ONTT confirms that neither the degree nor the pattern of visual loss can be used to distinguish typical optic neuritis from other unilateral optic neuropathies. At presentation patients had visual acuities ranging from $\geq 6/6$ to no perception of light (NPL). Their visual field loss was diffuse in 48% or focal nerve fibre bundle defects in 52% (altitudinal, arcuate, nasal step, central or centrocaecal, hemianopic or quadrantic). In adults, 14–48% may have subclinical acuity, field or colour abnormalities in the other eye on presentation. Bilateral involvement is more common in children. Approximately 10% of patients will later experience worsening of their symptoms in hot environments – Uhtoffs phenomenon due to interference of axonal conduction. By contrast, the rate of visual loss is an important distinguishing feature. A patient with typical optic neuritis experiences progressive visual loss over several days to one week, and recovery beginning by 1 month. Sudden, non-progressive visual loss is characteristic of vascular disease, whilst loss progressing over weeks or months suggests a compressive optic neuropathy.

3. *Pain.* Over 90% of patients in the ONTT experienced ocular or orbital pain. Typically, the pain is exacerbated by eye movement, and it frequently precedes the onset of visual symptoms. The presence of pain is not diagnostic but the absence of it may suggest an alternative diagnosis to demyelinating optic neuropathy and should therefore initiate investigation – see below. Similar pain occurs much less frequently with other inflammatory or infectious optic neuropathies, anterior ischaemic optic neuropathy and Leber's hereditary optic neuropathy.

4. *Photopsia.* Thirty per cent of patients experience photopsia which can take the form of flashing black squares/light or showers of sparks which are often precipitated by ocular movement.

5. *Colour.* Red desaturation may be much worse than the visual acuity measured.

6. *Fundoscopy.* Optic disc swelling occurs in only a third of patients with typical optic neuritis. Mild peripheral periphlebitis and only a few cells in the vitreous or anterior chamber may be present, but marked intraocular inflammation is atypical. Such patients should be investigated for other inflammatory diseases.

In summary, a typical episode of demyelinating optic neuritis presents between the ages of 16 and 50 years with symptomatic unilateral loss of vision that progresses over few days to one week, a relative afferent pupil defect, colour desaturation, reduced bright light appreciation, periocular pain that is exacerbated by eye movement, and a normal optic disc in 65% without any marked intraocular inflammatory findings. At 5 weeks 93% of patients have shown signs of optic nerve function recovery.

Patients who do not present with typical features of demyelinating optic neuritis should have a detailed history taken, looking for evidence of current or previous neurological or systemic disease. Particular attention should be given to previous thrombotic episodes, respiratory disease, skin rashes and joint problems. A family history of eye disease may be significant, particularly for Leber's hereditary optic neuropathy. The range of possible investigations is extensive and should be guided by the history.

7. Investigations. The Humphrey 24:2 programme is the field analysis recommended but this may be impossible if the patient has a dense central scotoma. Fields should be done on presentation and 6/52 later if acuity permits.

In a typical case there is no need for the ophthalmologist to perform an MRI scan. It does not give any information about the outcome of optic neuritis, they do not predict MS disability and the decision to 'treat' should not be based on the number/size of 'presumed' demyelinating plaques. Visual-evoked potentials are not needed for diagnosis in the acute setting. They are useful in helping form the diagnosis of multiple sclerosis in a patient who may have had asymptomatic optic neuritis.

A CT orbital scan or gadolinium-enhanced MRI scan of brain and orbits may be appropriate in certain 'atypical cases' to help rule out compressive or infiltrative causes. A chest X-ray may show signs of sarcoidosis, tuberculosis, or a systemic vasculitis.

Patients with an atypical clinical picture should have screening tests for systemic inflammatory disease (full blood count, erythrocyte sedimentation rate, C reactive protein, renal and liver function tests, serum angiotensin converting enzyme, anti-nuclear antibodies, anti-neutrophil cytoplasmic antibodies, syphilis serology). If Leber's hereditary optic neuropathy is suspected mitochondrial DNA should be analysed. Cerebrospinal fluid should be examined for cytology, protein, and oligoclonal bands.

Treatment

Many people have easy access to information on the prognosis of optic neuritis from the Internet and may ask about the link with multiple sclerosis and interferon treatment. At the very least, you will need to provide information about the chances of good visual recovery etc. It may be reasonable to warn the patient that further ophthalmological or neurological episodes could occur. It is not mandatory to discuss the link with multiple sclerosis (MS). This is only necessary if the link is volunteered by the patient.

The ONTT compared treatment with intravenous methylprednisolone 250 mg four times a day for 3 days followed by oral prednisolone 1 mg/kg/day for 11 days (ONTT steroids), with oral prednisolone 1 mg/kg/day for 14 days, and on oral placebo. At 1 year there was no difference in visual function, but those patients treated with intravenous methylprednisolone experienced a more rapid visual recovery. Patients in the intravenous treatment group also had a reduced rate of developing multiple sclerosis, if their MRI scans had a multiple signal abnormalities. However, at 3 years, this apparent protective effect was found to have worn off. Unexpectedly, treatment with oral prednisolone alone was associated with an increased rate of optic neuritis in the fellow eye compared to the other two groups and is not frequently used alone now. They found that the T2 MRI scan had the greatest predictive score for the future development of MS.

There is currently a lot of debate regarding the early treatment of optic neuritis in order to prevent the onset of clinically definite MS and some people are advocating earlier more aggressive treatment. The purpose of the CHAMPS study (Controlled High Risk Subjects Avonex Multiple Sclerosis Prevention Study) was 'to determine if the Interferon beta-1a drug Avonex may delay the occurrence of a second attack in patients with acute monosymptomatic syndromes and positive brain MRI scans consistent with MS'. From 50 centres in Canada and the USA, 383 patients, aged 18–50 years, with a monosymptomatic event less than 3 weeks old and two 'MS-like' MRI lesions were given intravenous methylprednisolone 250 mg four times a day for 3 days followed by oral prednisolone 1mg/kg/day for 11 days and weekly Avonex or placebo. The trial was stopped early as it was found that at 3 years, the treatment group had a reduced rate of developing clinically definite MS, fewer new brain lesions and fewer enlarging and enhancing lesions. Many neurologists would have liked the trial to continue as these findings do not tell us anything regarding future disability of MS. Different imaging techniques such as magnetic resonance spectrography may help better correlate the findings of an MR scan and symptomatic disability of an individual which is currently poor with regard to T2-weighted MRI scans. The results of the ETOMS study (Early Treatment Of Multiple Sclerosis), which used a different interferon beta-1a drug, Refib, and looked at mono/poly-symptomatic events within 3 months, are still awaited. Currently these treatments are expensive and it is not known how long treatment should be continued in order to see a lasting clinical benefit.

In atypical cases, as some patients have a steroid-responsive or steroid-dependent optic neuropathy, a trial of intravenous methylprednisolone (usually 1 g for 3 days) should be considered unless there is evidence of an infectious aetiology.

Prognosis

Over 90% get Snellen visual acuity better than 6/9. In those patients whose vision descends to NPL, 64% achieve 6/9 or better eventually. In those patients who have less than 6/60, 6% are still <6/60 at 6 months. A quarter have a recurrent episode within 5 years, and a half of these occur in the first year. With subsequent events visual recovery decreases. Less than 1% has visual acuity less than 6/9 in both eyes at 5 years. Uhtoff and Pulfrich phenomenon and red desaturation may persist.

Further reading

De Stefano N *et al.* Evidence of axonal damage in the early stages of multiple sclerosis and its relevance to disability. *Archives of Neurology* 2001; **58:** 65–70.

Frohman E. To treat or not to treat. The new therapeutic dilemma of idiopathic monosymptomatic demyelinating syndromes. *Archives of Neurology* 2000; **57:** 930–2.

Jacobs L. Intramuscular interferon beta-1a therapy during a first demyelinating event in multiple sclerosis. *New England Journal of Medicine* 2000; **343:** 898–904.

Optic Neuritis Study Group. The clinical profile of optic neuritis. Experience of the Optic Neuritis Treatment Trial. *Archives of Ophthalmology* 1991; **109:** 1673–8.

Optic Neuritis Study Group. The 5-year risk of MS after optic neuritis. Experience of the ONTT. *Neurology* 1997; **49:** 1404–13.

O'Riordan J. The prognostic value of brain MRI in clinically isolated syndromes of the CNS. A 10 year follow-up. *Brain* 1998; **121:** 495–503.

Related topics of interest

Multiple sclerosis and the visual system (p. 164); Optic atrophy (p. 208).

ORBITAL BLOWOUT FRACTURES

Brian Leatherbarrow

The term pure orbital blowout fracture is used to describe a fracture of the orbital floor, the medial orbital wall or both, with an intact bony orbital margin. The term impure orbital blowout fracture is used when such fractures occur in conjunction with a fracture of the orbital rim e.g. as part of a zygomatic complex fracture. The most common site for a blowout fracture to occur is in the posteromedial aspect of the orbital floor, medial to the infraorbital neurovascular bundle where the maxillary bone is very thin. As the lamina papyracea is also very thin, the medial orbital wall is also prone to fracture.

Problem

Blowout fracture is common but easy to miss. There is debate about the indications, timing and type of surgical intervention.

Background

There are two mechanisms thought to be responsible for pure orbital wall blowout fractures: the backward displacement of the globe caused by a blunt non-penetrating injury, which raises the intraorbital pressure sufficiently to cause a fracture and a transient deformation of the orbital rim transmitting the force of injury directly to the orbital wall.

The weak areas of the orbital walls provide some means of protection to the globe and orbital tissues, permitting these to expand into the maxillary antrum and/or ethmoid sinus. Although a rupture of the globe can complicate such fractures, this occurrence is rare. Conversely, any patient who has suffered blunt trauma sufficient to cause a ruptured globe has an orbital wall blowout fracture until proven otherwise. Such a fracture is commonly overlooked. In addition a high index of suspicion should be maintained for the presence of a blowout fracture in any patient who has sustained blunt periorbital trauma. Any patient who has sustained blunt orbital trauma should undergo a complete ophthalmic examination as the incidence of ocular injuries has been reported as 14–30%. The possibility of a globe rupture must always be considered and excluded before a forced duction test is performed.

Clinical features

The patient's clinical signs will depend on the timing of the examination in relation to the traumatic episode. A patient presenting some months after the traumatic event may have enophthalmos as the only physical sign. In the immediate post-trauma period, eyelid ecchymosis and haematoma are usually present, but may be absent in the so-called 'white eyed blowout fracture'. Subcutaneous or subconjunctival emphysema may be present if the fracture creates a communication with an air-filled sinus. Neurosensory loss in the distribution of the infraorbital nerve is almost pathognomonic and includes altered sensation in the ipsilateral cheek, upper teeth or tip of the nose. This occurs when the fracture extends along the infraorbital groove or canal injuring the infraorbital nerve. It is not present in all patients. Limitation of ocular motility may exist but does not prove that a fracture has occurred. Limitation in up-gaze is the commonest sequelae of a floor fracture. Limitation of abduction in the presence of a medial orbital wall blowout fracture is less commonly seen. The mechanisms, which may be responsible for limitation of ocular motility, are: entrapment of connective tissue septa or an extraocular muscle within the fracture, haematoma and/or oedema in the orbital fat adjacent to the fracture, haematoma or contusion of an extraocular muscle(s), palsy of an extraocular muscle(s) due to neuronal damage and/or Volkmann's ischaemic contracture of an entrapped extraocular muscle.

Enophthalmos can result from an enlarged orbital volume and varies from insignificant to cosmetically disfiguring. Fat atrophy contributes little if anything to the enophthalmos. It may be masked by orbital haematoma/oedema/air which can cause early proptosis. Hypoglobus is seen in the presence of extensive orbital floor blowout fractures. Very rarely, the globe may come to lie within the maxillary antrum or even within the ethmoid sinus. Enophthalmos results in decreased support of the upper eyelid, which leads to a secondary pseudoptosis and an upper eyelid sulcus deformity.

Any proptosis or enophthalmos should be measured using a Hertel exophthalmometer. Any vertical displacement of the globe should also be measured and recorded. The eyelids and periorbital tissues should be palpated for subcutaneous emphysema and for any orbital rim fractures. The malar eminences should be palpated and any depression noted. The patient should be asked to open and close his/her mouth to ensure there is no associated pain or trismus. Such signs and symptoms are suggestive of a zygomatic complex fracture. A record of the extent of any infraorbital sensory loss should be made.

A full orthoptic assessment should be performed including a Hess chart, a monocular and binocular visual field assessment. A forced duction test and an active force-generation test are useful in differentiating extraocular muscle paralysis from tissue entrapment. A patient with tissue entrapment will often experience pain on attempted globe movement in the direction of restriction.

A CT scan should be performed in an axial plane with coronal and sagittal reconstructions. A plain skull X-ray is of little use. CT demonstrates the relationship of the soft tissues to the fracture sites and permits an evaluation of any secondary effects of trauma (e.g. retrobulbar haemorrhage, intraoptic nerve sheath haematoma, subperiosteal haematoma and retained orbital foreign bodies). A CT scan is also useful in assessing complications such as orbital cellulitis and orbital or subperiosteal abscess.

Treatment

Patients should be urged not to blow their nose or to hold the nose when sneezing. The role of antibiotic prophylaxis is controversial. If the CT scan shows evidence of chronic sinusitis antibiotics should be prescribed to prevent a secondary orbital cellulitis.

A number of different specialties compete for the treatment of patients with a blowout fracture and opinions differ concerning the indications for surgery, the timing of surgery, the surgical approach and the use of orbital implant materials.

1. Indications. In general the indications for the surgical repair of a blowout fracture are: unresolving soft tissue entrapment with disabling diplopia, enophthalmos greater than 2 mm, or CT scan evidence of a large fracture.

Patients with diplopia may be observed for a period of up to 2 weeks. If the diplopia resolves and the fracture is small, no surgical intervention is required. There is an important exception to this. Young patients with marked tissue entrapment and a linear fracture on CT (a 'trapdoor' fracture) are at risk of developing an ischaemic contracture unless the tissue entrapment is released very early. This is an indication for very early surgery within 2 days of the injury. Such patients may also suffer problems as a consequence of stimulation of the oculocardiac reflex with nausea, vomiting and severe bradycardia. There may be residual diplopia even after a successful repair of the fracture if there has been extraocular muscle or neuronal damage. Spontaneous improvement may occur over a period of weeks to months. Diplopia can, however, occur in the presence of normal extraocular muscles but with a large fracture and a markedly displaced globe. This is due to a change in the line of muscle pull. Such patients have clinically significant enophthalmos and the decision to proceed with a surgical repair is made on this basis.

It is reasonable to defer operative decisions on the basis of the degree of enophthalmos for 2–3 weeks to determine, in consultation with the patient, whether or not the enophthalmos is cosmetically significant once periorbital oedema has settled. Extensive defects, particularly involving both the orbital floor and medial wall, suggest a high chance of progressive unsightly enophthalmos and support the decision for surgical intervention. The patient must be fully informed of the risks and potential complications of such surgery.

2.   Surgery.   If surgery is elected, a forced duction test should be performed under general anaesthesia before surgery is commenced, and should be repeated once all the entrapped tissue has been freed from the fracture and again after placement of the orbital implant. An orbital floor blowout fracture is usually approached via a lower eyelid incision, which can be made through the skin or the conjunctiva. The former is usually subciliary, although alternatives exist.

The infraorbital nerve is at risk from injury during the dissection as are the infraorbital artery and vein. All margins of the fracture should be exposed and prolapsing structures repositioned in the orbit. Overly aggressive dissection posteriorly risks damage to the optic nerve and other orbital apical structures. Once the prolapsing orbital contents have been lifted out of the fracture site, an implant is placed over the fracture site ensuring that all margins are covered and that no tissue is allowed to herniate from the orbit again. Fixation of an implant is usually unnecessary. If the fracture is so large that there is no posterior support, the implant should then be cantilevered over the fracture with microplates, which are fixated below the inferior orbital margin with screws.

We recommend that the periosteum be closed with 5/0 vicryl, avoiding the orbital septum. The skin is closed with continuous 7.0 vicryl suture. We apply a compressive dressing for an hour and then check the visual acuity and pupil reactions hourly for the first 12 hours. Postoperative eyelid massage is commenced the day after surgery to prevent wound contracture and any eyelid retraction. Prophylactic broad-spectrum antibiotics are prescribed for 7 days postoperatively. The patient must be instructed not to blow the nose for 6 weeks postoperatively.

3.   Complications.   Complications of surgery include visual loss due to intraoperative damage to the globe and/or optic nerve, postoperative orbital haemorrhage and compression of the optic nerve by misplacement of the orbital implant. The sudden occurrence of an orbital haematoma postoperatively may require an emergency orbital decompression with a lateral canthotomy and inferior cantholysis at the bedside.

It is important to warn patients that it is not uncommon for diplopia to be worse in the first few weeks following surgery. It is important however, to ensure that further inadvertent tissue entrapment has not been caused by misplacement of the orbital implant. For this reason the forced duction test must be repeated after placement of the orbital implant.

Lower eyelid retraction may be caused by incorrect closure of the periosteum over the infraorbital margin with inadvertent incorporation of the orbital septum, or adhesions of the orbital septum to the infraorbital margin. A lower lid entropion may occur after contracture of the wound following a transconjunctival approach to an orbital floor fracture. Extrusion of an orbital implant may occur early or late after surgery for a blowout fracture. It may even be seen many years after surgery. It may occur for a number of reasons: infection, the use of an oversized implant or inadequate closure of the periosteum along the inferior orbital margin. Although an infection must be treated with systemic antibiotics, the implant will usually require removal. Late problems with sinusitis may occur.

Patients should be warned about the potential for sensory loss in the distribution of the infraorbital nerve. Identification of the nerve may be difficult in the late management of large orbital floor fractures. Undercorrection of enophthalmos may be seen where there has been significant orbital fat atrophy although this is rare. A persistent orbital volume deficit is usually due to herniation of the posterior aspect of an orbital floor implant into the maxillary antrum due to an inadequately supported implant. It is also seen in cases where a medial wall fracture has not been repaired at the time of an orbital floor fracture repair.

Protopsis/hyperglobus may be seen where an oversized orbital implant has been used. The fellow eye should be uncovered during surgery for comparison of the relative eye positions. Lower lid lymphoedema is seen following inferior orbital rim incisions, which should be avoided.

Chemosis is more commonly seen following a transconjunctival approach to the orbital floor. It may require the temporary placement of a lower eyelid Frost suture with the use of frequent topical lubricants.

Further reading

Bailey WK, Kuo PC, Evans LS. Diagnosis and treatment of retrobulbar haemorrhage. *Journal of Oral and Maxillofacial Surgery* 1993; **51**: 780–2.

Berkowitz RA, Putterman AM, Patel DB. Prolapse of the globe into the maxillary sinus after orbital floor fracture. *American Journal of Ophthalmology* 1981; **91**: 253–7.

Dutton GN, Al-Qurainy I, Stassen LFA, Titterington DM, Moos KF, El-Attar A. Ophthalmic consequences of mid-facial trauma. *Eye* 1992; **6**: 86–9.

Fleishman JA, Beck RW, Hoffinan RO. Orbital emphysema as an ophthalmological emergency. *Ophthalmology* 1984; **91**: 1384–91.

Gilbard SM, Maffee MS, Lagouros PA, Langer BG. Orbital blowout fractures: the prognostic significance of computed tomography. *Ophthalmology* 1985; **92**: 523–8.

Helveston EM. The relationship of extraocular muscle problems to orbital floor fractures: early and late treatment. *Transactions of the American Academy of Ophthalmology* 1977; **83:** 660–2.

Jordan DR, Allen LH, White J *et al.* Intervention within days for some orbital floor fractures: the white-eyed blowout. *Ophthalmic Plastic Reconstructive Surgery* 1998; **14:** 379–90.

Jordan DR, White GL, Anderson RL, Thiese SM. Orbital emphysema: a potentially blinding complication following orbital fractures. *Annals of Emergency Medicine* 1988; **17:** 853–5.

Lindberg JV. Orbital emphysema complicated by acute central retinal artery obstruction. *Annals of Ophthalmology* 1982; **14:** 742–9.

Lipton JR, Page AB, Lee JP. Management of diplopia on downgaze following orbital trauma. *Eye* 1990; **4:** 535–7.

Lyon DB, Newman SA. Evidence of direct damage to extraocular muscles as a cause of diplopia following orbital trauma. *Ophthalmic Plastic Reconstructive Surgery* 1989; **5:** 81–91.

McGurk M, Whitehouse RW, Taylor PM, Swinson B. Orbital volume measured by a low-dose CT scanning technique. *Dento-Maxillo-Facial Radiology* 1992; **21:** 70–2.

Milauskas AT, Fueger GF. Serious ocular complications associated with blowout fractures of the orbit. *American Journal of Ophthalmology* 1966; **62:** 670–2.

Putterman AM. Management of orbital fractures: the conservative approach. *Survey of Ophthalmology* 1991; **92:** 523–8.

Putterman AM, Stevens T, Urist MJ. Nonsurgical management of blowout fractures of the orbital floor. *American Journal of Ophthalmology* 1974; **77:** 232–9.

Ruttum MS, Harris GJ. Orbital blowout fracture with ipsilateral fourth nerve palsy. *American Journal of Ophthalmology* 1985; **100:** 343–4.

Sires BS. Orbital trapdoor fractures and oculocardiac reflex. *Ophthalmic Plastic Reconstructive Surgery* 1999; **15**(4): 301–2.

Smith B, Lisman RD, Simonton J, DellaRocca R. Volkmann's contracture of the extraocular muscles following blowout fracture. *Plastic Reconstructive Surgery* 1984; **74:** 200–9.

Soll DB, Poley BJ. Trapdoor variety of blowout fracture of the orbital floor. *American Journal of Ophthalmology* 1965; **60:** 269–72.

Westfall CT, Shore JW. Isolated fractures of the orbital floor: risk of infection and the role of antibiotic prophlaxis. *Ophthalmic Surgery* 1991; **22:** 409–11.

Wilkins RB, Havins WE. Current treatment of blow-out fractures. *Ophthalmology* 1982; **89:** 464–6.

Wojno TH. The incidence of extraocular muscle and cranial nerve palsy in orbital blowout fracture. *Ophthalmology* 1987; **94:** 682–7.

PHAKOEMULSIFICATION MACHINES (THE NEW GENERATION)

Helen C. Seward & Sarah-Lucie Watson

There is an increasing number of Phakoemulsification machines now available, offering benefits of new programmes and different handpiece styles. They enable the surgeon to use higher vacuum levels and provide improved anterior chamber stability thus allowing greater control and safety when removing nuclei of various densities.

Problem

Burst mode, power pulse, effective Phako time, postocclusion surge, dual linear, angled, flared and ABS tips are some of the recent additions to the Phako language. It is important to understand the terminology and mechanisms of these systems to maximize their benefits.

Burst mode

Burst mode Phako provides fixed power with a variable interval in the application of that power. Burst mode can be controlled either by the surgeon or the panel. With surgeon control, the burst width (i.e. the length of time the ultrasonic burst is on, adjustable from 30 to 500 microseconds) and the ultrasound power are fixed by the programme. The surgeon controls the ultrasound off time which decreases as the foot travels downward on the pedal. The ultrasound is continuous at the end of the footpedal excursion (position 3).

With panel control of burst mode there is a single burst of pre-set length and power which is activated by entry to foot position 3. By returning to foot position 2 and re-entering foot position 3, a second burst occurs. Burst mode is available on the Alcon Legacy™ and Allergan Sovereign™ machines.

Effective Phako time (EPT)

This quantifies the total amount of ultrasound energy delivered to the eye taking into account percentage of power and the total elapsed time, (e.g. 1 minute of Phako time at 20% power is equivalent to 12 seconds EPT).

Phakoemulsification tips

Phako tips now come in a huge variety of designs and angulations. The zero degree tip provides excellent occlusion and is designed primarily for Phako chop surgeons whose technique requires frequent complete occlusions. A 45° tip provides good cutting power. A 30° tip is also available. Standard tips have a 1.1 mm overall diameter. Micro tips with an 0.9 mm overall diameter are said to provide improved chamber stability but are slower to create a vacuum at the tip. Flared tips are now available both on the standard and the micro tip improving the holding power and cutting efficiency. The surge which occurs on occlusion break varies with different tips. The ABS tip has the least surge on occlusion break. Mackool™ tips have an additional inner sleeve for added thermal protection. They are also available in the flared ABS design.

The ABS tip (Alcon) is a Phako tip with a small 0.18 mm hole (the ABS port) drilled in the side wall of the tip approximately 4–5 mm from the tip end. There is virtually no flow through the ABS port when the primary port is unoccluded. When occlusion occurs, irrigation fluid is drawn through the ABS port automatically reducing the aspiration flow rate in relation to the amount of fluid drawn through the ABS port. This allows vacuum to build in a smoother manner and the vacuum created will be approximately 10% less than the pre-set level. When the primary port is fully occluded the ABS port becomes fully active and provides continuous flow. This flow reduces the surge after an occlusion break and improves anterior chamber stability even with utilization of high vacuums.

Dual linear control

Dual linear control enables a surgeon to have simultaneous linear (or proportional) control of two functions: Phako power and aspiration. This is achieved with a pedal that moves in two planes: pitch (up/down) and yaw (side to side). Thus the surgeon can use the pedal in standard 3 position Phako mode and by moving the pedal into the yaw position, aspiration can be increased. In use the surgeon sets a minimum and maximum Phako power and a minimum and maximum aspiration (vacuum on venturi, vacuum or flow on Concentrix™). Thus flow can be kept low for sculpting and delicate manoeuvres, and increased to obtain good followability following cracking. The Sovereign™ machine from Allergan provides a heel or toe based foot pedal, depending on the surgeon's preference.

Computers in Phako machines

Computers both within the Phako machines and in the handpiece greatly help in providing a stable anterior chamber. The Allergan Sovereign™ has a device called the INTELLESIS sensor which incorporates an aspiration line diaphragm which moves in precise synchronization with the vacuum pressure variations at the tip. This on-board fluidics computer monitors and stabilizes conditions 50 times per second and controls the movement of the peristaltic pump. The digital-controlled peristaltic pump can rotate forwards linearly and backwards for controlled release greatly reducing surge.

The Phako handpiece also contains a computer which monitors the handpiece performance by reviewing up to 50 factors for optimization of the ultrasonic vibration, 500 times per second. The handpiece contains a four crystal design which adjusts for changing nuclear density at the tip reducing the Phako power. The vertically mounted Sovereign™ pump constantly purges air bubbles from the aspiration tubing providing greater accuracy.

Laser Phako

Recently, exciting advances have taken place with the development of lasers used in cataract surgery. The two most successful lasers include the NdYag laser system (Dodick Photolysis) and the Erbium laser system (Phakolase, Aesculap-Meditec Co). These procedures can be performed through small incisions (1.4 mm) and transmit much less energy into the eye. They appear to provide good protection of the corneal endothelium, do not heat up the anterior chamber and there is no risk of corneal burns. The Dodick system requires a bimanual technique (2×1.4 mm incisions opposite one another). The high vacuum (up to 400 mmHg) venturi aspiration device reduces operating time. The Phakolase system is used with a peristaltic irrigation/aspiration and bidirectional foot pedal which allows independent adjustment of aspiration and laser power. Harder nuclei require increased surgical time. Currently these systems are more expensive than routine Phako.

Conclusion

The new generation of Phako machines allow a more efficient use of Phako power whilst using vacuum levels which we would not have considered 10 years ago. This combination results in shorter, effective Phako times, quicker surgery and quieter eyes the next day. It also puts the onus on us, as surgeons, to understand the modalities available on the machines to maximize benefits to our patients.

Acknowledgements

I would like to thank Alcon, Allergan, and Bausch and Lomb for their invaluable assistance with the technical data included in this topic.

PHAKOMATOSES

Robert H. Taylor & Peter Shah

The phakomatoses (greek : birthmark) are a group of disorders predominantly affecting the skin, nervous system, and eyes amongst other organs. All are characterized by hamartomatous lesions.

Problem

Early diagnosis is essential to identify those patients who are at risk of the damaging sequelae from disease progression. Within each condition, there are a wide variety of clinical presentations of which the clinician should be aware. Many patients who have a phakomatosis will present to an ophthalmologist as the first specialist physician.

Neurofibromatosis

Neurofibromatosis is traditionally divided into type 1 and type 2 although there may be other subtypes (e.g. segmental, orbital). See Neurofibromatosis.

Tuberous sclerosis (Bourneville disease)

This condition is transmitted by autosomal dominant inheritance, with high penetrance and variable expressivity. Tuberous sclerosis (TS) is due to abnormalities in one of at least two genes: *TSC1* at 9q34 which makes the protein hamartin or *TSC2* at 16p13 which makes tuberin. Like most genes for the phakomatoses, these genes are felt to have tumour suppressor roles. TS has a prevalence of at least 1 in 10 000. Fifty per cent of cases are new mutations. Sixty per cent are diagnosed by 10 years of age. Epilepsy is present in 90% and commonly presents as infantile spasms. Mental impairment is present in 60% of patients but less common with mutations in *TSC1*. Adenoma sebaceum (present in 70–90%) is a highly vascularized angiofibroma in the malar distribution of the face that may easily be confused with cystic acne. The ash leaf sign, a hypopigmented naevus which may have a shape reminiscent of an ash leaf and fluoresces under Wood's (ultra-violet) light, is present in 15–50% of affected patients. The shagreen patch is an area of thickened skin, somewhat like the skin of an orange, often in the lumbar area. Vitiligo may occasionally be present. Intracranial lesions include cortical sclerotic areas that calcify, diffuse fibrillary gliosis and subependymal giant-cell astrocytomas (tubers), often in the walls of the lateral ventricles. Other organ system involvement includes renal cortex tumours (80%), myocardial rhabdomyomas (50%), pulmonary connective tissue overgrowth leading to shortness of breath, periungual and subungual fibromas, and bony lesions (40%).

The cardinal ocular manifestation is retinal astrocytic hamartoma which occur in 50% of cases. These lesions often begin as translucent nerve fibre layer tumours that can be difficult to detect, have a predilection for retina posterior to the equator, and may be confused with retinoblastoma. The lesions can increase in size with age and calcify. When involving the optic nerve or immediate peripapillary area, the tumour often takes the form of an elevated multilobed whitish 'mulberry-type' lesion. Hypopigmented spots of the iris and retina may be seen. Papilloedema can occur secondary to gliomas. Sixth cranial nerve palsy may occur from raised intracranial pressure.

Sturge–Weber syndrome (encephalotrigeminal angiomatosis)

Sturge–Weber syndrome has no known inheritance and is considered not a true phakomatosis by some authorities. Current theories suggest that it is due to a non-heritable somatic mutation. The characteristic cutaneous vascular malformation, the port wine mark, affects one or more divisions of the trigeminal nerve. Hypertrophy of the skin and hemiface occur with age unless laser treatment is begun early. The vascular malformation may occasionally cross the midline and can affect the trunk. In 10% of patients, the lesions are bilateral. This is associated with more severe central nervous system involvement and a higher risk for glaucoma.

Meningeal angiomas are ipsilateral to the port wine mark and commonly affect the parietal and occipital regions. Calcification produces the 'railroad track' sign on CT scan. Seizures usually occur early in life, with 50% presenting before 7 months of age. Epilepsy is usually treated medically although surgical approaches (including hemispherectomy – with attendant homonymous visual field loss) have been described. Mental impairment often occurs but is not obligatory.

Ocular features: ipsilateral glaucoma occurs in about 50% of patients, particularly if the upper lid is involved in the vascular malformation. Glaucoma may present in infancy as a typical congenital/infantile glaucoma, in mid childhood due to increased episcleral venous pressure (prominent episcleral venous plexus), or in adulthood as an idiopathic open angle glaucoma. Serial screening for glaucoma is extremely important for at risk patients (port wine mark involving the eyelids). Cavernous haemangiomas of the choroid, which may be extensive or patchy, are present in 40% of cases. If a choroidal haemangioma is present, the patient has a 90% chance of developing glaucoma. The hemangioma itself does not usually cause complications although retinal vascular tortuosity is sometimes seen. Leakage, cystic degeneration of the retina and exudative detachment are rare. Heterochromia iridis may be present due to prominent iris vascularization. Visual defects due to compression of the anterior visual pathway may occasionally be related to meningeal angiomas.

Care needs to be exercised at intraocular surgery, as patients with choroidal haemangiomas are prone to expulsive haemorrhages. Post-operative choroidal effusions are common after anterior segment surgery particularly when hypotony occurs (e.g. following glaucoma filtration or seton surgery).

Von Hippel–Lindau disease (angiomatosis retinae and cerebelli)

The inheritance of von Hippel–Lindau (VHL) syndrome is autosomal dominant, with incomplete penetrance and delayed expressivity. The abnormal gene is on the short arm of chromosome 3 (3p26). The incidence is approximately 1 per 36 000 per year. Skin involvement is not a major feature of this syndrome. All tumours are found with increasing frequency with increasing age. The most common are retinal capillary angiomas, cerebellar haemoangioblastomas and renal cell carcinoma. Haemangioblastomas nearly always occur in the cerebellum, but have been documented in the medulla, pons and spinal cord. Cerebellar haemangioblastomas are present in 38% at age 30 and 70% at 60. Renal cell carcinomas are present in 10% at age 30 and 69% at age 60. VHL is the most common cause of this familial tumour. Cysts occur in the kidneys, adrenal glands, liver, epididymus and lungs. Phaeochromocytomas occur in less than 10%, but are more common in some pedigrees. Syringomyelia and syringobulbia can occur.

Retinal capillary angiomas are present in 50% (figures vary) and are commonly multiple and bilateral. Initially they can appear similar to a microaneurysm, then enlarge to a red (disc-sized or greater) vascular mass, with prominent feeder vessels. Lipid exudation can occur and may lead to an exaggerated response at the macula. Retinal bleeding may be followed by vitreous haemorrhage, with secondary gliosis, traction retinal detachment and blindness. Early detection of retinal capillary angiomas is essential as treatment with laser photocoagulation or cryotherapy can readily be accomplished. Careful serial retinal examinations and fluorescein angiography are essential.

Hypertensive retinopathy may occur in association with phaeochromocytoma and should not be confused with the effects of retinal angiomas. Raised intracranial pressure from posterior cranial fossa haemangioblastomas may cause papilloedema.

Early detection of cerebellar haemangioblastomas and visceral tumours allows optimum surgical management. The Cambridge Screening Protocol provides criteria for serial examination and investigation of affected patients with (VHL) disease and at-risk relatives (Moore, 1991).

The VHL Family Alliance is a support group based in Brookline, Massachusetts.

Louis–Bar syndrome (ataxia telangiectasia)

This is a rare autosomal recessive condition with the abnormal gene localized on the short arm of chromosome 11 (11q23, *ATM* gene). It is characterized by progressive cerebellar ataxia, oculocutaneous telangiectasia, immunodeficiency, chromosomal instability, predisposition to malignancy and early death. Ataxia is noted soon after the child starts walking. Conjunctival telangiectatic vessels are present early in the course of the disease and become more pronounced with increasing age. Other telangiectasia occur on the ears, palate, face and extensor surfaces. Frequent sinus and pulmonary infections result from a deficiency in serum immunoglobulins and reduced T-cell function, as a result of thymic underdevelopment. Lymphoma and lymphoid leukaemia are also more common in these patients. Follicular keratosis, seborrhoeic dermatitis and secondary cutaneous infections occur. Other features include mental and growth retardation, choreoathetosis, dysarthria drooling, and dry, coarse hair and skin.

Ocular associations include the conjunctival changes, an inability to initiate saccades (progressive oculomotor apraxia) and later pursuit movements. Total ophthalmoplegia can occur late in the course of the disorder. The lesions are supranuclear and vestibular ocular movements are intact. Cerebellar oculomotor signs may also occur. Other non-allelic variants have been reported such as the autosomal recessive ataxia-telangiectasia-like syndrome mapped to 9q34 and another variant at 9p13.

Wyburn–Mason syndrome

This condition is characterized by vascular hamartomatous lesions between the arterial and venous circulations, with no intervening capillary bed. Vascular hamartomas are usually found close to the optic disc. Midbrain, basofrontal and posterior fossa lesions are associated with ipsilateral retinal arterio-venous malformations. The cranial lesions are usually asymptomatic, but may cause haemorrhage or epilepsy.

The ocular lesions are sometimes termed racemose haemangiomas and are usually unilateral. Most are asymptomatic and rarely bleed. They present as extremely large dilated and tortuous vascular loops off of the optic nerve. Vision may be reduced particularly if they result in a vascular steal.

Klippel–Trenaunay–Weber syndrome

This is an autosomal dominant condition with variable expressivity. A cutaneous vascular lesion, usually affecting one or more limbs, is present at birth, with varicosities or cutis marmarata and asymmetric local hypertrophy of bone and soft tissues. Cutaneous vascular lesions may occasionally have sufficiently high blood flow that they compromise cardiac function.

Ophthalmic findings include orbital varix, strabismus, heterochromia iridis, coloboma, glaucoma, and angiomas of the choroid. Ocular involvement is uncommon.

Cutis marmarata telangiectasia congenita

This is another vascular disorder which may be associated with brain and eye involvement is. This is a disorder perhaps on the spectrum of the phakomatoses. It is not heritable and probably also represents a somatic or mosaic mutation.

Further reading

Awad AH, Mullaney PB, Al-Mesfer S, Zwaan JT. Glaucoma in Sturge–Weber syndrome. *Journal of AAPOS* 1999; **3(1):** 40–45.

MacDonald IM, Bech-Hansen NT, Britton WA Jr, Green J 2nd, Paterson M, Stone J. The phakomatoses: recent advances in genetics. *Canadian Journal of Ophthalmology* 1997; **32(1):** 4–11.

Maher ER, Moore AT. Von Hippel–Lindau disease. *British Journal of Ophthalmology* 1992; **76:** 743–745.

Miller NR. In: Walsh and Hoyt's Clinical Neuro-Ophthalmology, 4th edn. Baltimore: Waverly Press, 1988; 1747–827.

Moore AT, Maher ER, Rosen P, Gregor Z, Bird AC. Ophthalmological screening for von Hippel–Lindau disease. *Eye* 1991; **5:** 723–728.

Northrup H. Tuberous sclerosis complex: genetic aspects. *Journal of Dermatology* 1992; **19:** 914–919.

Roach ES, Smith M, Huttenlocher P, Bhat M, Alcorn D, Hawley L. Diagnostic criteria: tuberous sclerosis complex. Report of the Diagnostic Criteria Committee of the National Tuberous Sclerosis Association. *Journal of Neurology* 1992; **7:** 221–224.

Taylor AMR, Jaspers NGJ, Gatti RA. Fifth International Workshop on Ataxia Telangiectasia. *Cancer Research* 1993; **53:** 438–441.

Truhan AP, Filipek PA. Magnetic resonance imaging. Its role in the neuroradiological evaluation of neurofibromatosis, tuberous sclerosis and Sturge–Weber syndromes. *Archives of Dermatology* 1993; **129:** 219–226.

Related topics of interest

Dermatology and the eye 1: local lid disease (p. 82); Dermatology and the eye 2: systemic diseases (p. 86); Neurofibromatosis (p. 180).

POSTERIOR UVEITIS

Helen Devonport

Strictly speaking the term posterior uveitis refers to inflammation of the posterior uvea (choroiditis), but generally the term encompasses choroiditis, retinitis, retinal vasculitis and when present, associated vitritis. Posterior uveitis *per se* is unusual and normally co-exists with a degree of anterior chamber activity i.e. a panuveitis.

Problem

Multiple aetiologies exist for posterior uveitis, some of which are associated with serious systemic disease, making accurate and speedy diagnosis essential. Though some types of posterior uveitis are self-limiting, others necessitate the use of systemic therapeutic agents with potentially serious adverse effects.

Background

1. Idiopathic specific posterior uveitis entities are a group of conditions each with characteristic clinical findings to which a name has been given but in which the aetiology remains unclear. These conditions include birdshot choroidopathy, serpiginous choroidopathy, sympathetic ophthalmitis and a further subset of conditions known as the white dot syndromes. These include multiple evanescent white dot syndrome (MEWDS), multifocal choroiditis (POHS-type picture with vitritis), punctate inner choroiditis (PIC), acute retinal pigment epitheliitis, acute posterior multifocal placoid pigment epitheliopathy (APMPPE) and subretinal fibrosis and uveitis syndrome.

2. Idiopathic non-specific posterior uveitis refers to posterior uveitis, occurring with no clear aetiology that does not fit the pattern of any of the named uveitis entities. The term idiopathic retinal vasculitis is used in a similar way when vasculitis predominates.

3. Non-infectious systemic diseases are a group of conditions of which sarcoidosis is the most commonly identified. Posterior uveitis is reported in 30% of sarcoid patients with ocular involvement. The most common finding is a segmental retinal vasculitis with associated panuveitis, but there may also be optic disc involvement or choroiditis. Other non-infectious systemic diseases include systemic lupus erythematosus (SLE), polyarteritis nodosum (PAN), multiple sclerosis (MS), Behçet's syndrome, Vogt–Koyanagi–Harada syndrome (VKH) and Wegener's granulomatosis.

4. Infectious systemic disease. In viral posterior uveitis the clinical picture depends not only on the infecting organism, but also on the immune status of the host. Varicella zoster, herpes simplex and cytomegalovirus (CMV) cause retinitis and have each been implicated in retinal necrosis. In the immunocompetent host the resulting clinical picture is that of acute retinal necrosis (ARN), but progressive outer retinal necrosis (PORN), is described in the severely immunocompromised host. Classic CMV retinitis is most commonly seen in HIV infection.

Toxoplasmosis is the most common cause of parasitic posterior uveitis. In the UK and USA, 50–75% of cases of posterior uveitis are attributable to reactivation of toxoplasmic retinochoroiditis. Toxocara is another cause of childhood posterior parasitic uveitis and may give rise to a chronic panuveitis, posterior pole granuloma or peripheral granuloma. The latter may be asymptomatic and only be detected on routine examination in later life. Onchocerciasis is associated with a chorioretinitis and optic atrophy.

Syphilis, both acquired and congenital can be responsible for focal or diffuse spirochete chorioretinitis. *Borrelia burgdorferi*, the organism responsible for Lyme disease may also give rise to retinal vasculitis, neuroretinitis, chorioretinitis or optic neuropathy.

Responsible fungal organisms include *Histoplasma, Candida* and *Aspergillus. Histoplasma* infection does not occur in the UK, and so the term presumed ocular histoplasmosis syndrome (POHS) has been used to describe cases of multifocal choroiditis with an identical clinical picture, but in whom there is no evidence of infection. Ocular candidiasis occurs as a result of candidaemia in the immunocompromised, intravenous drug abusers and patients with long-term intravenous lines. Initial foci involve the choroid, but soon invade the retina and then the vitreous, giving rise to characteristic vitreous 'puff balls'. Cryptococcal endophthalmitis is rare, but has been reported in immunocompromised hosts. *Pneumocystis carinii* infection, seen in patients with HIV, may involve the choroid.

Tuberculosis may also give rise to a multifocal choroiditis.

5. Masquerade syndromes. A number of malignancies may give rise to symptoms and signs similar to those of posterior uveitis. These include choroidal metastases, uveal melanoma and intraocular lymphomas such as CNS non-Hodgkin's lymphoma, systemic non-Hodgkin's metastatic to the eye and Hodgkin's lymphoma. In children retinoblastoma and leukaemia may mimic posterior uveitis. Cancer-associated retinopathy is a paraneoplastic syndrome which may be mistaken for posterior uveitis.

Clinical features

Patients may present with reduced vision and/or floaters.

A degree of anterior activity may be seen. Secondary cataract may be present as a result of disease or treatment (e.g. steroid).

Vitritis may be present to varying degrees. The severity of the vitritis can be graded according to the degree to which retinal detail is obscured when viewed with an indirect ophthalmoscope. Posterior vitreous detachment (PVD) may result. More localized inflammatory collections within the vitreous may be seen as 'snow balls'. Snow balls and snow banking are also seen in intermediate uveitis (or pars planitis).

Retinitis, as seen for example in CMV, is characterized by retinal infiltrates, which have a white cloudy appearance with indistinct margins, and may obscure retinal vessels. There may be associated retinal haemorrhages or cotton wool spots. Cystoid macular oedema is frequently seen as a complication in many types of uveitis and is responsible for reduced visual acuity. Retinal detachment, may be exudative, tractional or rhegmatogenous.

Retinal vasculitis is characterized by sheathing of retinal venules, peripheral narrowing or obliteration and in some cases, retinal neovascularization. In sarcoidosis, characteristic findings are of a peripheral segmental periphlebitis. In Behçet's syndrome, although the vasculitis predominantly affects retinal veins (periphlebitis), arterioles may also be involved. The ischaemia induced by the vasculitis may be associated with cotton wool spots.

Small hemispherical mounds of retinal pigment cells are called Dalen–Fuchs nodules. They are seen in sympathetic uveitis and VKH.

Areas of active choroiditis appear as greyish yellow lesions with reasonably well demarcated borders, over which retinal vessels pass undisturbed. Pale atrophic chorio-retinal lesions with surrounding hyperpigmentation represent old inactive disease. Choroidal neovascularization may occur as a late complication of choroiditis.

Screening with multiple investigations has a low diagnostic yield and a carefully taken history and appropriate examination are more important in reaching a diagnosis. A full blood count, including a differential white cell count for eosinophilia, erythrocyte sedimentation rate, urea and electrolytes, chest X-ray, serum angiotensin-converting enzyme and syphilis serology are recommended with additional tests when clinically indicated.

Treatment

Treatment is aimed at controlling inflammation, preventing visual loss and minimizing complications of both the disease and its therapy. In some types of posterior uveitis e.g. MEWDS, APMPPE and non-sight-threatening toxoplasmosis, inflammation is self limiting and no treatment is required. Infectious causes of posterior uveitis are treated with appropriate antimicrobial agents, often with the addition of corticosteroids.

Corticosteroids remain the mainstay of medical treatment in posterior uveitis. Periocular corticosteroids, given either as an orbital floor or posterior subtenons injection are useful in uniocular disease or when there are contraindications to systemic corticosteroids, but must not be used in those with glaucoma or a history of steroid-related raised intraocular pressure. Systemic steroids are initiated at maximal doses and then reduced to the minimum required to control inflammation. In cases of therapeutic failure or where the maintenance corticosteroid dose is high, a second immunosuppressive agent is indicated. Cyclosporin is the most commonly used, but others include azathioprine, methotrexate and cyclophosphamide. All of these have potentially serious adverse effects. Mycophenolate mofetil and FK506 (Tacrolimus) have also been used.

Removal of secondary cataract should be delayed until the eye has been free from active inflammation for 3 months and systemic corticosteroid cover may be necessary. Vitrectomy may improve vision when there is significant residual vitreous opacity and may also improve disease control in younger patients. Vitrectomy may be indicated for repair of secondary retinal detachment. In some conditons, e.g. POHS, PIC, choroidal neovascular membranes affecting the fovea can be surgically removed.

Laser therapy is indicated for choroidal neovascularization (e.g. in POHS) and for retinal neovascularization when there is ischaemia present (e.g. in Behçet's syndrome).

Further reading

Gasch AT, Smith JA, Whitcup SM. Birdshot retinochoroidopathy. *British Journal of Ophthalmology* 1999; **83**(2): 241–9.

Guex-Crosier Y, Rochat C, Herbert CP. Necrotising herpetic retinopathies. A spectrum of herpes virus-induced diseases determined by the immune state of the host. *Ocular Immunology and Inflammation* 1997; **5**(4): 259–65.

McClusky PJ, Towler HM, Lightman S. Management of chronic uveitis. *British Medical Journal* 2000; **320**: 555–8.

Stavrou P, Linton S, Young DW, Murray PI. Clinical diagnosis of ocular sarcoidosis. *Eye* 1997; **11**(3): 365–70.

Tabbara KF. The differential diagnosis of posterior uveitis. *Bulletin de la Societe Belge D'Ophthalmologie* 1997; **267**: 199–201.

Related topics of interest

Behçet's disease (p. 19); Sarcoidosis (p. 276); Toxoplasmosis (p. 330); Uveitis: who and what to investigate (p. 337).

POSTOPERATIVE ENDOPHTHALMITIS

David E. Laws

The incidence of infective endophthalmitis after routine cataract surgery is reported to be between 0.33% and 0.02%. The incidence of infective endophthalmitis is probably falling. In a retrospective series of 19 269 patients nine developed postoperative endophthalmitis.

Problem

The eye is particularly at risk from infection. The retina is extremely sensitive to the effects of invading micro-organisms and their toxic products. The vitreous has a relatively large avascular volume. It is inaccessible to parenteral antibiotics and contains many substrates for bacterial growth. The healing process, while appropriate for many tissues, causes scarring which can result in further damage in the eye. These factors combine so that some organisms can overwhelm the eye in hours. Due to the low incidence, studies aimed to identify interventions to reduce the incidence of infection therefore require large numbers to demonstrate clinical benefit.

Background

Genetic testing of organisms cultured from the eye indicate that the patient's own flora is the main source of infection. The value of routine preoperative lid or conjunctival culture is debatable because the results vary from day to day. The situation is different in the presence of clinical signs of infection, particularly where risk factors exist such as diabetes. The lids should be inspected for signs of blepharitis and lid scrubbing instituted preoperatively if present. If there are golden crusts on the lid margin Staphylococcal blepharitis should be suspected, swabs taken and antibiotic therapy instituted. Gentle pressure over the lachrymal sac may cause regurgitation in patients with nasolachrymal obstruction. This is best dealt with prior to undertaking intraocular surgery. Evidence of infective conjunctivitis is a contraindication to operating until treated.

Antibiotic prophylaxis

The conjunctival sac cannot be sterilized but the bacterial count can be reduced. Administration of an antibiotic just prior to surgery will reduce the bacterial load and more recent studies have shown that the incidence of endophthalmitis is also reduced. Evidence for the optimal route of administration is lacking but many antibiotics attain therapeutic concentrations in the anterior chamber after topical administration. The best agent to use is also the subject of debate. This is not only on the basis of efficacy but also because of problems with resistance caused by antibiotic prophylaxis for such an uncommon event as endophthalmitis. An ideal antibiotic would be one which is effective but which is not likely to be required in sight- (or life-) threatening disease. These are difficult criteria to meet. Chloramphenicol, gentamicin, cephalosporins and quinolones are all used but definitive evidence regarding the best choice for endophthalmitis prophylaxis is awaited.

Surgical preparation

Aqueous povidone iodine 5% (not alcohol solution or detergent scrub) can be instilled into the eye and used to clean the lid margins as part of the operative prep. It has the advantage of being effective against both spores and vegetative organisms. The optimal effect is after the solution has been left in place for a few minutes. This is the most cost-effective method proven to reduce the incidence of endophthalmitis.

Adhesive drapes which cover the lashes and lid margins by folding under the upper and lower lids may also be helpful. Any mucus in the conjunctival sac should be removed.

Instrumentation and technique

Wherever practical, single-use items should be used during surgery. Reusable items have been associated with outbreaks of endophthalmitis and must be approved for the sterilization process used by the theatre in which they are to be used. Particular care should be taken with reusing items, such as tubing, in which it is difficult to demonstrate that all surfaces are sterile. This is especially relevant to instruments used during phakoemulsification procedures. Shorter surgical time, no complications and smaller wounds are also associated with a lower infection risk. Around 14% of aqueous cultures will demonstrate growth at the end of a cataract procedure so instrumentation within the eye should be kept to a minimum. Wound closure avoiding a fistula and using monofilament sutures will reduce the chance of bacterial ingress postoperatively.

Clinical features

Endophthalmitis may present early in the postoperative period, a few weeks later or months after surgery depending on the organism. Late infection, sometimes years after surgery, can occur in a filtering bleb. Suspicion of endophthalmitis should be raised if the inflammatory response is greater than expected for the surgery undertaken. Accurate diagnosis is a matter of urgency as the condition can rapidly progress to blindness.

Acute postoperative endophthalmitis usually presents within a few days of surgery with reduced vision, discharge and photophobia but pain is the most important symptom. The lids may be swollen with marked conjunctival inflammation. The presence of an afferent pupillary defect and inaccurate light projection are poor prognostic signs. Slit lamp examination will demonstrate cells in the anterior chamber or hypopyon and corneal opacity may be present. Poor visibility of the iris, and membrane formation on the lens are also features of more severe disease. Early endophthalmitis causes retinal periphlebitis. Opacity in the vitreous cavity will cause loss of the red reflex when advanced. Chorioretinal thickening and vitreous densities may be observed on ultrasound.

When bacteria are isolated after cataract surgery over 90% of isolates are Gram-positive cocci particularly in the presence of corneal opacity, diabetes and wound problems. Severe vitritis precluding fundal view is a risk factor for Gram-negative organisms. In acute endophthalmitis the causative organisms are usually *Staphylococcus aureus* or *Streptococcus* species. *Staphylococcus epidermidis* infection may be less severe and present with inflammation persisting for longer than expected postoperatively. This presentation may be delayed even further if topical steroids are used postoperatively. Fungal or *Propionibacterium acnes* induce a chronic postoperative endophthalmitis that may present several months after surgery. The former is characterized by a profound vitritis and the latter by granulomatous keratoprecipitates with white plaques on the posterior capsule, which can mimic a Soemmering ring.

Infection of filtering blebs can be seen years after surgery. The causative organisms are usually *Haemophilus* or *Streptococcus* species. Thin, avascular blebs, as commonly found after the use of cytotoxic agents, are most at risk from infection. Isolated bleb infection does not always progress to endophthalmitis.

Infection after trauma repair is caused by a different group of organisms as they are taken into the eye by the injury rather than from the patient's own flora. In a rural setting anaerobes or fungi may be found. If soil may have contaminated the object which perforated the eye, then coverage for bacteroides is especially important.

Microbiology

Accurate determination of the infecting organism is invaluable. It will provide a guide to appropriate therapy and antibiotic sensitivities. Anterior chamber samples alone are frequently culture-negative while the vitreous yields growth in about 65% of postoperative endophthalmitis cases. Where possible both anterior chamber and vitreous samples should be obtained before commencing antibiotic therapy. Prior notification of the microbiology services will enable the sample to be immediately plated out increasing the chance of identifying the organism. Cultures on blood agar, chocolate agar, thioglycolate broth and Sabouraud media should be taken. If anaerobes such as *Propionibacterium acnes* are suspected additional anaerobic media should be used and the capsular bag should be sampled. Gram staining is commonly undertaken but rarely alters management.

The vitreous sample may be taken by passing a 23-gauge needle through the pars plana, 3.5 mm from the limbus so that it is visible in the pupil and aspirating 0.2 ml. In children, a larger bore needle would be needed to aspirate the vitreous. An alternative (and more commonly performed) method is to undertake a three port pars plana vitrectomy to obtain the sample. The latter technique has the theoretical advantage of obtaining a larger volume for culture and placing less traction on the retina. However, the Endophthalmitis Vitrectomy Study (EVS) did not demonstrate any difference in the complication or culture rate between the two techniques. The practical implication of this is that if there is difficulty with access to vitrectomy, vitreous sampling by needle should not be delayed.

Treatment

Once infective endophthalmitis has been diagnosed effective therapy requires adequate levels of appropriate therapeutic agents in the vitreous cavity. The Endophthalmitis Vitrectomy Study was a multicentre randomized study involving 420 subjects with endophthalmitis within 6 weeks of cataract surgery. The main objectives of the study were to identify any benefit of early vitrectomy, the role of intravenous antibiotics and to determine which other factors affect the outcome of endophthalmitis patients.

1. Therapeutic vitrectomy. The EVS found that if the presenting visual acuity was equal to or better than 'count fingers' in the affected eye early vitrectomy did not confer any additional benefit. Below this level of acuity reducing the infective load with vitrectomy increased the number of people achieving 6/12 or better by a factor of three. The number of subjects in this group developing severe visual loss was also reduced from 47% to 20% by early vitrectomy.

2. Intravenous antibiotics. The EVS did not show any additional benefit from the use of intravenous antibiotics in bacterial endophthalmitis. Animal experimental models of endophthalmitis have been successfully treated with systemic quinolone antibiotics but not against a wide range of organisms.

3. Intravitreal antibiotics. Ocular toxicity and the infective organism determine the choice of therapeutic agent. All Gram-positive isolates in the EVS and several other studies were susceptible to vancomycin. Teicoplanin is less toxic than vancomycin but is also less effective against some coagulase negative *Staphylococci*. Gram-negative isolates were equally sensitive to amikacin and ceftazidime in the EVS. The quinolone antibiotics while achieving excellent vitreous penetration and effective at low concentrations are slightly less effective against Gram-positive organisms and resistance is emerging. The third-generation quinolones such as sparfloxacin attain even greater levels in the vitreous. Gentamicin is effective against Gram-negative bacteria but is reported to cause retinal toxicity (macular infarction) at therapeutic levels. Fungal infection after trauma can be treated with amphotericin B.

The timing and composition of repeat intravitreal injection is controversial as retinal toxicity may be exacerbated, particularly if aminoglycosides are used. Failure to respond at 48 hours is often treated by repeat intravitreal injection, which may be altered in the light of antibiotic sensitivities.

Intravitreal dose of antibiotics (in 0.1 ml)	
Vancomycin	1 mg
Gentamicin	0.2 mg
Amikacin	0.4 mg
Ceftazidime	2.0 mg
Ciprofloxacin	0.2 mg

4. Topical and periocular antibiotics. Topical and periocular antibiotics do not usually achieve therapeutic levels in the vitreous but may be helpful treating organisms situated more anteriorly.

5. Steroid treatment. The inflammatory response in the eye can cause opacification and traction on the retina. Systemic administration or injection of steroid has unproven value in reducing this response and should be avoided in suspected cases of fungal infection. Animal experimental data support the use of intravitreal steroids in bacterial infection.

6. Intraocular lens. Removal of an intraocular lens should be considered in endophthalmitis but is not usually required. Adherent inflammatory material can be removed if vitrectomy is performed.

Conclusion

Endophthalmitis may be mistaken for postoperative inflammation and the diagnosis delayed. If the diagnosis is seriously considered vitreous samples must be obtained before therapy is started in the hope of identifying the causative organism. The constantly changing pattern of antibiotic resistance will mean that the optimal antibiotics will change over time. If intravitreal antibiotics are to be used, hospital pharmacists using typewritten protocols and sterile technique most safely make them up.

Further reading

Han DP, Wisniewski SR, Wilson LA, Barza M, Vine AK, Doft BH, Kelsey SF. The Endophthalmitis Vitrectomy Study: Spectrum and susceptibilities of microbiologic isolates. *American Journal of Ophthalmology* 1996; **122:** 1–17.

Han DP, Wisniewski SR, Kelsey SF, Doft BH, Barza M, Pavan PR. Microbiologic yields and complication rates of vitreous needle aspiration versus mechanized vitreous biopsy in the Endophthalmitis Vitrectomy Study. *Retina* 1999; **19:** 98–102.

Johnson MW, Doft BH, Kelsey SF, Barza M, Wilson LA, Barr CC, Wisniewski SR. The Endophthalmitis Vitrectomy Study. Relationship between clinical presentation and microbiologic spectrum. *Ophthalmology* 1997; **104**(2): 261–72.

Royal College of Ophthalmologists. *Management of Endophthalmitis.* Occasional update. Issue 1. 1996.

The Endophthalmitis Vitrectomy Study Group: Results of the Endophthalmitis Vitrectomy Study: A randomized trial of immediate vitrectomy and of intravenous antibiotics for the treatment of postoperative bacterial endophthalmitis. *Archives in Ophthalmology* 1995; **113:** 1479–96.

PRIMARY INTRAOCULAR LYMPHOMA

Panagiota Stavrou

Primary intraocular lymphoma is a component of the non-Hodgkin's lymphoma of the central nervous system (CNS). Hodgkin's lymphoma rarely causes ocular disease. However, two clinically distinct forms of non-Hodgkin's lymphoma frequently involve the eye: primary lymphoma of the CNS and systemic lymphoma.

Problem

Primary CNS lymphoma with ocular involvement, masquerading as chronic uveitis, has been increasingly recognized. Although it is rare, its diagnosis is important because of the risk of visual loss and its high mortality when associated with CNS involvement. The diagnosis remains difficult and requires a high degree of suspicion. Most cases remain misdiagnosed as idiopathic uveitis for several months or years.

Background

The primary non-Hodgkin's lymphoma of CNS is a large B-cell lymphoma which arises within the brain, spinal cord, leptomeninges or the eye and may then spread throughout the CNS. These tumours were often incorrectly called reticulum cell sarcomas; but they are neither sarcomas nor comprised of reticulum cells. Systemic spread outside the CNS occurs rarely and has been reported in 7–8% of autopsies. In contrast, systemic non-Hodgkin's lymphoma almost always arises outside the CNS. Involvement of the eye occurs through the choroidal circulation. Unlike patients with non-Hodgkin's lymphoma of CNS, patients with systemic lymphoma often have signs and symptoms of an underlying malignancy and pose less of a diagnostic dilemma.

Primary CNS lymphoma can be difficult to diagnose especially in patients who exhibit ocular or leptomeningeal involvement without symptomatic mass lesions in the brain. In a series of 32 patients with histologically proved intraocular lymphoma, CNS involvement occurred in 18 patients (56%); ocular symptoms preceded CNS symptoms in 82% of these patients. The mean time between the onset of ocular symptoms and the onset of CNS symptoms was 29 months (range, 7–108 months). Disease was limited to the eye in 22% of patients. Over the past decade the number of reported primary CNS and intraocular lymphomas has risen in both immuno-compromised and healthy individuals. This increase is not well understood and cannot be explained by changes in tumour classification, the increased prevalence of the acquired immune deficiency syndrome, or the increased number of organ transplantations or other causes of immunosuppression. The median age of presentation is 50 to 60 years, although it has also been reported in children; a slight male predominance has been found in some series.

Clinical features

Primary CNS lymphoma with ocular involvement, typically presents a diagnostic challenge, masquerading as uveitis, vitritis or chorioretinitis. Patients often complain of floaters and blurred vision. Ocular pain and conjunctival hyperaemia are rare. Ocular examination reveals decreased visual acuity, mild anterior segment inflammation and vitritis. Vitreous cells are typically large and are formed into thick sheets with a distinctive appearance on slit-lamp biomicroscopy. Whitcup and associates also described the following fundoscopic findings on 12 patients with primary intraocular lymphoma and chorioretinal lesions: subretinal yellow infiltrates, punctate retinal lesions, retinal vasculitis, perturbation of the retinal pigment epithelium, macular oedema and a macular star. Atypical presentations have also been reported, including a haemorrhagic retinal vasculitis mimicking viral retinitis. The vitritis is initially 'responsive' to steroid therapy because not all vitreous cells are malignant but rather 'reactive' lymphocytes or histiocytes.

The most common abnormality on fluorescein angiography is punctate hyperfluorescent lesions predominantly involving the posterior pole. These lesions represent window defects and appear to correspond to tumour infiltrates at the level of the retinal pigment epithelium. In some cases, distinct retinal lesions cannot be seen on clinical examination and are only visible on fluorescein angiography. Hypofluorescent as well as hyperfluorescent lesions are noted on some angiograms, and may even show blocked fluorescence late in the angiogram.

Diagnosis

Diagnosis of primary CNS and intraocular lymphoma is made by identifying malignant large B lymphocytes in the eye, brain and cerebrospinal fluid, however, these cells are few, friable and difficult to recognize. In patients with primary CNS lymphoma and intraocular involvement the diagnosis still depends on vitreous cytology. Although prompt and appropriate handling of specimens can improve the diagnostic yield, misdiagnosis still occurs despite properly prepared specimens. In a series of patients whose condition was diagnosed as primary CNS lymphoma, 30% had a previous false-negative vitreous biopsy specimen and more than one third of patients had false-negative cerebrospinal fluid specimens. It has also been shown that previous steroid therapy can limit the diagnostic yield of vitreous cytology. Examination of the vitreous for lymphoma requires review by an experienced cytopathologist. Typical lymphoma cells are characterized by large, pleomorphic cells with scanty cytoplasm and round, oval, bean-shaped or clover leaf-shaped nuclei. Hypersegmented nuclei with prominent nucleoli often are diagnostic. Usually few of these characteristic lymphoma cells are present in the vitreous specimen. Immunohistochemical-stained sections showing B-cell markers with either a kappa or lambda light chain monoclonal response are critical to confirm the diagnosis. It has also been shown that there is compartmentalization of the lymphoid tumour cells with the majority of cells infiltrating the retina staining for B-cell markers and the majority of cells infiltrating the choroid staining for T cells. The cause of this compartmentalization remains unclear.

Whitcup *et al.* showed that levels of interleukin (IL)-10 in the vitreous of patients with primary intraocular lymphoma exceeded those of IL-6. They also showed that malignant cells were significantly more likely to be present in cerebrospinal fluid when levels of IL-10 exceeded those of IL-6. However, in 1999, Akpek and associates showed that an elevated IL-10 to IL-6 or IL-10 to IL-12 ratio are not always associated with intraocular-CNS lymphoma as they may also be found in patients with non-neoplastic uveitis.

Gene rearrangement

Clonal heavy chain immunoglobulin gene rearrangement and *bcl-2* gene translocation have been reported in systemic B-cell lymphoma. The *bcl-2* gene expression is restricted in tissues characterized by apoptotic cell death, and translocation of this gene is believed to be the fundamental event in the oncogenesis of several haematologic malignancies including non-Hodgkin's lymphoma. In this tumour, the *bcl-2* gene, located on chromosome 18, is involved in the t (14;18) chromosomal translocation that brings the *bcl-2* gene into juxtaposition with the immunoglobulin H (IgH) promoter located on chromosome 14. Successful amplification of the rearranged *IgH* gene in both frozen and formaldehyde-fixed and paraffin-embedded samples has been achieved by polymerase chain reaction in microdissected specimens. Therefore, rearrangement of the *IgH* gene can serve as molecular marker for primary CNS lymphoma.

Diagnostic approach

The currently suggested diagnostic approach in patients with suspected intraocular involvement due to primary CNS lymphoma is to perform a CT scan or an MRI of the brain with or without gadolinium and a lumbar puncture. The suspicion of intraocular lymphoma is based on the findings of a characteristic vitritis in an older patient with deep retinal lesions on fundus examination or fundus angiography and a visual acuity which is often better than expected based on clinical examination. Neurologic symptoms at the time of presentation also support a diagnosis of possible intraocular lymphoma. All patients should undergo a neurological workup, including radiological imaging of the brain and examination of the cerebrospinal fluid. Although contrast-enhanced CT and MRI scans are useful in determining CNS lesions they fail to detect subarachnoid or ocular involvement. Occasionally, repeat lumbar punctures are performed with at least 10 ml of cerebrospinal fluid sent for cytopathologic examination. As the lymphoma cells are fragile, it is important that samples be immediately hand carried to the cytology laboratory for processing. If neurologic workup is negative, sarcoidosis should also be excluded. Some have suggested that even if focal CNS lesions are noted on neuroradiological studies, a full vitrectomy should be performed on the eye with the most severe vitritis or poorest visual acuity as the initial diagnostic procedure. If the cerebrospinal fluid is positive for lymphoma, it is unnecessary to perform a vitrectomy.

Treatment

In a large series including primary CNS lymphoma in 248 immunocompetent patients the mean survival time was 12 months. The lesion was single in 66% of patients and supratentorial in 87% of them. Prognostic factors related to favourable outcome were age younger than 60 years, radiation therapy, radiation combined with chemotherapy and chemotherapy consisting of anthracycline. This study suggested the following sequence of management: stereotactic biopsy sampling, chemotherapy with an anthracycline- or methotrexate-based regimen followed by cranial irradiation. Another study showed that the addition of chemotherapy to radiation therapy for the initial treatment of primary CNS lymphoma significantly improved disease-free survival to a median of 41 months and contributed to overall survival. Repeat intravitreal injections of methotrexate and thiotepa have also been used with encouraging results in patients with intraocular lymphoma which recurred following radiotherapy and repeated systemic chemotherapeutic regimens.

It has been reported that most patients with primary CNS lymphoma involving the eye die within 1 to 5 years from diagnosis.

Further reading

Akpek EM, Maca SM, Christen WG, Foster CS. Elevated vitreous interleukin-10 level is not diagnostic of intraocular-central nervous system lymphoma. *Ophthalmology* 1999; **106:** 2291–5.

Fen Shen D, Zhuang Z, LeHoang P, Böni R, Zheng S, Nussenblatt RB, Chan CC. Utility of microdissection and polymerase chain reaction for the detection of immunoglobulin gene rearrangement and translocation in primary intraocular lymphoma. *Ophthalmology* 1998; **105:** 1664–9.

Freeman LN, Schachat AP, Knox DL *et al.* Clinical features, laboratory investigations, and survival in ocular reticulum cell sarcoma. *Ophthalmology* 1987; **94:** 1631–9.

Hochberg FH, Miler DC. Primary central nervous system lymphoma. *Journal of Neurosurgery* 1988; **68:** 835–53.

Whitcup SM, de Smet MD, Rubin BI *et al.* Intraocular lymphoma: clinical and histopathologic diagnosis. *Ophthalmology* 1993; **100:** 1399–406.

Whitcup SM, Stark-Vancs V, Wittes RE *et al.* Association of interleukin 10 in the vitreous and cerebrospinal fluid and primary central nervous system lymphoma. *Archives of Ophthalmology* 1997; **115:** 1157–60.

REFRACTION IN CHILDREN

David E. Laws & Robert H. Taylor

Correcting refractive error in adults is most often undertaken to alleviate visual symptoms. However, a history of blurred vision is not often forthcoming in children, even with large refractive errors. Paediatric refraction is also undertaken against a backdrop of visual development and ocular growth during which time emmetropia is not always the normal state.

Problem

Refraction in children has aims and difficulties that vary from adults. A clear understanding of the benefit of correcting a given refractive error must be obtained before subjecting a child to spectacle wear.

Animal studies have raised concerns that prescription of spectacles in infants may alter the normal growth of the eye towards emmetropia. This is controversial in humans and some studies have indicated that when the animal model of spectacle compliance mimics that of children, with at least some part of the day without correction, the effects on eye growth are not seen. This story is still unfolding at the time of writing.

Background

Normal refractive development in infancy is characterized by a wide distribution of refractive error centred around low hypermetropia. This pattern progresses towards emmetropia with a narrow distribution in later childhood. A different pattern emerges in adolescence with a subset becoming myopic giving a negative skew or possibly bimodal distribution.

In addition to treating blur, refractive error and its correction in children may be of diagnostic value (see table), be required to aid visual development (amblyopia) or to control accommodation in strabismus.

Clinical features

Refraction is best undertaken early in the examination, as it is less threatening than other activities, such as slit-lamp examination or some forms of fundoscopy. It is not performed in isolation and can only be interpreted with knowledge of the medical history and acuity. Welcoming the child directly by their first name is best practice and it is useful to have a reasonable stock of toys at hand. Often the first task of the refractionist is to allay the fears of the parents as well as the child. Only after all are relaxed can the best results be obtained. If the child will not settle striking up a conversation with the parents can be calming and reassure that nothing untoward is going to suddenly happen. Small children are best examined after feeding. Before starting show them what the instruments do. The lights on an ophthalmoscope or the rotating slit beam of a retinoscope may fascinate small children. Once underway a swift and dextrous examination will usually be rewarded by compliance. It should not be forgotten that the retinoscopy reflex is also an excellent method of assessing the clarity of the media.

Conditions associated with myopia

- Connective tissue disorders
  - Marfan's syndrome
  - Ehlers Danlos
  - Pseudoxanthoma elasticum
  - Sticklers
- Prematurity and cryotherapy for ROP
- Retinal disorders
  - Retinitis pigmentosa
  - Albinism
  - Congenital stationary night blindness
- Chromosomal disorders
  - Down syndrome
- Metabolic
  - Homocystinuria

Conditions associated with astigmatism

- Nystagmus
- Prematurity
- Periocular developmental disorders
  - Ptosis
  - Limbal dermoid
  - Periocular haemangioma

Conditions associated with hypermetropia

- Lebers amaurosis
- Microphthalomos
- Chromosomal disorders
  - Down syndrome

Cycloplegic retinoscopy is the most commonly performed method having the advantage of exerting some control over accommodation and facilitating fundoscopy. Cyclopentolate 1% is used in children at term and 0.5% below. Prior administration of a topical anaesthetic such as proxymetacaine reduces the discomfort and allows the cycloplegic agent to work more rapidly. Atropine is also an effective cycloplegic but side effects preclude its routine use. Atropine and cyclopentolate refraction has been compared in several studies with conflicting results. Atropine refraction in most papers gives greater hypermetropia and allowance for this effect may be made depending on the reason for giving spectacles. If, for example, control of accommodation in esotropia is required the full prescription can be given. No allowance is made for the effects of cycloplegia if cyclopentolate is used.

The child is encouraged to look directly at the retinoscope light and, in the absence of significant latent nystagmus, the fellow eye is occluded which also reduces any convergence effort. In children younger than approximately 3 years refraction is performed using hand-held lenses or a retinoscopy rack. After this age half-frame paediatric trial spectacles can be used. The least negative lens that neutralizes is taken as the endpoint. If no clear movement of the light reflex is discernible without a lens in place repeating with + or − 5 diopter lens will help identify high ametropia. Once neutralization is observed, moving nearer or further from the patient will cause the reflex to reverse confirming the endpoint. If the child is sleeping or under anaesthetic, care must be taken that the refraction is on axis, as small differences in alignment will result in significant artefactual astigmatism. It is often worth quickly repeating these findings when the child is awake if possible.

If astigmatism is present, find the most negative axis first, then confirm the axis position, before moving more positive to find the cylinder power. If the axis is oblique, it may be prudent to check the sphere power again now the axis is known.

Near (Mohindra) retinoscopy avoids the use of cycloplegic agents and was developed for mass screening of refractive errors. It is performed in a darkened room using the retinoscope as the fixing target with the assumption that this induces tonic accommodation of about 0.75D in older children and 1.25D in infants. The retinoscope reading is taken after the initial fluctuations in accommodation have settled. This technique also has the advantage that an accommodative target can subsequently be introduced and accommodation measured in children where this is thought to be a problem.

A detailed examination of the fundus is essential in every child attending an eye clinic. This is best performed through a dilated pupil and can be undertaken at the same time.

Autorefraction can provide objective data but both coaxial and eccentric systems are currently insufficiently sensitive to routinely prescribe. Photoscreeners have the advantage that the image produced can also detect strabismus and media opacity but they also have a significant false-negative error rate when used for population screening. Subjective refraction can be performed with children aged about 8 and above. If a previous refraction is available both eyes should be fogged with +1.5D at the beginning of the test to reduce accommodation.

Treatment

If one considers that spectacles are prescribed to treat blurred vision, amblyopia or control accommodation and that there may be myopia, hypermetropia, astigmatism or anisometropia and that several of these can coexist in the presence of other variables, it is obvious that each child must be considered individually. A pragmatic approach is to ask yourself if the problem is sufficient to warrant wearing spectacles and if correcting the refractive error will help the problem.

The combination of hypermetropia and esotropia is common, and glasses are prescribed to control the accommodative element of the squint. Debate exists but errors greater than +1.5D are usually fully corrected in this situation. In the presence of a high accommodative convergence to accommodation (AC/A) ratio and potential fusion high executive bifocals are given. In the absence of esotropia, hypermetropia over +4 in a child 18 months or older would normally be corrected. It may be unnecessary to prescribe the full amount. In these cases careful follow up must be arranged as accommodation may be stimulated because of the clearer image, an esotropia develops, and the full cycloplegic correction is now required. Warning parents of this possibility is helpful.

Spectacles are also prescribed if anisometropia is greater than 1D and amblyopia is suspected based on fixation patterns or visual acuity. In pure anisometropic amblyopia improvement in acuity can occur over many months after glasses are prescribed without resorting to occlusion therapy.

If the child is myopic and acuity is reduced the weakest prescription should be given that corrects the acuity. The use of a postcycloplegic subjective test can be useful in older children. Myopic correction should also be considered to help control exotropia. Astigmatism greater than 1.5D may lead to meridional amblyopia and is usually corrected after 1 year of age.

Nystagmus is commonly associated with refractive errors, particularly astigmatism. These patients particularly benefit from accurate refraction which can be both difficult and time consuming. The use of cycloplegic refraction in older children can make the measurement easier.

Care must be taken when dispensing children's glasses; their needs can be different from adults. Spectacle frames must be robust with side arms that can be subjected to a reasonable amount of forced abduction. Glass lenses should be avoided in all children in view of the risk of potential injury. Certain groups of children deserve special consideration when prescribing spectacles, such as those with light sensitivity (e.g. albinism or achromats), who will benefit from at least one pair of tinted prescription lenses. The back vertex distance should be recorded if the error is greater than 5 diopters. Separate glasses for near or a reading addition should not be forgotten in aphakia or those with reduced accommodation (to be anticipated in children with Down syndrome or developmental delay). Some children may have poor head control and look at a computer screen with upgaze. A traditional bifocal will be useless and two pairs are recommended. Pseudophakic children seem to benefit from varifocal lenses. Children with craniofacial deformity require careful fitting of frames which may need to be expertly assessed and specially manufactured. Children with only one seeing eye should be advised to wear protective (polycarbonate) glasses.

Conclusion

Once used to the physical sensation of wearing spectacles, correct glasses are often worn well. Intolerance should lead to reconsideration of the need for glasses or an error in the prescription or dispensing. One possible exception is the child with a manifest esotropia with accommodative element and amblyopia, who has one good eye with minimal refractive error. For these children, both patching and glasses wear may be problematic.

Further reading

Angi, MR, Pillotto, E. Photorefraction for the detection of amblyogenic defects: past and present. In: Infant Vision. Vital-Durand F, Atkinson, J & Braddick, OJ (ed.) Oxford University Press. Oxford 1996.

Celebi S, Aykan U. The comparison of cyclopentolate and atropine in patients with refractive accommodative esotropia by means of retinoscopy, autorefractometry and biometric lens thickness. *Acta Ophthalmologica Scandinavica* 1999; **77**(4): 426–9.

Goldstein, JH, Schneekloth BB. Atropine versus cyclopentolate plus tropicamide in esodeviations. *Ophthalmic Surgery & Lasers* 1996; **27**(12): 1030–4.

Kawamoto K, Hayasaka S. Cycloplegic refractions in Japanese children: a comparison of atropine and cyclopentolate. *Ophthalmologica* 1997; **211**(2): 57–60.

Mohindra, I. A non-cycloplegic refraction technique for infants and young children. *Journal of the American Optometric Association* 1977; **48**(4): 518–23.

Saunders *et al.* 'Emmetropisation in human infancy: rate of change is related to initial refractive error' *Vision-Res.* 1995; **35**(9): 1325–8.

Related topics of interest

Child with strabismus work-up (p. 45); Congenital nystagmus (p. 69); Diplopia work-up (p. 105); Esotropia, convergence and accommodation (p. 113); Exotropia, divergence and accommodation (p. 118); Visual impairment in children (p. 341).

REFRACTIVE SURGERY

Paul Chell

Ametropia is common. Myopia alone accounts for up to 10% of the population. The standard treatment for ametropia is spectacles. Spectacles are considered by some to be inconvenient and cumbersome. Intrinsic optical aberrations may be intolerable. Improved techniques and outcomes in refractive surgery have led to greater numbers of patients seeking this alternative to spectacle wear. This is particularly so in patients who are unable to wear contact lenses, or who choose to avoid them.

Problem

The main problem with refractive surgery is that it is not risk free.

Background

The main risks in refractive surgery come from poor patient selection, surgical complications and postoperative complications. The patient must be seen not as two eyes but as a whole and their expectations carefully assessed. Their knowledge, no matter how well researched, will be limited. Often they will have decided to go ahead with surgery before consultation, having performed the risk assessment from a standpoint of limited knowledge. It is therefore incumbent on the surgeon to ensure the patient has accurate data on both the risks and benefits of refractive surgery. This aspect of care takes time, but is an essential part of modern refractive surgery. Full evaluation of the eyes and the best option for the patient can only be achieved by a specialist with considerable experience in the field of corneal, lens and refractive surgery.

Treatment

The treatments for myopia include laser-assisted in-situ keratomileusis (LASIK), surface photorefractive keratectomy (S-PRK), radial keratotomy (RK), intrastromal corneal rings (ISCR), phakic intraocular lens (posterior and anterior chamber) and small incision clear lensectomy with insertion of intraocular lens.

Surface-photorefractive keratectomy (S-PRK)

After removal of the corneal epithelium the excimer laser reshapes the stromal bed. The delivery systems vary between different machines, but the reshaping profile is similar. The corneal curvature is reduced in the central treatment zone relative to the pretreatment curvature, thus reducing the vergence power of the cornea. Early systems had intrinsic problems due to small treatment zone size (3.5 to 4.5 mm) with resultant halos and glare. Current systems are more sophisticated and not only have larger treatment zones (5.5 to 6.6 mm) but also have outer blend zones. The other major problems with early treatments were central islands. Modern machines have within their software integral anticentral island modalities.

The major drawbacks of S-PRK are haze-regression reactions, pain following treatment and prolonged visual recovery. Haze-regression reactions occur simultaneously with the vision becoming hazy along with myopic regression. The more myopic the treatment the more likely are haze-regression reactions. Haze-regression reactions can be mild or severe enough to regress to the original refraction with dense corneal scarring. The scarring usually fades with time. As a rule of thumb, severe haze-regression reaction occurs in 2% at −2.00, 8% at −4.00 and 16% at −8.00. This keratocyte response does not occur with LASIK. The cause is unknown but may be related to epithelial growth factors and/or the removal of Bowman's layer in S-PRK. These complications lead to lower thresholds for choosing LASIK. Initially LASIK started at −6.00 DS, but now the starting point for many surgeons is −3.00 DS, and some prefer all their patients to have LASIK.

Laser-assisted in-situ keratomileusis (LASIK)

LASIK utilizes old and new technology and began in 1989. The 1960s microkeratome and keratomileusis techniques of Barraquer (Bogotá) were combined with newer excimer laser techniques (popularized by S-PRK) and the LASIK procedure was born. The surgeons responsible for early development were Lucio Buratto (Milan) and Iannis Pallikaris (Crete). Using a modern microkeratome a flap of anterior cornea is fashioned, leaving a short segment attached that acts as a hinge. The flaps are generally 8.5 to 9.5 mm in diameter and 160 to 200 µm thick. The laser is applied to the exposed stroma. The flap is replaced. The main advantages are rapid recovery in unaided acuity and absence of haze-regression reactions. It is almost painless postoperatively and carries similar risks of infection (1:2000) to S-PRK. Because of the rapidity in recovery many surgeons perform bilateral simultaneous LASIK, avoiding the problems of anisometropia between treatments.

The main drawbacks with LASIK are flap problems. These occur in 1–5% of LASIK procedures. These may vary from mild wrinkling or interface foreign bodies to severe damage or even loss. Incomplete passes of the microkeratome are best left and retreated at a later date, usually successfully. Flap melts are rare but have been reported and require further flap surgery if affecting the axial zone. For this, flaps may be repositioned vertically or horizontally but should not be rotated. Epithelial in-growth not requiring intervention is common. Severe forms requiring intervention are rare (<1%).

Accuracy is optimal up to −6.00 DS, good up to −8.00 DS and falls off over −10.00 DS. Patients should be counselled accordingly. Above −12.00 DS, the depth of ablation requires a smaller treatment zone in normal thickness corneae, and this combined with lower refractive accuracy makes LASIK suitable up to about −10.00 to −12.00. Retreatment with LASIK is much easier than S-PRK and is usually performed at 3 months when the refraction has stabilized, the flap can easily be re-lifted and further excimer laser applied. Normal postoperative flap risks apply.

Contact lenses should be removed prior to assessment and surgery: soft lenses for 2 weeks, gas-permeable 4 weeks and hard 6 weeks. This allows the cornea to return to its natural curvature prior to assessment and treatment. Topography is essential and many cases of previously undiagnosed keratoconus will be discovered. Pachymetry is mandatory and at least 33% of the corneal thickness should remain after flap and ablation are summed, to prevent late ectasia and myopic shift. Manifest refraction must be accurate and should include duochrome and +1.00 DS blur tests to prevent overcorrection. If monovision is required then this should be tried, wherever possible, with contact lenses first. Up to 30% of patients will not tolerate the −1.75 D of residual myopia in the nondominant eye. The best test for eye dominance is the swinging +2.00 blur test for distance over fully corrected eyes. This is carried out by swinging a +2 lens between the two eyes and asking the patient to choose which option has better vision. The +2 lens is in front of the nondominant eye.

Other procedures

Radial keratotomy is rarely performed since the advent of excimer laser. Intrastromal corneal rings are under development, as are phakic intraocular lenses. Clear lens extraction in myopia carries a 5% risk of retinal detachment over 5 years.

Hyperopia

The same LASIK principles apply for hyperopia but the laser treatment increases the vergence power of the treatment zone by increasing the central corneal curvature. Results are less accurate than for myopia and the treatment zone is smaller leading to an increased risk of halos and glare. Most surgeons will treat up to +4.00 DS to +6.00 DS. In the presbyope, clear lens surgery may be better with either a monofocal or a multifocal lens implant. The accuracy of biometry is a problem in hyperopia and there is also a risk of aqueous misdirection syndrome, choroidal effusion syndrome and malignant glaucoma.

Further reading

Buratto L. *Corneal topography*. Slack incorporated, 1996.
Claoué C. *Laser and Conventional Refractive Surgery*. BMJ Publishing Group, London, UK, 1996.
Machat JM. Excimer laser refractive surgery. Slack incorporated, Thorofare, NJ, USA, 1996.
Thornton SP. Radial and astigmatic keratotomy. Slack incorporated, Thorofare, NJ, USA, 1994.

RETINAL DYSTROPHIES

S.J. Talks & Peter Shah

There are a wide variety of inherited retinal dystrophies that can cause severe visual loss. They are characterized by slow and progressive retinal degeneration. In recent years much has been learned about their aetiology and there is new hope for treatment in the future.

Problem

Retinal dystrophies often present at a young age and can cause life-long progressive visual impairment. Such a diagnosis has implications for the whole family and continued visual support and social support may be needed. An accurate diagnosis should be the aim of management as this enables the clinician to give a more accurate prognosis and also helps with genetic counselling. Many patients are keen to be kept up to date on the progress of research in the field of retinal dystrophies.

Background

Using a classification based on phenotypic appearance, the retinal dystrophies can be divided into: macular dystrophies, cone–rod dystrophies and peripheral retinal degenerations. Recent research is now allowing many of these diseases to be reclassified on the basis of the molecular genetic abnormality. Interestingly the phenotypic and genetic classifications do not always segregate clearly together. One gene can be responsible for many phenotypes and one phenotype may result from many different genes. The mode of inheritance of the retinal dystrophies can be autosomal dominant, autosomal recessive, X-linked recessive or mitochondrial.

Examples of genes which if abnormal can lead to retinal dystrophies include :

1. Phototransduction pathway.

- *Rhodopsin*   Retinitis pigmentosa – (>100 mutations) or congenital stationary night blindness;
- *Transducin*   CSNB PDE   RP, CSNB;
- *RETGC1*   Leber congenital amaurosis, cone–rod dystrophy;
- *GCAP1*   cone dystrophy, cone–rod dystrophy;
- *arrestin*   Oguchi disease.

2. Structural proteins.

- *Peripherin/RDS*   AD RP, AD macular dystrophy, AD cone–rod dystrophy, AD pattern dystrophy, AD central areolar choroidal dystrophy;
- *XLRS1*   X-linked retinoschisis.

3. RPE-photoreceptor metabolism.

- *ABCR*   AD Stargardt disease, cone–rod dystrophy, RP, role in ARMD;
- *TIMP3*   AD Sorsby fundus dystrophy;
- *RPGR*   X-linked recessive RP;
- *Bestrophin*   AD, Best disease (vitelliform macular dystrophy).

Clinical features

The age of onset may help diagnosis. For example, RP, Best and Stargardt disease can start in childhood. Pattern dystrophy usually presents in mid life and Sorsby's dystrophy in later life. However, the effect on vision can be very variable and may remain unnoticed for some time.

A careful analysis of the visual symptoms is very useful. Night blindness suggests rod involvement, however, initial problems in dim light which then improve are often due to a cone problem. Vision which is better in a dim light suggests a cone dystrophy. Decreased visual acuity and colour vision point to macular involvement.

Mode of inheritance may also help with diagnosis. Family members need to be examined as there is often phenotypic variation which may help pin down a diagnosis. Family members may not know they are affected, and one must be sensitive to this when they are examined and counselled particularly if children are to be investigated. Carriers may also be affected (e.g. X-linked RP and choroideraemia).

The clinical pattern of abnormality is often the best clue to a diagnosis. The macula, peripheral retina, retinal vessels and optic disc all need to be examined. For example, the retinal vessels will be narrow and the optic disk pale in RP, but normal in choroidaraemia and Stargardt. A macular lesion in association with a peripheral flecked retinal appearance is likely to be Stargardt's disease or fundus flavimaculata. However, in some cases the phenotypic appearance can only suggest a range of diagnoses. For example, a Bull's eye appearance at the macular could be chloroquine maculopathy, a macular dystrophy, a cone dystrophy or a cone–rod dystrophy. It is also important to remember that the retinal appearance may be normal, despite the presence of a retinal dystrophy.

Perimetry may demonstrate peripheral field loss or macular scotomas. Some patients may be asymptomatic for these losses.

In some cases fluorescein angiography may help the diagnosis. In particular a dark choroid is very suggestive of Stargardt disease, and slow choroidal filling is seen in Sorsby dystrophy. Fluorescein angiography may also be useful in the management of associated complications of the dystrophies such as choroidal neovascularization (which can occur in many dystrophies) and cystoid macular oedema.

1. ***Electrodiagnostic tests*** can objectively measure the function of the macula (pattern ERG), cones (30 Hz flicker ERG), rods (scotopic ERG) specifically. Some disease may have characteristic abnormalities, e.g. in vitelliform macular dystrophy the EOG is severely subnormal in all stages of the disease in affected patients, and is also subnormal in carriers with apparently normal fundi. Characteristic inversion of the 'b' wave is seen in CSNB.

2. ***Genetic tests*** are not widely available outside of research labs and in many cases would be difficult to do on a routine basis due to the wide range of gene mutations involved. However, it is possible that different testing strategies will become possible soon. In some dystrophies most affected individuals in the United Kingdom are due to one mutation (e.g. 181 mutation in TIMP3 in Sorsby's dystrophy) thus making testing more practical.

3. Treatment. There are no specific treatments to slow the retinal degenerative process at the present time for almost all dystrophies. Visual support needs to be given by low vision aids and appropriate registration of visual impairment. Advice on schooling, work, driving, prognosis and genetics may be needed. Patient support groups can be of great help, particularly for conditions that are relatively rare. There are as yet no specific treatments which can alter the cause of these diseases, with a few exceptions: such as the use of a phytanic acid-free diet which may help in Refsum disease. Research work is progressing rapidly on the use of growth factors and other mediators to slow the rate of cell death, gene therapy to supply working copies of the faulty genes, retinal transplantation and the use of artificial vision.

Further reading

Gregory-Evans K, Bhattacharya SS. Genetic blindness: current concepts in the pathogenesis of outer retinal dystrophies. *TIG* 1998; **14:** 103–8.

Chong NHV, Bird AC. Management of inherited outer retinal dystrophies: present and future. *British Journal of Ophthalmology* 1999; **83:** 120–2.

http://www.sph.uth.tmc.edu/RetNet/

Related topics of interest

Night blindness (p. 182); Retinitis pigmentosa (p. 265).

RETINAL VEIN OCCLUSION

Paul Dodson & Marie D. Tsaloumas

Retinal vein occlusion (RVO) can occur in all ages: 51% occur in patients aged 65 years or older, but 10–15% occur in patients under the age of 45 although it is very rare in childhood. Both central retinal vein occlusion (CRVO) and branch retinal vein occlusion (BRVO) are less common amongst African-Caribbean and Asian (Indo-Pakistani) races in the UK. The visual prognosis is dependent on the type of retinal vein occlusion (CRVO or BRVO), the severity of initial insult, underlying medical and ocular conditions, ocular sequelae and recurrence.

Problem

There is no standardized ocular or medical intervention that can reverse retinal vein occlusion once it has occurred, therefore ocular management is aimed at preventing and dealing with complications and medical management is aimed at identifying underlying medical risk factors to possibly prevent a recurrence.

Background

It is now recognized that an important primary event is damage of the wall of the venous vasculature, with cellular proliferation in the venous endothelium. The mechanism underlying initial endothelial swelling is multifactorial and is likely to reflect the differing aetiologies of RVO. Whether retinal arteriolar abnormalities are responsible for venous occlusion at the site of arteriolar venous crossing (e.g. BRVO) has been much debated, but experimental and other long-term follow-up data suggests that primary retinal venous disease is a separate entity. Histologically, thrombus formation is probably a secondary event and may be responsible for final occlusion of the retinal vein. Platelet function abnormalities and thrombophilic disorders may underlie this process.

Mechanisms of visual loss:

1. ***Ischaemic.*** Visual loss may result from either direct foveal involvement in the RVO, or indirectly from the complications of the RVO (vitreous haemorrhage from retinal neovascularization, traction retinal detachment and neovascular glaucoma).

2. ***Exudative.*** Breakdown of the blood–retinal barrier causes macular oedema and lipid exudation.

Underlying ocular conditions may include raised intraocular pressure (IOP), trauma, orbital lesions and tumours. Major underlying medical conditions include hypertension, diabetes mellitus and hyperlipidaemia, with rarer causes due to hyperviscosity/hypercoagulability syndromes, inflammatory disease and thrombophilic disorders. Patterns of underlying conditions vary according to age (e.g. in young patients thrombophilic and lipid disorders are more common) and race. The contraceptive pill has been implicated in young female patients but current evidence does not incriminate hormone replacement in postmenopausal women.

Table 1. Aetiological conditions in retinal vein occlusion

	Systemic	Local
Common	Hypertension	Glaucoma
	Hyperlipidaemia	Trauma
	Diabetes mellitus	Orbital lesions
	Smoking	
Rarer	Chronic renal failure	
	Myeloma and Waldenstrom's macroglobulinaemia	
	Inflammatory disease/systemic vasculitis – Behçet's disease, polyarteritis nodosa, sarcoidosis, Wegener's granulomatosis, Goodpasture's syndrome, SLE.	
	Thrombophilic disorders – protein S, C, factor V Leiden, antithrombin 3 deficiency, and activated protein C resistance abnormalities.	
	Oestrogen containing oral contraceptive	
	Secondary causes of hypercholesterolaemia, diabetes and hypertension e.g. acromegaly, Cushing's syndrome, hypothyroidism	

Clinical features

Patients usually present with painless loss of vision of varying severity although occasionally it can be an asymptomatic finding. Routine ocular examination is performed with attention to the following details: visual acuity, presence of a relative afferent pupil defect (RAPD), presence of rubeosis iridis (including gonioscopy), IOP measurement and detailed fundal examination.

BRVOs usually occur at arteriovenous crossings with the arteriole positioned anterior to the vein. The changes of venous occlusion are limited to either the superior or inferior retina. The resultant visual acuity is determined by the location of the BRVO in relation to the fovea and the presence of a collateral circulation. Macular branch vein occlusion is a subgroup of BRVO, where the occlusion is limited to a smaller venous tributary draining a sector of the macula. Macular BRVO is treated as a BRVO. Occasionally it may be mistaken for diabetic maculopathy. Clinically BRVO is characterized by flame haemorrhages, dot and blot haemorrhages, cotton wool spots and retinal oedema in the sector of the retina drained by the affected vein. Chronic retinal changes are characterized by venous sheathing, exudates, collateral vessels (which must be differentiated from new vessels), cystoid macula oedema and retinal pigment epithelial changes. Extensive retinal ischaemia (five disc diameters or more of retinal non-perfusion) can result in new vessel formation from the retina or rarely from the optic nerve.

Characteristic fundus appearance of CRVO consists of dilated tortuous retinal veins, a swollen optic disc, intraretinal haemorrhages, cotton wool spots and retinal oedema, all of varying severity depending on whether the CRVO is *non-ischaemic* or *ischaemic* type. Papillophlebitis, where the changes are mainly confined to the optic disc can be seen in the younger age group and may have an inflammatory basis. Non-ischaemic CRVO is characterized by better visual acuity at baseline, and fluorescein angiography demonstrates prolonged circulation time rather than non-perfusion. It must be differentiated from ocular ischaemia. Chronic changes include sheathing of veins, absorption of the haemorrhages, disc collaterals and macular disturbances. Anomalous patterns of venous drainage may give rise to hemicentral (hemispherical) retinal vein occlusion (HRVO) which is considered a variant of CRVO.

Other diseases may have a similar clinical appearance to RVO and include: accelerated hypertension, diabetes mellitus, slow-flow retinopathy, peripapillary telangiectasia, anterior ischaemic optic neuropathy, lupus retinopathy and cytomegalovirus retinitis.

A number of parameters can be used to predict new vessel formation:

- Relative afferent papillary defect and severely reduced visual acuity.
- Fundus fluorescein angiography (FFA). Showing more than 10 disc diameters (DD) of capillary closure (significant ischaemia) or 5–10 DD (borderline ischaemia).
- Retinal signs including cotton wool spots (more than 10 indicate significant ischaemia and five to 10 borderline) or deep dark haemorrhages (haemorrhagic infarcts).
- Iris rubeosis (more common in the more elderly population with CRVO).

Up to one third of CRVO eyes with an initial non-ischaemic picture will convert to the ischaemic form usually within the first 4 months 13% at 6 months, and 18% by 18 months.

Treatment

This is based on the findings of the Central and Branch Retinal Vein Occlusion Study Groups. The diagnosis of branch retinal vein occlusion is by clinical examination. Macular oedema and proliferative complications may require laser therapy. Randomized clinical studies have recommended argon laser treatment of macular oedema if the foveal vasculature is intact, and vision is between 6/12 and 6/60. Therapy should be delayed until 3–6 months following the initial event to permit maximum spontaneous resolution of oedema and intraretinal blood. Fluorescein angiography should be carried out prior to therapy to identify the leaking capillaries and to assess the presence of macular ischaemia which may limit or contraindicate laser treatment. Those with severe visual loss (<6/60) are unlikely to benefit. Proliferative complications are an indication for laser treatment to the area of ischaemic retina (usually sector photocoagulation). Laser can also be considered where angiography reveals large areas of nonperfusion (5 DD or more). Patients should be reviewed within 6 weeks of the event with results of investigations and follow-up is up to 2 years or until it is obvious that the condition has stabilized or resolved, e.g. collateral vessel formation.

A new surgical interventional technique for the acute occlusion involves surgical decompression of the BRVO via an arteriovenous crossing, termed sheathotomy.

For CRVO, treatment is aimed at preventing neovascularization. Any elevation of intraocular pressure in the affected or fellow eye should be treated. Grid laser treatment for macular oedema does not benefit visual acuity and is not undertaken. Rather, adequate panretinal scatter photocoagulation should be performed as soon as possible in the presence of disc or iris neovascularization and can be considered for very ischaemic CRVOs before frank neovascularization develops. Close follow up of ischaemic CRVOs is necessary to monitor for rubeosis iridis in order to prevent neovascular glaucoma.

If there is no evidence of neovascularization the first review should be around 4 weeks, depending on clinical findings and results of routine investigations. If laser photocoagulation or FFA is indicated, the haemorrhages should have resolved sufficiently to allow these procedures to be carried out. If there is an unequivocal RAPD, and severe reduction in visual acuity and a 'blood and thunder' haemorrhagic retinal appearance, pan-retinal photocoagulation (PRP) should be performed avoiding areas of retinal haemorrhage. Monthly follow-up is advised. The intermediate group (>10 and <40 DD of closure on FFA) do not require laser treatment unless early rubeosis develops. Fluorescein angiography should be performed to identify the intermediate group. In nonischaemic CRVO (or <10 DD of closure on FFA), trials of PRP vs. no PRP have shown no difference in visual outcome. Corneal oedema and a small pupil may prevent PRP in patients with neovascular glaucoma. In borderline cases, one should err towards photocoagulation. Do not miss the therapeutic window.

Once nonischaemic CRVO is stable, there is no evidence to date that laser improves the visual outcome of macular oedema. There is usually a minor improvement in visual acuity with time. Recently there has been interest in the technique of laser-induced chorioretinal venous anastomosis for nonischaemic CRVO to establish a collateral circulation before irreversible macular changes occur.

At further review (about 3 months), gonioscopy for new vessels should be undertaken and IOP should be checked. If the PRP has insufficient uptake, do further laser. Serial checks for RAPD are needed and if conversion to an ischaemic type occurs consider PRP. If at any time, retinal new vessels are seen, or neovascular glaucoma occurs, then immediate PRP is indicated. Retinal cryotherapy may be considered if there is a poor fundal view. Medical treatment of the raised intraocular pressure is rarely useful and cyclodiode laser to the ciliary body should be considered. For most patients, a total follow-up period of 2 years is advisable.

Medical management of patients presenting with RVO includes a full history and examination as well as appropriate investigations (see Table 2). These include investigations for all patients and more specialised investigations appropriate to clinical indication.

Medical management should be targeted at four areas:

- to maximize visual outcome or reversal of RVO – e.g. pre-occlusive RVO may reverse;
- to ameliorate excess cardiovascular morbidity and mortality associated with RVO;
- to achieve cardiovascular risk factor treatment as guided by national guidelines;
- prevent recurrence in the fellow eye, and thus prevent potential disastrous visual outcome.

Table 2. Initial medical investigations for patients presenting with RVO

All patients
    Full blood count and ESR (plasma viscosity)
    Urea, electrolytes, creatinine, liver function tests
    Blood glucose
    Lipid profile (random cholesterol and HDL cholesterol)
    Plasma protein electrophoresis
    ECG
    Thyroid function

More specialized according to clinical information
    Chest X-ray
    Thrombophilia screen
    Cardiolipin, lupus anticoagulant
    C-reactive protein
    Serum angiotensin-converting enzyme
    Auto-antibodies – rheumatoid/ANA/DNA/ANCA
    MRI – orbital and brain scan

Trials of medical treatments to improve retinal venous flow (anticoagulants, streptokinase, clofibrate, antiplatelet drugs and haemodilution) have been disappointing, either due to lack of efficacy or to adverse events. However, the studies are incomplete and recent reports open the possibility of streptokinase therapy in acute RVO (within hours), steroids in younger patients and haemodilution.

There is an increase in vascular causes of death (cardiac and cerebral) in patients with RVO. Management of cardiovascular risk factors should be according to the joint guidelines of the British Hypertension, Hyperlipidaemia and Diabetic Associations. Suggested targets and a summary are shown in Table 3. This will commonly result in patients being treated with dual antihypertensive therapy, a statin and aspirin. Several series have demonstrated that recurrence of retinal vein occlusion may occur in up to 15% of patients over a 5-year period. Available data support the concept that recurrence of retinal vein occlusion may be reduced by medical treatments of underlying cardiovascular risk factors with addition of aspirin/persantin therapy. Conventional management of rarer conditions underlying RVO (e.g. myeloma, collagen inflammatory diseases, thrombophilic disorders) should be referred and managed by appropriate specialists.

Table 3. Suggested targets and cardiovascular risk management in patients with RVO

1.	Measure BP, serum cholesterol, HDL cholesterol, and ECG. Record presence of diabetes, smoking, age and sex.
2.	Calculate overall cardiovascular risk according to Framingham equation.
3.	>15% CHD risk (10 year)
	Systolic BP ≤ 140 mmHg
	Cholesterol < 5 mmol/l $^+$
	Glycosylated haemoglobin <7%
4.	<15% CHD risk (10 year)
	Systolic BP and glycosylated haemoglobin as above.
	Cholesterol >6.5 mmol – lifestyle advice, check for genetic hyperlipidaemia.*

(* Genetic hyperlipidaemia should be managed appropriately.)

Further reading

The Central Vein Occlusion Study Group. Natural history and clinical management of central retinal vein occlusion. *Archives of Ophthalmology* 1997; **115:** 486–91.

Hayreh SS, Zimmerman MB, Podhajsky P. Incidence of various types of retinal vein occlusion and their recurrence and demographic characteristics. *American Journal of Ophthalmology* 1994; **117:** 429–41.

Keenan JM, Dodson PM, and Kritzinger EE. Management of retinal vein occlusion. *British Journal of Hospital Medicine* 1993; **49:** 268–73.

Risk factors for branch retinal vein occlusion. The Eye Disease Case–control Study Group. *American Journal of Ophthalmology* 1993; **116:** 286–96.

Related topics of interest

Behçet's disease (p. 19); Diabetic maculopathy (p. 97); Diabetic retinopathy (p. 100); Sarcoidosis (p. 276).

RETINITIS PIGMENTOSA

S.J. Talks & Peter Shah

Retinitis pigmentosa (RP) is one of a large group of inherited retinal dystrophies characterized by slow progressive retinal degeneration. It affects about 1:3500 people in the population.

Problem

The diagnosis of RP has serious implications and so the assessment needs to be accurate. Although there is no treatment that as yet can alter the underlying retinal degenerative process, the patient should have access to: advice on visual prognosis, genetic counselling, visual rehabilitation and low vision assessment, registration for visual disability and social support services. Many patients are also keen to know about information on progress in RP research. There are many RP-associated syndromes which require specific management (e.g. Refsum's disease and a phytanic acid-free diet).

Background

RP inheritance is dominant (10–25%), recessive (60%) or X-linked recessive (5–18%). Less commonly, and usually in association with other findings, RP may be due to a mitochondrial DNA abnormality. An accurate family history is very important as the mode of inheritance has implications for likely prognosis and enables accurate genetic counselling. X-linked cases tend to have a worse prognosis. If possible, all family members should be examined. In X-linked families female carriers may also be affected, but not usually as severely as males in the same family and usually at a later age. In some dominant families there is variable expression or incomplete penetrance and the condition may have appeared to have skipped a generation. Electrodiagnostic tests may be helpful in this situation. Singleton cases are often presumed to be recessively inherited but this is not always correct. The chance of autosomal recessive disease is increased if the parents are consanguineous. In autosomal recessive RP, siblings may be affected but their children are not at risk unless they have a partner who is a carrier (also more likely in consanguineous relationships). RP-like pigmentation can develop in a number of conditions that may not be progressive and are not inherited. These include: retinal detachment, posterior segment trauma, drug-induced (e.g. phenothiazine use), central retinal artery occlusion, and inflammatory conditions such as AZOOR and DUSN. A unilateral RP appearance is likely to be due to an acquired cause, although inherited RP can be asymmetric. In these cases, electroretinographic (ERG) testing and serial follow up are necessary.

Clinical features

RP typically presents in late childhood or early adulthood with night blindness, progressing to profound visual loss in middle or later life. However, some patients may not be aware of visual loss until central vision is affected. Occasionally patients may present with central visual loss due to macular oedema. Some patients are asymptomatic but found to have peripheral visual field loss or retinal pigmentation on routine screening. A few may have associated symptoms such as hearing loss in Usher's syndrome. The classical findings in RP are bilateral 'bone-spicule' pigmentation of the fundus, narrowed retinal vessels and an optic disc with 'waxy' pallor. However pigmentary changes may be sparse, or not found in the early stages of the disease. Other ocular findings may include: posterior subcapsular cataract, scanty vitreous cells, cystoid macular oedema, epiretinal membrane, Coats'-type telangiectasia with exudative leakage. Cystoid macular oedema can present at any stage.

Atypical forms of RP include: RP sine pigmenti, retinitis punctata albescens, Leber's congenital amaurosis, paravenous retinochoroidal atrophy and sector RP. Mid-peripheral scotomas lead to marked visual field constriction and tunnel vision in severe cases. Electrodiagnostic tests are essential if the diagnosis is uncertain, are useful to measure remaining retinal function and can help with follow up. The scotopic ERG will be reduced reflecting reduced rod function. The 30 Hz flicker ERG may also be reduced reflecting some cone loss and the EOG may be reduced as the retinal pigment epithelium is also affected. Molecular genetic tests are not readily available at present. A large number of genetic defects have been found in a variety of genes associated with RP. In a large family where a specific mutation has been found then other members could be screened.

Treatment

Acetazolamide (500 mg daily as a single slow-release tablet) can help cystoid macular oedema. Cataract surgery may be of benefit although it can exacerbate macular oedema. Small PSC can be particularly disabling in the patient with severely constricted visual fields. Care must be taken during cataract surgery in RP patients to reduce the risk of photic maculopathy from incident operating microscope light by the use of appropriate surgical techniques and microscope filters. Counselling, low vision aids assessment and blind registration may be necessary in some patients. Self-help groups, such as the British RP Society can put families in touch with other people with RP.

Possible future treatments include slowing cell death either with growth factors or genetic regulation of apoptosis, replacement or reparative gene therapy in which cells are transfected with a functioning copy of the faulty gene, DNA-based or repair mechanism, retinal cell transplantation and electronic forms of visual processing are all techniques which are under active research.

Further reading

Bird AC. Retinitis pigmentosa. In: *Genetic Eye Disease*. T. Elias (ed.) OUP, 1998.
Heckenlively JR. *Retinitis Pigmentosa*. JB Lippincott company, Philadelphia, 1988.

Related topics of interest

Night blindness (p. 182); Retinal dystrophies (p. 256).

RETINOBLASTOMA

Massoud Fouladi & Harry Willshaw

Retinoblastoma (RB) is the commonest ocular malignancy of childhood and is fatal unless treated. In the United Kingdom the incidence of RB is between 1/20 000 and 1/23 000 live births, causing about 3% of all childhood cancers. Males and females are equally affected. Based on evaluation by the UK Childhood Cancer Research Group (UKCCRG) it is now possible to provide accurate empiric counselling for affected families. The incidence of bilateral involvement ranges between 25% and 40%. Approximately 10% of all affected children will have a positive family history, though between 8 and 14% of familial cases will only be unilaterally affected. Conversely 3% of unilaterally affected parents will go on to have affected children, of whom more than 90% have bilateral tumours.

Problem

Despite the high survival rate for RB (90%), there are a number of concerns about conventional, conservative retinoblastoma treatment, and particularly the impact of radiotherapy on facial growth and CNS development in such young children. However, the identification of a significant second, nonocular tumour risk in treated obligate gene carriers and the development of effective chemotherapy regimens that avoided the use of alkylating agents, has triggered the search for a chemotherapeutic approach to treatment.

Clinical features

RB can be classified on clinical or histological bases. The vast majority of children present in the first two years of life, but the diagnosis should be entertained throughout the first decade. Bilaterally affected children present earlier than those who are unilaterally affected (mean 8 months) and the most common presenting complaint is a white/yellow pupillary reflex. Other modes of presentation include strabismus, buphthalmos, iris rubeosis, unexplained severe uveitis, pseudohypopyon, heterochromia and, extremely rarely, raised intracranial pressure when a 'trilateral retinoblastoma' presents with CNS pathology before the ocular disease has been identified. Amongst European and North American patients, presentation with extraocular spread is extremely rare, but in series from developing countries orbital spread or distant metastases are more common at presentation, and the survival rates are correspondingly poor.

1. Clinical classification. The classification introduced by Reese and Ellsworth in 1964 is the most widely used clinical classification, though a more comprehensive classification suggested by Murphree in 1996 is being adopted in many centres. Both take into account the observable clinical parameters of tumour size, location, vitreous involvement and associated retinal detachment. In addition, the Murphree classification takes account of the presence of glaucoma, anterior segment disease and lens touch. The more advanced tumours, Reese–Ellsworth groups IV and V, or Murphree groups D2, E and F are likely to be considered for enucleation.

2. *Histopathological classification.* There are two main patterns of RB growth. Endophytic tumours tend to grow forward into the vitreous and exophytic tumours grow into the subretinal space. Histologically RB is a more or less differentiated malignant tumour of primitive retinal cell, which contains large hyperchromatic nuclei and scanty cytoplasm. Attempts at cell differentiation in some tumours result in 'Flexner–Wintersteiner rosette' formation seen as columnar cells uniformly arranged in a sphere around a lumen containing primitive outer segments of photoreceptors. Other features include pseudorosette formation and the development of fleurettes. RBs typically undergo calcification as the tumour growth outstrips its blood supply and this calcification can be seen on CT scanning. If an eye containing RB is enucleated, histopathological examination is needed to define the extent of any optic nerve invasion, choroidal invasion, anterior segment involvement and scleral or extrascleral extension.

The major difficulty arises in distinguishing between retinoblastoma and Coats' disease, parasitic granulomata, some instances of persistent hyperplastic primary vitreous (though the eye in PHPV is usually microphthalmic), and retinal dysplasias. The late onset, diffuse infiltrating tumour, which typically fails to calcify, may also be mistaken for an intermediate uveitis.

Though retinoblastoma affects 45% of the offspring of obligate gene carriers (90% penetrance for the gene), at a molecular level it requires both alleles of a tumour suppressor gene to be damaged before the tumour(s) can develop. Therefore, in known familial cases and the offspring of bilateral sporadic cases, the transmitting parent must be heterozygous for the gene mutation, transmitting the abnormal allele to 50% of their offspring. Thereafter, a second mutagenic event affecting a retinal precursor cell will result in malignant transformation. Since single events are relatively common, these heterozygotes typically show early onset, bilateral and multifocal tumours. In the absence of a germinal mutation, a developing retinal cell must suffer two exogenous 'hits' and, therefore, such tumours tend to be of later onset, unilateral and unifocal. It is now clear that in those unilateral tumours without germ-line mutation the two alleles are also lost, but in this instance it is within the tumour alone rather than all body cells, and hence the affected child does not show the same predisposition to develop other malignancies in later life.

The gene locus for retinoblastoma susceptibility was identified as being on the long arm of chromosome 13 in the early 1960s, later located at the 13q14 region. The *Rb1* gene was defined as a large, 180 kb gene with 27 exons encoding an mRNA transcript of 4.7 kb. Its protein product p110RB1 is involved in regulating the normal cell cycle (acting as a tumour suppressor gene). Loss of this protein allows unrestrained cellular proliferation.

Treatment

The management of RB should be undertaken by a multidisciplinary health care team. Assessment of the affected child to confirm the diagnosis is followed by disease staging and identification of any metastatic spread. Treatment of ocular and metastatic tumour in the affected child must be linked to genetic counselling for the family and early identification of any subsequently affected family members. Close relatives of children with RB should also be screened since these relatives may show evidence of regressed retinomas, and because they are also at increased risk of developing RB themselves.

At presentation a detailed history must be taken, followed by an examination under anaesthesia (EUA) with fully dilated pupils to define the full extent of the tumour. EUA must include scleral indentation, to identify any peripheral lesions, and a fundal drawing is made together with indirect video recording or digitalized imaging of the tumour.

Fundus fluorescein angiography is rarely necessary but may occasionally be used to differentiate RB from other conditions. CT scans are particularly useful for identifying calcification within the tumour that is rare in lesions simulating RB. It can also be used to identify intracranial extension and 'trilateral' tumours. Bone marrow aspiration, lumbar puncture and bone scan investigations must be undertaken in patients with definite or suspected optic nerve involvement or with evidence of extraocular spread. Any attempt to biopsy the RB tumour should be avoided since this can lead to extraocular extension.

The survival rate for RB has improved dramatically since it was first described. At present over 90% of children survive thanks to early diagnosis and aggressive treatment. The challenge for any new treatment modality is not only to improve the survival rate, but also to reduce the complications associated with existing modes of treatments. Over the years there has been increasing emphasis on preserving sight in affected eyes whilst still eradicating the tumour.

Enucleation alone is curative for most children with unilateral disease and in many children with bilateral disease in whom the worst affected eye can be enucleated. Enucleation is performed with a minimal manipulation technique and an attempt is made to obtain at least 8–12 mm of optic nerve. In recent years, hydroxyapatite or medpor orbital implants have been successfully used to improve long-term cosmetic results.

The introduction of external beam radiation (EBR) in the 1960s significantly improved the chance of preserving sight whilst maintaining the high cure rate for RB. Unfortunately, EBR has been reported as carrying a 35% risk of second malignancy during the 30 years following treatment (in bilaterally affected patients). There are also cosmetic and functional consequences associated with EBR including defects of the bony orbit, dry eyes and subsequent ocular surface disease, cataract and hypopituitarism. Many of these problems persist despite fractionating the radiotherapy into 20 or more doses.

Historically, chemotherapy was used only in cases with extraocular extension of RB, but in recent years it has been introduced as a primary treatment in combination with focal therapy. This development has reduced the need for EBR and enucleation in many patients with RB. The most commonly used chemotherapeutic agents are vincristine sulphate, etoposide and carboplatin. It has been observed, however, that many retinoblastomas demonstrate the phenomenon of multiple drug resistance (MDR). A surface p-glycoprotein is induced by the chemotherapy which in turn actively pumps the chemotherapy agents out of RB cells. This p-glycoprotein can be 'switched off' experimentally with cyclosporin-A, and clinically it has been possible to treat effectively some postchemotherapy recurrences by introducing cyclosporin A into the therapeutic regimen.

The modality of local treatments varies between centres but the most commonly used are laser treatment, cryotherapy and plaque brachytherapy. Successful treatment is assumed when the tumour becomes completely calcified, or is replaced by a flat chorioretinal scar.

Spread of RB either locally beyond the sclera, or to a distant site, carries a poor prognosis. These patients are treated with a combination of chemotherapy and EBR.

Further reading

Gallie BL, Budning A, DeBoer G *et al.* Chemotherapy with focal therapy can cure intraocular retinoblastoma without radiation. *Archive of Ophthalmology* 1996; **114:** 1321–30.

Harbour JW. Overview of RB gene mutation in-patients with retinoblastoma: implications for clinical genetic screening. *Ophthalmology* 1998; **105:** 1442–7.

Murphree AL, Villablanca JG, Deega III WF *et al.* Chemotherapy plus local treatment in the management of intraocular retinoblastoma. *Archives of Ophthalmology* 1996; **114:** 1348–56.

Parkes SE, Amoaku WMK *et al.* Thirty years of retinoblastoma (1960–1989) changing patterns of incidence. *Paediatric Perinatal Epidemiology* 1994; **8:** 282–91.

Reese AB, Ellsworth RM. Management of retinoblastoma. *Annals New York Academy of Science* 1964; **114:** 958–62.

Sheilds CL, De Potter P, Himelstein BP *et al.* Chemoreduction in the initial management of intraocular retinoblastoma. *Archives of Ophthalmology,* 1996; **114:** 1330–8.

RHEGMATOGENOUS RETINAL DETACHMENT: ASSESSMENT

Theodoros Potamitis & Robert H. Taylor

A rhegmatogenous RD occurs as a result of a break in the neurosensory retina. It occurs at a rate of 1:10 000 per annum in the general population. Once a retinal break forms, fluid can pass into the subretinal space, separating the retina from the retinal pigment epithelium. At presentation, 10% of patients with a rhegmatogenous RD will also have an asymptomatic RD in the contralateral eye.

Problem

It is important to identify the patient with RD early and to identify the cause of the RD. It is also important to identify the patient at risk of a retinal detachment and provide prophylactic treatment in cases of retinal breaks. The timing of surgery and surgical approach is sometimes controversial. In addition a RD must be differentiated from retinoschisis and choroidal effusion/detachment. Differentiating these may be possible with a combination of clinical examination, ultrasonography and fundus fluorescein angiography.

Background

1. ***Pathophysiology.*** The vitreous consists of collagen fibrils and hyaluronic acid molecules within an aqueous gel. Its volume reduces with increasing age accompanied by the appearance of lacunae or liquid pockets in the gel. When one of these fluid pockets connects with the pre-retinal space, a posterior vitreous detachment (PVD) ensues. Retinal tears can occur due to vitreo–retinal traction at the time of vitreous detachment. Tears are, therefore, usually situated at the site of strongest vitreo–retinal adhesion, that is the vitreous base and areas of abnormal vitreo–retinal attachment, such as lattice degeneration. Once the vitreous and retina have fully separated there is no further risk of traction and therefore no further risk of new retinal tears. Retinal tears are present in 15% of symptomatic PVDs, and 50% of these will have more than one tear. Vitreous haemorrhage occurs in about 13–19% of acute PVDs and the incidence of retinal tears is 70% in these eyes. Myopes have a higher frequency of PVD at younger ages.

2. ***Pre-existing retinal findings.*** Lattice degeneration is characterized by an area of liquefying vitreous, overlying an area of thinned retina, with abnormal vitreo–retinal attachment. Clinically it appears as well demarcated areas of thin retina. A lattice type pattern of white lines is often present, often associated with pigmentary changes. Snail track degeneration is a variant of lattice, with a similar appearance, however the prominent feature is circumferential criss-cross white lines tracking in the retina. Lattice degeneration is present in approximately 7% of the population and is usually bilateral. Myopic eyes have a higher prevalence of lattice and it becomes increasingly common with increasing axial length. Diffuse chorioretinal atrophy may develop in highly myopic eyes and may be associated with the development of atrophic retinal holes. About 40% of eyes with a RD have lattice. Atrophic holes are present in 31% of patients with lattice and retinal tears frequently occur along the posterior border of the lattice following an acute PVD.

White without pressure is an appearance of the retina similar to the translucent grey appearance induced by indenting the retina (white with pressure). Giant retinal tears (a tear in the retina of more than 3 clock hours) may develop in eyes with white without pressure.

3. At-risk patients. Myopes have 42% of all RDs but make up 10% of the population. Up to 1.4% of patients who have had uncomplicated extracapsular surgery will develop RD. Laser posterior capsulotomy increases the incidence to 2.3%. RD may occur up to 20 years following surgery for congenital cataract.

Blunt ocular trauma may cause a retinal break or dialysis. A dialysis is an avulsion of the neurosensory retina from its attachment at the ora serrata. Unlike a retinal tear, the vitreous remains attached to both the proximal and distal edges of the break, giving rise to a relatively stable configuration. RD is therefore slow to progress. Retinal breaks have been found in up to 18% of patients with hyphaemas. Penetrating injury to the posterior segment may also damage the retina directly leading to RD, or may result in vitreous incarceration leading to tractional RD.

Other risk factors for RD include a group of diseases characterized by an optically empty vitreous, white bands attaching to the retina (vitreous veils), lattice and moderate myopia. These include Wagner syndrome, Marshall syndrome, Jansen syndrome and Stickler syndrome.

Other inherited conditions with a high risk of RD include Ehlers–Danlos syndrome, Goldmann–Favre syndrome, Marfan syndrome, spondyloepiphyseal dysplasia, coloboma and homocystinuria.

4. Acquired infections and retinal detachments. RD is seen in around 20% of patients with cytomegalovirus retinopathy in association with HIV infection. Vitrectomy with silicone oil is usually required for its management. It is estimated that up to 5% of AIDS patients are likely to develop a RD.

Acute retinal necrosis is a condition thought to result from infection with either the varicella zoster virus or the herpes simplex virus. RD occurs late in the course of the disease. The incidence of this complication may be reducing as a result of intensive therapy with systemic acyclovir and retinal photocoagulation.

Clinical features

The three 'Fs' of retinal detachment are floaters, flashing lights and field loss. Floaters may be caused by a PVD giving rise to opacities on the posterior vitreous face (e.g. Weiss ring), blood in the vitreous from damage to a retinal vessel at the time of PVD or retinal opercula, and condensation of the collagen fibrils in the mid-vitreous. Photopsia is present in about one third of patients with an acute PVD and occurs as a result of traction on the retina. Mechanical stimulation caused by the movement of a detached retina can also be a cause. The field loss is usually an enlarging peripheral defect (which may vary with postural changes). Other symptoms of RD include macular phenomena, such as metamorphopsia, or reduced central vision from macular detachment.

Examination findings include pigment (tobacco dust) in the anterior vitreous, which, in the absence of previous surgery, inflammation, retinal degeneration, or injury, is diagnostic of a retinal break. The intraocular pressure is often lower in an eye with a RD compared to the contralateral eye. There may be mild anterior uveitis.

A detached retina has a pale appearance due to the retinal oedema and because it is separated from the retinal pigment epithelium. It becomes corrugated and the subretinal fluid (SRF) can move with postural changes. In patients suspected of RD, bilateral retinal examination with indentation is mandatory. A drawing is made of the position of the retinal breaks and the distribution of any SRF. The position of the holes may be deduced in part from the distribution of the SRF (Lincoff's laws), with fluid initially lying inferior to the most superior break, and more fluid being on the side of the retinal break. If distribution of the fluid does not correlate with the position of the retinal breaks, a search for other breaks should be made or other conditions considered (e.g. exudative detachments).

A pigment demarcation line may develop in longstanding RD. In 23% of these patients, adhesions form that will hinder the progression of the detachment. In the remaining 77% the detachment may advance. The presence of such a line should, therefore, not influence surgical planning. Retinal cysts may occur in RDs of more than 1 year.

In the patient with a media opacity and a RD, the following are useful: afferent pupil defect, lower intraocular pressure on that side, inaccurate projection of light and B-mode ultrasound scan.

1. **Proliferative vitreoretinopathy.** Signs of proliferative vitreoretinopathy (PVR) are present in 10% of RDs. Glial or pigment epithelial cells may cause fibrosis on the surface of the detached retina, the posterior vitreous face and may also cause subretinal fibrosis. Signs of PVR include vitreous haze, wrinkling of the retina, rolled edges of retinal holes, tortuosity of the blood vessels, retinal rigidity, fixed folds, sub-retinal bands and funnelled detachments. Predisposing conditions for PVR include large holes, previous RD surgery, excessive cryotherapy, longstanding RDs and vitreous loss at cataract surgery.

2. **Differential diagnoses.** Retinoschisis is usually inferotemporal, bilateral and common in hypermetropic eyes. A schisis is suggested by the absence of tobacco dust in the vitreous, the absence of a pigment line, the presence of an absolute scotoma, non-shifting fluid and prominent white with pressure. If there is an inner and outer leaf break a retinal detachment may ensue.

Exudative retinal detachment should be excluded by examining for shifting fluid and a smooth detachment, with no corrugated appearance. By definition retinal breaks are absent. Look very carefully for a solid mass (e.g. a choroidal melanoma). This may become apparent by altering the posture of the patient in order to view the choroid.

Choroidal detachments do not demonstrate shifting fluid and commonly follow hypotony. They rarely extend posterior to the equator as they are limited by the vortex veins. Ultrasound appearance is diagnostic. A choroidal detachment may co-exist with RD.

A tractional retinal detachment is caused by a fibrous process in the vitreous cavity. It may cause a concave traction detachment in the absence of a retinal break. There is usually a demonstrable cause such as proliferative diabetic retinopathy. A combined rhegmatogenous and traction RD may occur if a break occurs in a traction retinal detachment.

Treatment

Asymptomatic lattice degeneration as a coincidental finding during routine examination is not an indication for prophylactic treatment because the risk of treatment outweighs the risk of retinal detachment. Lattice degeneration in the fellow eye of an eye with a RD should be treated. Treatment in these cases may be with photocoagulation or cryotherapy. Opinions vary as to the correct management of asymptomatic atrophic holes with no subretinal fluid or vitreous traction, but patients should be warned of the symptoms characteristic of RD. White without pressure in the fellow eye of a giant retinal tear requires prophylactic treatment.

Patients who have had blunt trauma require thorough examination of their peripheral retina. This may not be possible until the inflammation from the trauma has settled. RDs occurring as a result of a traumatic dialysis are usually delayed by several months, particularly in children.

The aim of RD surgery is to close the retinal breaks, relieve vitreo–retinal traction, appose the retina to the retinal pigment epithelium and create a scar around the breaks thus closing them. If the RD is shallow, retinal breaks can be closed by indenting the sclera to appost the RPE and retina using buckling techniques. If the RD is bullous the excess subretinal fluid is drained through the sclera and the volume deficit is replaced by using an intraocular gas (SF6 or C_3F_8) or silicone oil. The high surface tension of the gas bubble does not allow fluid to enter the subretinal space. By posturing the patient so that the break is uppermost, the bubble rises to tamponade the hole thus preventing further accumulation of SRF. Any remaining SRF should be removed by the RPE pump provided the retinal breaks remain closed. Vitreo–retinal traction in the region of the break is relieved by suturing an explant onto the sclera creating an internal indent and pressing the RPE against the retina. There are two ways of applying tissue damage to create scarring (retinopexy): laser or cryotherapy. Indirect laser treatment has the advantage of inducing no scleral damage and creating greater than physiological retinal adherence within 48 hours of application. It requires clear media and the complete drainage of subretinal fluid with the apposition of the retina to the retinal pigment epithelium in order to achieve good laser uptake. Cryotherapy causes scleral inflammation and requires 10 days in order to achieve the same retinal adherence as laser treatment but it can be applied through less clear media and in the presence of subretinal fluid.

Further reading

Leaver P. Expanding the role of vitrectomy in retinal detachment surgery. *British Journal of Ophthalmology* 1993; **77**: 197.

Yoser SL, Forster DJ, Narsing AR. Systemic viral infections and their retinal and choroidal manifestations. *Surv Ophthalmol* 1993; **37**(5): 313–52.

Gartry DS, Chignell AH, Franks WA, Wong D. Pars plana vitrectomy for the treatment of rhegmatogenous retinal detachment uncomplicated by advanced proliferative vitreoretinopathy. *British Journal of Ophthalmology* 1993; **77:** 199–203.

Crapotta JA, Freeman WR, Feldman RM, Lowder CY, Ambler JS, Parker CE, Meisler DM. Visual outcome in acute retinal necrosis. *Retina* 1993; **13**(3): 208–13.

Lincoff H, Kreissig I. Finding the hole in the pseudophakic eye with detachment. *American Journal of Ophthalmology* 1994; **117**(4): 442–6.

Snead MP, Payne SJ, Barton DE, Yates JRW, Al-Imara L, Pope FM, Scott JD. Stickler Syndrome: Correlation between vitreoretinal phenotypes and linkage to Col 2A1. *Eye* 1994; **8**(6): 609–14.

Benson WE. Retinal Detachment: Diagnosis and Management. 2nd edn. 1988. JB Lippincott Company, East Washington Square, Philadelphia, Pennsylvania 19105.

Gilbert C, Mcleod D. d-ace surgical sequence for selected bullous retinal detachments. *British Journal of Ophthalmology* 1985; **69:** 733–6.

Scott JD. Surgery for retinal and vitreous diseases, 1st edn, London: Butterworth-Heinemann, 1998.

Related topics of interest

HIV and the eye (p. 127); Vitrectomy (p. 353).

SARCOIDOSIS

Philip I. Murray

Sarcoidosis is a multisystem granulomatous disorder of unknown aetiology. Although the most common clinical manifestations are bilateral hilar lymphadenopathy, pulmonary infiltration, skin and eye involvement, its clinical course can be variable and unpredictable and may mimic other diseases. An acute onset with erythema nodosum and hilar lymphadenopathy leads to a benign self-limiting course that can often be shortened by corticosteroid therapy. An insidious onset is usually followed by progressive pulmonary fibrosis and organ damage. This may be modified but not necessarily prevented by corticosteroids. Granulomata can be distributed throughout the body without causing significant organ dysfunction or may be concentrated in one or more organs with striking clinical effects. Ocular involvement is seen in 25% to 50% of patients with systemic sarcoidosis and can precede involvement of other organs by years.

Problem

A knowledge of the epidemiology, aetiology, diagnosis, extraocular and ocular involvement, and treatment is important in understanding this disease.

Background

The prevalence of sarcoidosis is thought to vary from 10/100 000 to 100/100 000 with an overall incidence of 6 to 10 per 100 000. There is a higher incidence in women, ranging from 1.1 to 1.7 times than in men. The highest incidence is between the ages of 20 and 35 years, and some populations show a small increase in the 50–60-year-old group, especially in women. Studies suggest an 8–15-fold increased incidence in the African-Caribbean population in the USA. Recent epidemiological studies have also shown a higher incidence in Asian immigrants than in the indigenous population in the UK. In a group of patients whose initial presentation related to the chest, 54.2% were found to have intraocular involvement when examined by an ophthalmologist.

No study has yet shown a consistent relationship with a causative agent in sarcoidosis. Atypical mycobacteria have been implicated/suggested. The immunopathogenesis is thought to be mediated via antigenic activation of alveolar macrophages and T lymphocytes, which release cytokines and chemotactic factors that promote an inflammatory response in the lungs. There is an increase in CD4+ T helper cells. These in conjunction with activated macrophages secrete cytokines that result in the formation of epithelioid granulomas.

Clinical features

The definitive diagnosis of sarcoidosis is the finding of noncaseating epithelioid cell granulomas, in the presence of supporting clinical and/or radiological findings, without evidence of infection. The typical granuloma consists of whorls of epithelioid cells surrounding multinucleated giant cells. Mononuclear cells, fibroblasts and lymphocytes may be found in the periphery of these nodules, with surrounding areas of fibrosis.

Other diagnostic tests for sarcoidosis include serum angiotensin-converting enzyme (ACE) levels and Gallium scanning. Raised ACE has been associated with active sarcoidosis and appears to be a sensitive biochemical marker of disease activity. ACE is a dipeptidyl carboxypeptidase that catalyses the conversion of angiotensin I to angiotensin II and increases the degradation of bradykinin. It is primarily synthesized by endothelial cells of pulmonary capillaries and epithelial cells of proximal renal tubules but also by macrophages under certain conditions of stimulation, such as in sarcoidosis. Children have higher mean ACE activity than adults; it progressively increases from 4 to 13 years, then decreases to adult levels by 18 years.

ACE levels are elevated in 50–80% of patients with active sarcoidosis. Other conditions associated with raised ACE are leprosy, berylliosis, mycobacterial infection, silicosis, histoplasmosis, lymphangiomyomatosis, Farmer lung, Gaucher disease, primary biliary cirrhosis and Hodgkin's disease. Hypercalcaemia occurs in only 17% of ocular sarcoidosis patients. The Baarsma co-efficient calculates a predictive value of 83% for sarcoidosis if ACE exceeds 40 u/l and lysozyme exceeds 10 mg/ml.

An abnormal chest X-ray (CXR) is found in about 93% of patients with sarcoidosis and ocular involvement. The CXR may be staged as follows: stage 0 – normal (8%), stage 1 – bilateral hilar lymphadenopathy (BHL, 37%), stage 2 – BHL with associated parenchymal disease (34%) and stage 3 – parenchymal disease in the absence of BHL (21%). Spontaneous resolution occurs in 80% of stage 1 patients, 50–60% of stage 2 cases, and in 30% of stage 3. Pulmonary involvement has a 74% incidence of hilar lymphadenopathy and less commonly parenchymal infiltration is noted on X-ray. Many of these patients are asymptomatic but some experience dry cough and breathlessness. A high resolution CT scan of the chest is the imaging of choice, particularly in the older patient. Pulmonary function tests may show a characteristic restrictive deficit, but may be normal even if there are pulmonary infiltrates radiographically. Transbronchial biopsy may yield tissue containing the definitive histology (63–91%) and is frequently performed because of the high yield and relative safety of the procedure. Supportive evidence comes from the analysis of the brochoalveolar lavage fluid, which shows increased lymphocytes and an increased CD4/CD8 ratio in active alveolitis.

Gallium[67] scanning generally demonstrates enhanced uptake due to the activated T and B lymphocytes and macrophages as opposed to the epithelioid cells in the granuloma. Gallium uptake is not specific for sarcoidosis, but the uptake in the lacrimal and parotid glands (Panda appearance) together with pulmonary and mediastinal uptake (lambda sign) is highly suggestive of sarcoidosis.

Cutaneous anergy is well recognized in sarcoidosis and the Mantoux test may be negative in patients who have had a BCG vaccination and therefore would be expected to have a positive Mantoux test. The Kveim Siltzbach Test is now rarely performed because of the theoretical transmission of HIV.

Sarcoidosis can also directly affect the heart muscle causing conduction defects, pericarditis, cardiomyopathy and congestive cardiac failure. Pulmonary involvement can lead to cor pulmonale.

Erythema nodosum is a nodular, subcutaneous inflammation that presents mainly on the lower extremities as red papules and tender lesions and occasionally seen on the upper extremities and face. It is an acute hypersensitivity reaction, non-granulomatous and self-limiting, seen predominantly in women in the second and third decade who express HLA-B8. The granulomatous skin lesions of sarcoidosis are mobile, non-tender nodules on the lower limbs. Biopsy of these lesions is diagnostic. Lupus pernio is a chronic progressive cutaneous sarcoidosis that most commonly affects the face and ears.

Arthritis affecting large joints is most common in acute sarcoidosis and rarely becomes chronic. Phalangeal cysts may also be seen and chronicity leads to destruction of involved joints.

Liver involvement is detected by biopsy in 60% of the cases but liver failure and cirrhosis are very rare. Intrahepatic cholestasis is also rare and predominant in African-Caribbeans. Splenomegaly and lymphadenopathy are more frequent findings in 10 and 28% of patients respectively.

Neurosarcoidosis affects 5% of the patients but increases to 37% in those with retinal periphlebitis. Cranial nerve palsies (mainly affecting the VII nerve), peripheral neuropathy, myopathy and aseptic meningoencephalitis can result. Often the presentation may mimic a space-occupying lesion. Heerfordt's syndrome (uveoparotid fever) is an uncommon presentation of parotid and submaxillary gland enlargement, facial nerve palsy and uveitis. A lumbar puncture and high-resolution imaging are required to define the extent of the disease. Although contrast-enhanced CT and MRI scans are useful in determining CNS lesions they may fail to detect subarachnoid or ocular involvement. MRI, particularly gadolinium-enhance T1-weighted images, is the preferred technique for evaluating CNS sarcoidosis. Sarcoidosis primarily involves the leptomeninges and the enhancement follows the contour of the brain extending into the sulci. The basal portion of the brain is the commonest location to be involved. About 1–5% of patients have optic nerve involvement and granulomatous involvement is best demonstrated using fat-suppressed, gadolinium-enhanced MRI. Cerebrospinal fluid examination may be normal in 50%, and a raised CSF ACE level found in 50% of patients with neurosarcoidosis. Oligoclonal IgG bands may also be found.

Mickulicz's syndrome comprises the diffuse swelling of most or all lacrimal and salivary glands usually secondary to sarcoidosis. An enlargement of the lacrimal gland is seen in 7–26% of the affected patients.

Ocular involvement

Ophthalmic involvement is reported in most series to be between 25–50%. It is often bilateral, can be highly symmetrical. In 7–17% of patients with ocular involvement, sarcoid granulomas are seen in the palpebral conjunctiva. The demonstration of non-caseating granuloma in a conjunctival biopsy specimen can be diagnostic but blind conjunctival biopsy does not give a high positive yield.

The most common ocular manifestation is anterior uveitis, which occurs in 60%. Two-thirds of these patients will have a chronic granulomatous uveitis, with large mutton-fat keratic precipitates. In the other one-third the uveitis is acute, usually bilateral and symmetric and may be associated with erythema nodosum and BHL. Iris nodules occur in only 11% and when large can mimic tumours. Posterior synechiae are often seen. Complications such as cataract or glaucoma are seen in 8–17% and 11–23% of the cases, respectively. There is an increasing incidence with increasing duration of chronic granulomatous disease. Phakoemulsification with intraocular lens implant is successful in the majority of these patients as long as the inflammation is adequately controlled in the pre-, peri- and postoperative periods. The glaucoma can be secondary to pupillary block or trabecular meshwork damage.

Posterior segment involvement occurs in about 25% of patients with ocular sarcoidosis, and in only 5% is the posterior segment affected without anterior segment involvement. Vitreous infiltrate, opacities (snowballs) and haemorrhage may also occur.

Retinal involvement may include periphlebitis, cystoid macular oedema, neovascularization, choroidal nodules and pigment epithelial changes. An intermediate uveitis with snowballs is the presenting feature in 18% of the cases. All intermediate uveitis patients should be investigated to exclude underlying sarcoidosis. Many patients will have patchy peripheral retinal venous sheathing, highlighted by fluorescein angiography though the classic 'candle wax dripping' is not common or pathognomonic. Branch vein occlusion may occur as a complication of the retinal vasculitis. Neovascularization occurs in approximately one-fifth of patients with posterior segment disease and in three-quarters of these it involves the optic disc. Neovascularization occurs due to ischaemia from peripheral vascular closure or as a direct result of the inflammation. Fluorescein angiography is vital and laser ablation should be carried out to any ischaemic areas while the active inflammation is treated medically. Cystoid macular oedema is the commonest cause of visual loss in this group of patients.

Choroidal nodules vary in size and probably represent granulomas. Small, deep, yellow lesions are probably choroidal granulomas that resolve and cause secondary pigment epithelial alteration seen in 36% of patients with posterior segment disease. They are similar in appearance to Dalen–Fuchs' nodules in sympathetic ophthalmia. Occasionally, a subretinal neovascular membrane may develop.

The optic nerve has been found to be involved in 7.4% of cases of ophthalmic sarcoidosis. Optic nerve swelling may occur for a variety of reasons. There may be papilloedema from raised intracranial pressure due to cerebral granuloma, papillitis due to optic nerve involvement in posterior uveitis or there may be an optic nerve granuloma, which is usually unilateral. The overall incidence of CNS involvement in sarcoidosis is 8.7%, but in patients with posterior segment disease, the CNS is affected in 19.6–35%.

Treatment

The combination of active ocular disease with inactive systemic disease is common. In general, the disease requires treatment only if there are significant symptoms or evidence of progressive damage to the involved organ. Corticosteroids are the mainstay of therapy. Topical steroids and mydriasis are required for anterior uveitis. Posterior segment involvement requires periocular injections or systemic therapy. Most patients that require oral prednisolone respond well to treatment, but in some patients it is impossible to reduce the prednisolone to safe levels and additional immunosuppressive agents need to be added, such as azathioprine, cyclosporin and methotrexate.

Further reading

Jabs DA, Johns CJ. Ocular involvement in chronic sarcoidosis. *American Journal of Ophthalmology* 1986; **102:** 297–301.

Mayers M. Ocular sarcoidosis. *International Ophthalmology Clinics* 1990; **30:** 257–63.

Rothova A. Risk factors for ocular sarcoidosis. *Doc Ophthalmol* 1989; **72:** 287–96.

Stanbury RM, Graham EM, Murray PI. Sarcoidosis. *International Ophthalmology Clinics* 1995; **35:** 123–37.

Related topic of interest

Cataract surgery in uveitis (p. 33).

SCLERITIS

Philip I. Murray

Scleritis covers a spectrum of ocular disease that ranges from mild self-limiting episodes of inflammation to a painful, sight-threatening, destructive necrotizing process.

Problem

Scleritis can be a severe, destructive, blinding disease requiring immunosuppressive therapy. It may also be a manifestation of a potentially life-threatening systemic autoimmune disease.

Background

Classification of scleritis is based on the anatomical site and clinical appearance of the inflammation at presentation. The inflammation may be divided into anterior and posterior scleritis. Anterior scleritis is further sub-divided into diffuse, nodular and necrotizing with and without inflammation.

The average age of patients is around 50 years with a slight female predominance. The incidence of bilateral disease is about 30%. The diffuse and nodular forms of anterior scleritis occur more often, with ocular complications seen in all groups. Overall, visual loss occurs in 40% of patients but is more frequent in necrotizing and posterior scleritis. A recurrence of scleral inflammation is likely in about 35% of patients. Posterior scleritis is usually diffuse or nodular on B-scan and not necrotizing.

Clinical features

Anterior scleritis presents with pain and redness. The pain is often so severe that it can wake the patient at night. The extent of the scleritis is best seen macroscopically as it may be less obvious on slit-lamp examination. Scleral thinning from previous attacks may be present. Remember to lift the upper lid otherwise superior scleral disease may be missed (ptosis may be a clue). Occasionally, surgery may be a triggering factor (surgically induced necrotizing scleritis – SINS). Posterior scleral thickening is best diagnosed using B-scan ultrasound.

An associated systemic disease, such as a systemic vasculitis, autoimmune disease or lymphoma can be identified in 29% of patients. Overall, an associated disease is found in 25% of patients with a higher incidence occurring in those with necrotizing scleritis. Scleritis has been reported in association with a wide variety of conditions, the most frequent being a connective tissue or vasculitic disease. Of these, rheumatoid arthritis is the most common followed by Wegener's granulomatosis. In a small proportion of these patients scleritis may be the presenting feature. Patients older than 50 years have an increased risk of an associated systemic disease and are more prone to experience visual loss. Patients with associated systemic disease also require more aggressive therapy and more frequently have accompanying anterior scleritis.

Ocular complications include visual loss, scleral thinning, peripheral ulcerative keratitis (marginal infiltrates may be a presenting sign in patients with Wegener's granulomatosis), anterior uveitis (42% of scleritis patients in one series, associated with necrotizing disease, reduced vision, peripheral ulcerative scleritis and glaucoma), glaucoma, cataract, and a variety of fundal findings including disc and macular oedema, choroidal folds, circumscribed subretinal mass and choroidal and exudative retinal detachment.

Treatment

For mild disease, oral nonsteroidal anti-inflammatory drugs are the initial choice. Topical steroid drops are usually used as supplementary therapy rather than primary treatment. Failure of the inflammation to resolve or clinical evidence of more severe disease would require the introduction of oral corticosteroids. For those patients who fail to improve or who develop scleral necrosis, oral immunosuppressive agents, such as cyclophosphamide, azathioprine, cyclosporin or methotrexate are added and pulsed immunosuppression in the form of intravenous methylprednisolone and cyclophosphamide may be necessary. The response to therapy in patients with posterior scleritis can often be correlated with posterior scleral thickness seen on serial B-scan ultrasounds. All these therapies have potential serious side effects and treatment is best carried out in conjunction with a rheumatologist.

Further reading

McCluskey PJ, Watson PG, Lightman S, Haybrittle J, Restori M, Branley M. Posterior scleritis: clinical features, systemic associations, and outcome in a large series of patients. *Ophthalmology* 1999; **106:** 2380–6.

Sainz de la Maza M, Jabbur NS, Foster CS. Severity of scleritis and episcleritis. *Ophthalmology* 1994; **101:** 389–96.

Sainz de la Maza M, Foster CS, Jabbur NS. Scleritis-associated uveitis. *Ophthalmology* 1997; **104:** 58–63.

Tuft SJ, Watson PG. Progression of scleral disease. *Ophthalmology* 1991; **98:** 467–71.

SECONDARY GLAUCOMA

Peter Shah

In contrast to primary open-angle glaucoma, it is possible to identify specific factors causing raised IOP in the different types of secondary glaucoma. The importance of gonioscopy (including indentation gonioscopy) cannot be stressed too much. In many types of secondary glaucoma, specific treatment measures can be taken once the correct diagnosis has been made. Most of this section will focus on the causes of acquired secondary glaucoma in adults.

Background

A useful classification is to divide acquired secondary glaucomas into: (i) secondary open-angle and (ii) secondary closed-angle. Secondary open-angle glaucomas can be further subdivided into: (a) pretrabecular, (b) trabecular, and (c) post-trabecular causes. In some cases, more than one factor may be acting to increase the IOP. Secondary closed-angle glaucomas can be divided into: (a) those with pupil block and (b) those without pupil block.

Problem

There are a large number of causes of secondary glaucoma, and a careful history and thorough examination are necessary in order to detect the underlying pathological process. When managing patients with raised IOP and glaucomatous optic disc and visual field changes, one must identify those in whom the raised IOP is secondary to some other process.

Pretrabecular causes are characterized by a physical obstruction which prevents access to the drainage angle. Pathological processes which may obstruct the angle include fibrovascular membranes in neovascular glaucoma. The stimulus for neovascular glaucoma is usually posterior segment pathology, with resulting ischaemia. Vascular causes include retinal venous occlusions, diabetic retinopathy, central retinal arteriolar occlusion and carotid artery disease. Inflammatory causes include chronic uveitis and longstanding retinal detachment. Neoplastic disease of the choroid, including malignant melanoma and metastases, may also be associated with neovascular glaucoma. Other causes of secondary pretrabecular open-angle glaucoma include abnormal epithelial in-growth (associated with faulty apposition of wound edges after surgical or accidental injuries) and cellular proliferation of the endothelium in the irido-corneal endothelial (ICE) syndromes.

Trabecular causes can be broadly divided into those which either clog up, or those which alter the structure of, the trabecular meshwork. Examples of cellular material which can clog up the trabeculum include: red blood cells in hyphaema, white blood cells in uveitis, macrophages in phacolytic conditions, ghost cells in vitreous haemorrhage and neoplastic cells. The trabeculum may also become clogged by noncellular material, including fibrin, lens protein, pigment and pseudoexfoliative material. The physical structure of the drainage angle is altered in traumatic angle recession, trabeculitis, uveitis, scleritis and chemical injury (oedema of the trabecular meshwork). The angle may also be altered in conditions such as siderosis following an intraocular foreign body.

Post-trabecular causes tend to raise IOP by elevating the episcleral venous pressure. Examples of diseases which can do this include: carotico-cavernous fistula, cavernous sinus thrombosis, orbital tumours, dysthyroid eye disease, Sturge–Weber syndrome and superior vena caval obstruction.

Secondary closed-angle glaucoma with pupil block is found in conditions such as severe acute anterior uveitis with seclusio pupillae, intumescent cataractous lens, subluxed lens and pseudophakia. Secondary closed-angle glaucoma without pupil block can be found in such diverse conditions as malignant glaucoma following filtration surgery, intraocular tumours (including ciliary body tumour), after scleral buckling retinal detachment surgery, retinopathy of prematurity and persistent hyperplastic primary vitreous.

A critical component of the management of patients with secondary glaucoma is to identify the underlying cause. Management options will include the conventional medical and surgical treatments for glaucoma, but specific attention must be directed at the underlying cause of the elevated IOP. This is a broad and complex area and is covered in specialist texts.

Further reading

Lucas DR. Glaucoma. In: Lucas DR (ed.) *Greer's Ocular Pathology*. Oxford: Blackwell Scientific Publications, 1989; 213–26.

Related topics of interest

Carotico-cavernous fistula (p. 28); Iridocorneal endothelial syndrome (p. 146); Visual field testing (p. 348).

SHAKEN BABY SYNDROME

Alex V. Levin

The shaken baby syndrome (SBS) is a form of child abuse in which the perpetrator violently shakes an infant such that the child suffers all or some combination of eye, brain and skeletal injury. Victims are usually less than 2 years old but occasionally may be as old as 4 years. It is the unique anatomy of these young children that makes them particularly vulnerable to this type of injury. Retinal hemorrhages are the most common ocular manifestation.

Problem

When faced with a baby in the SBS age range who has retinal hemorrhages, the ophthalmologist may be asked to help ascertain if the child is a victim of SBS or whether the retinal hemorrhages could have resulted from alternate mechanisms.

Background

Infants have a relatively big head with weak cervical musculature, a brain which is not fully myelinized, incompletely fused cranial sutures in the first year or more, and relatively large volumes of cerebrospinal fluid. Likewise, the periosteum is perhaps less adherent to the shafts of long bones. The vitreous is more formed and cohesive as compared to adults. In addition, there are stronger attachments between the vitreous and the macula, retinal blood vessels and retinal periphery. All of these factors contribute to a particular susceptibility to shaking forces and the characteristic injuries that result.

From perpetrators we have learned that the force of shaking in SBS is beyond that which would be recognized as safe by any reasonable observer. It is extremely unlikely that resuscitative attempts of an unconscious child would produce violence in this range. Although blunt head trauma causes a rapid increase in accelerative-decelerative forces, and may exacerbate shaking injury, it is not required to severely injure or kill a baby.

Although the exact cause of all retinal hemorrhages is not known, theories such as the acute rise in intracranial pressure, the association with intracranial haemorrhage (Terson syndrome), increased intrathoracic pressure (Purtscher retinopathy), anoxia and anaemia have all been suggested to play a role but none of which seems to offer a unifying explanation. The entity of traumatic retinoschisis is an important indicator regarding causation. During an episode of shaking, the vitreous is also shaken. Its strong attachments to the macula may result in shearing of the retina in the macula to create a dome-like cavity which may be partially or completely filled with blood with the schisis at virtually any retinal layer. This phenomenon supports the concept that shaking creates unique forces in the eye and orbit which may explain why retinal haemorrhages seem to be particularly consistent with SBS. Traumatic retinoschisis has never been described in any other clinical entity in children within the SBS age range.

Although there are many causes of retinal haemorrhage in young children, most of these can be distinguished from haemorrhages of SBS based on history (or the absence of a satisfactory explanatory history), coincidental physical findings or the pattern of retinal haemorrhages within the retina. Yet some shaken babies, particularly those with just a small number of intraretinal haemorrhages confined to the posterior pole, may have a retinopathy indistinguishable in isolation from other disorders.

Retinal haemorrhaging due to normal birth is quite common. However, flame haemorrhages characteristically resolve within the first week of life while dot and blot haemorrhages usually resolve by 4 weeks and virtually always by 6 weeks. With the exception of traumatic retinoschisis, retinal haemorrhaging during the first 6 weeks of life during these timelines can be indistinguishable from SBS and therefore cautious interpretation is needed.

Physicians should avoid using the generic term 'retinal haemorrhages' as it holds little specificity. More importantly, one should document the number of retinal haemorrhages (e.g. less than 10, too numerous to count), their distribution (e.g. posterior pole, paravascular, extending to the ora), types of haemorrhages (e.g. flame, dot/blot, subretinal, preretinal) and the presence or absence of traumatic retinoschisis. In the absence of other clearly causative clinical scenarios, the picture of widespread retinal haemorrhaging at multiple retinal layers extending to the ora, even in the absence of traumatic retinoschisis, is virtually pathognomic of SBS.

Retinal haemorrhages are rarely found in association with accidental head trauma in children. In less than 3% of cases, almost always those in which there was a severe life-threatening accidental injury for which the suspicion of child abuse would never be raised (e.g. motor vehicle accidents), there may be a small number of intraretinal and preretinal haemorrhages confined to the posterior pole and even less commonly in the midperiphery. Several studies have shown that retinal haemorrhages almost never result from cardiopulmonary resuscitation. Retinal haemorrhages in children ≤ 4 years old do not result from seizures, sickle cell disease, diabetes or normal play.

Clinical features

Retinal haemorrhages occur in 50–100% of shaken babies. The exact number for a given series will depend on the population studied. There is a correlation between the overall severity of shaking injury and the severity of ocular findings. Retinal haemorrhages may present with a less specific picture such as a few scattered intraretinal haemorrhages in the posterior pole or there may be massive haemorrhaging throughout the retina. SBS is one of the few entities that can often cause preretinal, intraretinal and subretinal haemorrhaging of the same eye. There is also a higher incidence of haemorrhaging extending to the ora in SBS as compared to other entities, in particular as compared to accidental head trauma. Fine splinter haemorrhages around the optic nerve associated with papilloedema do not have the same diagnostic significance as other retinal haemorrhages not related to optic nerve swelling. Asymmetrical or unilateral retinal findings are well recognized in SBS and there appears to be no correlation between the laterality of the ocular findings and laterality of the brain injury.

Traumatic retinoschisis is seen in a minority of cases but when present is highly specific. It most often affects the internal limiting membrane or superficial retinal layers. To distinguish it from subhyaloid haemorrhage one should look for a haemorrhagic or hypopigmented arcuate edge to the schisis cavity or a paramacular fold in this region.

Other clinical characteristics of the SBS include rib fractures which may be multiple, at different stages of healing, and almost exclusively posterior or posterior/lateral. Typical long bone fractures include metaphyseal corner fractures or 'bucket-handle' fractures with or without haemorrhagic stripping of the periosteum of the shaft. Shaken babies are usually not multiply battered babies.

Intracranial injuries include subdural, subarachnoid, intraventricular and parenchymal haemorrhage. There may be contusions or lacerations to the surface of the brain from its movement within the cranial vault. Particularly characteristic findings on neuroimaging also include posterior interhemispheric subarachnoid haemorrhage or diffuse cerebral oedema (diffuse axonal injury) associated with occlusion/infarction of one or more of the major cerebral blood vessels. In the latter circumstance, the posterior fossa may remain perfused leaving a 'black brain' with a relatively radiodense cerebellum, called the 'reversal sign'. Skull fracture, or subgaleal haemorrhages seen at autopsy, would indicate that blunt head trauma also occurred.

Although survivors of SBS may demonstrate retinal scarring or detachment, visual loss, if not blindness, is more often due to optic atrophy or occipital cortical damage. Circumlinear folds in the macula, which are often quite hypopigmented, may be the only remaining sign of traumatic retinoschisis although irregularities of the macula and blunting of the foveal reflex may also occur. Survivors may also have neurologic compromise with brain atrophy on neuroimaging.

The primary goal of treatment in SBS is the preservation of life and the prevention of extensive brain injury. Skeletal injuries rarely require orthopaedic intervention. Likewise, ophthalmic surgery is rarely needed unless there is an extension of blood into the vitreous cavity which does not clear rapidly and could thus contribute to amblyopia. Removal of blood from the retinal schisis cavity is usually not necessary, and can be quite difficult particularly if the blood is sitting in a layer of the retina deeper than the internal limiting membrane.

Appropriate psychosocial intervention, including reporting of suspected child abuse to the appropriate agency, is a corner stone of management. The ophthalmologist may be asked to examine other children in the household to ensure their safety. Long-term visual therapy and low vision resources may also be needed.

Conclusion

Shaken baby syndrome is a potentially lethal form of child abuse. One of the major features is the presence of retinal haemorrhages. Although the haemorrhagic retinopathy is usually quite specific, and indicates that abusive shaking has occurred, the ophthalmologists must be able to recognize when the retinal appearance is more or less specific and be able to identify alternative diagnoses. However, in the presence of traumatic retinoschisis, characteristic brain or skeletal injury, or widespread haemorrhagic retinopathy, the ophthalmologist should document the findings clearly and report their suspicion of abuse.

Further reading

Caffey J. The whiplash shaken infant syndrome: manual shaking by the extremities with whip-lash-induced intracranial and intraocular bleedings, linked with residual permanent brain damage and mental retardation. *Pediatrics* 1974; **54**: 396–403.

Greenwald M, *et al.* Traumatic retinoschisis in battered babies. *Ophthalmology* 1986; **93**: 618–25.

Kivlin JD, Simons KB, Lazoritz S, Ruttum MS. Shaken baby syndrome. *Ophthalmology* 2000; **107**: 1246–54.

Levin AV. Retinal haemorrhage and child abuse. In: David TJ (ed.) *Recent Advances in Paediatrics* no. 18. London: Churchill Livingstone, 2000, pp. 151–219.

Ludwig S, Warman M. Shaken baby syndrome: a review of 20 cases. *Annals of Emergency Medicine* 1984; **13**: 51–4.

SIXTH (ABDUCENS) CRANIAL NERVE PALSY

Mike Burdon

Sixth cranial nerve palsy is the most common oculomotor paralysis.

Problem

The correct management of a sixth cranial nerve palsy is firstly to determine the cause of the palsy and secondly to treat the diplopia.

Background

The sixth cranial nerve nucleus lies in the lower pons, separated from the floor of the fourth ventricle by looping fibres of the seventh (facial) nerve. The nucleus contains motor neurons for the lateral rectus muscle and interneurons that ascend via the medial longitudinal fasciculus (MLF) to innervate contralateral medial rectus motor neurons. Thus, the sixth cranial nerve nucleus coordinates ipsilateral horizontal conjugate gaze.

The sixth cranial nerve fascicle passes through the medial lemniscus (contralateral touch and proprioception) and lateral to the corticospinal tract (contralateral motor pathway). The nerve exits the brainstem at the lower border of the pons. It then ascends in the subarachnoid space between the clivus and the brainstem, pierces the dura medial to the fifth (trigeminal) nerve, and passes anteriorly under the petroclinoid ligament to enter the cavernous sinus lateral to the internal carotid artery. The sixth cranial nerve enters the orbit through the annulus of Zinn to innervate the lateral rectus muscle.

Aetiology

Sixth cranial nerve palsy may occur as a result of disease anywhere along the course of the nerve. Other neurological signs may localize the site of the lesion. Nuclear or fascicular palsies may be caused by brainstem disease including infarction, demyelination and tumour. Although rare, Wernicke syndrome should not be forgotten. Within the subarachnoid space, the sixth cranial nerve may be affected by infiltrative, inflammatory or infectious disease, or compression by clivus or cerebropontine angle tumours. It may be stretched by supratentorial tumours or raised intracranial pressure. In the region of the cavernous sinus, the sixth cranial nerve may be affected by a basal skull fracture, an internal carotid artery aneurysm, a cavernous sinus thrombosis, a carotid-cavernous fistula, or a tumour (pituitary, meningioma, nasopharyngeal, metastatic). Orbital inflammation or tumour may also cause a sixth cranial nerve palsy.

'Non-localizing' sixth cranial nerve palsies are frequently due to microvascular disease (e.g. diabetes) but may follow viral illness or vaccination. Giant cell arteritis should be considered in older patients.

Differential diagnosis

Alternative causes of impaired abduction including thyroid eye disease, myasthenia gravis, fracture of the medial wall of the orbit, convergence spasm, Duane syndrome and Moebius syndrome. Mechanical disorders such as thyroid eye disease and orbital fractures typically have normal velocity abducting saccades. Convergence spasm causes miosis and blurring of distance vision. Duane's syndrome is characterized by narrowing of palpebral fissure on adduction. Patients with this syndrome rarely complain of diplopia, and usually have good stereopsis in their field of binocular single vision. Myasthenia gravis should be suspected if there is a history of variability in either the degree or direction of the diplopia, or if there is weakness or fatigue of other muscles, in particular the orbicularis oculi.

Clinical features

Patients complain of horizontal diplopia, greater for distance than near, that increases on ipsilateral gaze. They may adopt a head turn towards the affected side. Cover testing reveals an eso-deviation that is greatest when fixing with the affected eye. When fixing with the non-paretic eye there is an increase in the prism cover test measurement when gazing in the direction of the affected eye (lateral incommitance). The degree of duction deficit varies from very little to an inability to abduct beyond the midline. The abducting saccade may appear normal or grossly reduced.

Once other causes of impaired abduction have been excluded a full neurological examination is required to determine whether the sixth cranial nerve palsy is isolated or associated with other neurological deficits. Particular attention should be paid to: the optic discs (papilloedema), contralateral adduction (gaze palsy), other cranial nerve deficits, pupil abnormalities, ptosis (Horner's syndrome), and neurologic abnormalities of the contralateral limbs. Patients with other neurological deficits require immediate investigation beginning with neuroimaging.

Investigation

The investigation of an isolated sixth cranial nerve palsy is determined by the likely underlying aetiology. Microvascular disease is the most common cause of isolated sixth cranial nerve palsies in patients over the age of 50 years. The majority of such palsies will show at least partial recovery within 12 weeks. Adults below the age of 50 years and children are more likely to have an underlying neoplasm, inflammatory or infiltrative disease. Isolated sixth cranial nerve palsies are only infrequently caused by aneurysms. Therefore, patients who are less than 50 years old should undergo magnetic resonance imaging of the brain and further investigation, including cerebrospinal fluid examination and a vasculitis screen, if no intracranial mass is identified. Patients over the age of 50 years should be screened for vasculopathic risk factors (blood pressure, full blood count, glucose, lipid profile) and for giant cell arteritis. Patients in this age group should undergo further investigation if there is no sign of recovery by 12 weeks.

Patients with chronic sixth cranial nerve palsies (more than 6 months duration) should be reinvestigated looking in particular for infiltrative or neoplastic disease of the skull base and nasopharynx.

Treatment

The timing of treatment depends on the underlying cause. Initially, an eye patch or a base out fresnel prism will provide symptomatic relief from diplopia. Recovery of sixth nerve function following, for example, surgery to an intracranial tumour, often occurs over 6 months to a year. During this time ocular motility can be monitored by repeated prism cover tests, Hess charts and fields of binocular single vision. Strabismus surgery must be deferred until there is clear evidence that spontaneous recovery has ceased.

Injection of botulinum toxin into the ipsilateral medial rectus muscle has both a therapeutic and a diagnostic role in the management of sixth cranial nerve palsy that does not fully recover. Such an injection may have one of three possible outcomes. Firstly, where recovery has been incomplete because of contracture of the medial rectus, binocular single vision may be permanently restored. Secondly, the eye may be seen for a while to abduct beyond the midline. This indicates that the sixth nerve palsy is partial and can be treated surgically by a lateral rectus resection and a medial rectus recession. Thirdly, the eye may still be unable to abduct beyond the midline because of a complete sixth nerve palsy. In such circumstances horizontal muscle surgery is ineffective and vertical muscle transposition surgery should be performed instead. There is debate about whether to inject botulinum toxin in the first six months as spontaneous recovery is common and difficult to predict.

In young children, loss of fusion is rapid and suppression will lead to amblyopia. The timely optical realignment with fresnel prisms can re-establish fusion and prevent amblyopia. If amblyopia occurs this needs treating with occlusion or penalization.

Further reading

Foster RS. Vertical muscle transposition augmented with lateral fixation. *Journal of the American Association for Pediatric Ophthalmology and Strabismus* 1997; **1:** 20–30.

Moster ML, Savino PJ, Sergott RC, Bosley TM, Schatz NJ. Isolated sixth-nerve palsies in younger adults. *Archives of Ophthalmology* 1984; **102:** 1328–30.

Riordan-Eva P, Lee JP. Management of VIth nerve palsy – avoiding unnecessary surgery. *Eye* 1992; **6:** 386–90.

Rucker WC. The cause of paralysis of the third, fourth, and sixth cranial nerves. *American Journal of Ophthalmology* 1966; **61:** 1293–8.

SJÖGREN'S SYNDROME

Andrew Whallett, John Ross Ainsworth, John Hamburger &
Simon Bowman

Sjögren's syndrome (SjS) is characterized by a slow immune-mediated destruction of exocrine glands possibly triggered by a viral infection, such as Epstein–Barr virus, hepatitis C virus or cytomegalovirus. Infiltration of the lacrimal glands causes keratoconjunctivitis, and salivary gland involvement leads to xerostomia. Patients with SjS may have exocrine gland dysfunction elsewhere in the body, e.g. pancreas, sweat glands, gastrointestinal or respiratory tracts, vagina.

Problem

Sjögren's syndrome is a problem that may be overlooked. The condition should always be considered in those patients presenting with keratoconjunctivitis sicca. Referral to a rheumatologist or oral medicine specialist may be appropriate for management of the features associated with the condition.

Background

The prevalence of SjS is unknown; there are likely to be a large number of individuals with undiagnosed mild disease. There is a female preponderance (M:F = 9:1). The peak age of onset is in the fourth or fifth decade.

The condition is classified into primary or secondary SjS. In *primary* SjS, the disease occurs in isolation whereas in *secondary* SjS it is associated with other autoimmune conditions, such as rheumatoid arthritis or systemic lupus erythematosus (SLE). Polymyositis, scleroderma, primary biliary cirrhosis, chronic active hepatitis and coeliac disease are other less common associations.

Questions should always be asked to determine whether there are associated autoimmune features to suggest secondary SjS that may require referral for further management, such as:

- Have you any joint pain, swelling or stiffness? (arthritis)
- Have you had any facial swelling? (SjS, sarcoidosis)
- Have you had any rashes or skin reaction with the sun? (photosensitivity – SLE)
- Do your fingers change colour with the cold weather? (Raynaud's phenomenon – SLE, SjS, scleroderma)
- Does the skin over your face or fingers feel tight? (scleroderma)
- Do you have any skin itchiness, dark urine or pale motions? (primary biliary cirrhosis)
- Are your muscles painful or weak? (myositis)
- Do you have any shortness of breath? (pulmonary fibrosis)
- Do you have any pains in the stomach, diarrhoea or weight loss? (coeliac disease)
- Do you have mouth ulcers, migraine or hair loss? (SLE)

There is an increased risk of B-cell lymphoma particularly in patients with primary SjS with glandular swelling and hypergammaglobulinaemia. Swollen parotid, mandibular or lacrimal glands suggest primary SjS rather than keratoconjunctivitis sicca alone. Primary SjS is strongly associated with the presence of anti-Ro (in 85%) and anti-La (in 60%) autoantibodies. Serum immunoglobulins are raised in 80% of patients with primary SjS. Anti-Ro and anti-La are also associated with secondary SjS, except in SjS secondary to rheumatoid arthritis (RA) where the association is much weaker. SjS secondary to RA is virtually always associated with a positive rheumatoid factor. A significantly positive ANA (titre >1:40) is found in many connective tissue disorders found with SjS (e.g. SLE, scleroderma).

Clinical features

Keratoconjuctivitis sicca presents with gritty, burning eyes, photosensitivity or contact lens intolerance. Examination may reveal dilated bulbar conjunctival vessels, pericorneal injection and an irregular corneal surface. A punctate or filamentary keratitis is seen on slit-lamp examination. In the Schirmer tear test, less than 5 mm (< 3 mm if anaesthetic used) wetted suggests keratoconjunctivitis sicca. Traditionally, Rose Bengal was used to identify damaged corneal and conjunctival epithelium but now more often Lissamine Green is used. A deficiency in the mucin or lipid layer of the eye leads to a more rapid break-up of the tear film (i.e. abnormal tear film break-up time if <10 seconds).

To detect xerostomia, the unstimulated salivary flow rate is measured. Saliva is collected in a container for a 15-minute period. A volume of 1.5 ml or less over this time is consistent with clinical xerostomia.

For a diagnosis of SjS, keratoconjunctivitis sicca and/or xerostomia alone are not enough. Most patients with keratoconjunctivitis sicca have dry eyes due to other causes (e.g. post-menopausal, age-related gland loss or drugs such as anticholinergics). The 'San Diego criteria' are useful in clinical practice. All three criteria below must be satisfied for the diagnosis of SjS:

- keratoconjunctivitis sicca;
- xerostomia;
- either a characteristic minor salivary gland lip biopsy or characteristic autoantibodies (see below).

Treatment

The aim of therapy is to provide symptomatic relief and minimize the consequences of tear and saliva insufficiency by replenishing secretions. Tear drops, gels and ointments are commonly used. Topical acetylcysteine can be tried as a mucolytic. The lacrimal puncta can be plugged or occluded. Regular fluid intake, scrupulous oral hygiene and artificial saliva (sprays, gels, lozenges and pastilles) are useful in the management of xerostomia.

The role of muscarinic receptor stimulation (e.g. pilocarpine) and disease-modifying therapy in SjS is unclear and controlled studies are required. Immunosuppression for an underlying disorder associated with secondary SjS may be required. Referral to a rheumatologist or a SjS clinic is recommended.

Further reading

Fox RI, Robinson CA, Curd JG, Kozin F, Howell FV. Sjögren's syndrome: proposed criteria for classification. *Arthritis Rheum* 1986; **29:** 577–85.

Valesini G, Priori R, Bavoillot D *et al.* Differential risk of non-Hodgkin's lymphoma in Italian patients with primary Sjögren's syndrome. *Journal of Rheumatology* 1997; **24:** 2376–80.

Van Bijsterveld OP. Diagnostic tests in the Sicca syndrome. *Archives of Ophthalmology* 1969; **82:** 10–14.

STEM-CELL GRAFTING

Harminder Singh Dua

The scientific principles which define surgical approaches to the management of ocular surface disorders should be based on an understanding of stem cells of the corneal and conjunctival epithelium.

Problem

Stem cells are the progenitor cells that are responsible for cellular replacement and tissue regeneration. They are poorly differentiated, long-lived, slow-cycling cells that have a high capacity for self renewal and an increased potential for error-free division. Stem cells have a long life span, which might be equivalent to the life of the organism which harbours them. All cells except stem cells have a limited life span and are destined to die. Stem cells demonstrate a capability to divide in an asymmetric manner. When a stem cell divides, one of the daughter cells remains as a parent stem cell and serves to replenish the stem cell pool, whereas the other daughter cell is destined to divide and differentiate with the acquisition of features that characterize the specific tissue. These daughter cells are called 'transient amplifying cells' (basal corneal epithelial cells) and are less primitive than the parent stem cell. Transient amplifying cells divide more frequently than stem cells but have a limited proliferative potential and are considered the initial step of a pathway that results in terminal differentiation. They differentiate into 'postmitotic cells', spare (wing cells) and finally to 'terminally differentiated cells' (superficial squamous cells). Both postmitotic and terminally differentiated cells are incapable of cell division. Stem cells of the corneal epithelium reside in the limbus. The interpalisade (of Vogt) rete ridges are considered to be repositories of stem cells. Stem cells for the conjunctival epithelium reside maximally in the fornices. Stem cells for goblet cells and perhaps for conjunctival epithelium may also be scattered throughout the epithelial surface.

The aetiology of limbal stem-cell deficiency can be related to a hereditary aplasia of limbal stem cells as occurs in aniridia and congenital erythrokeratodermia. More often though, stem cell deficiency is acquired as a result of extraneous insults that acutely or chronically destroy limbal stem cells. These include chemical or thermal injuries, ultraviolet and ionizing radiation, Stevens–Johnson syndrome, advanced ocular cicatricial pemphigoid, multiple surgeries or cryotherapies, contact lens wear or extensive/chronic microbial infection such as trachoma.

Clinical features

The hallmark of limbal stem cell deficiency is 'conjunctivalization' of the cornea, the most significant clinical manifestation of which is a persistent corneal epithelial defect. Superficial corneal vascularization, scarring, calcification, ulceration, melting and perforation of the cornea are other features of limbal stem cell deficiency that develop over time. The clinical symptoms of limbal deficiency may include decreased vision, photophobia, tearing, blepharospasm, and recurrent episodes of pain (epithelial breakdown), as well as a history of chronic inflammation with redness.

The diagnosis of stem-cell deficiency remains essentially clinical. On slit-lamp biomicroscopic examination, conjunctivalized cornea presents a dull and irregular reflex. The epithelium is of variable thickness and translucent to opaque. Conjunctival epithelium on the cornea is more permeable than corneal epithelium and takes up fluorescein stain in a stippled or punctate manner. In cases of partial conjunctivalization of the cornea, fluorescein dye tends to pool along the junction of the sheets of corneal and conjunctival epithelial cell phenotypes. Loss of architecture of the limbal palisades of Vogt and vascularization are other common features. When damage is extensive, vascularization occurs in the form of fibrovascular pannus, which increases the thickness of the affected area of the cornea.

The presence of goblet cells on impression cytology specimen taken from the corneal surface is pathognomonic of conjunctivalization of the cornea. Other features such as squamous metaplasia or loss of cornea specific cytokeratins (CK 3/12) on immunohistology support the clinical diagnosis.

Treatment

All associated lid abnormalities, intraocular pressure problems and presence of cataract should ideally be dealt with prior to undertaking ocular surface restorative surgery. However, these eyes may suffer higher morbidity from all types of intraocular surgery and topical medication. Copious continuous lubrication is essential. Symblepharon correction with buccal mucosa graft should also precede stem cell grafting. At times, if a corneal graft procedure is being contemplated at the time of stem cell grafting, it can be combined with cataract extraction and lens implantation. When an intumescent cataract is associated with raised pressure, corneal grafting may become a necessity if a dense fibravascular pannus or corneal scar precludes visualization of the interior of the eye.

Most stem cell grafts do not survive in a dry (eye) environment. At times the injurious insult resulting in stem cell deficiency also results in a severe dry eye state. In such situations, if punctal occlusion and buccal mucosa grafts do not restore adequate moisture to the ocular surface, a keratoprothesis procedure should be considered.

1. Sequential sector conjunctival epitheliectomy (SSCE). In cases with partial, mild to moderate conjunctivalization of the cornea, without significant fibrovascular pannus, removal of the conjunctivalized epithelium is all that is required. This can be achieved at the slit-lamp under topical anaesthesia. SSCE can also be usefully combined with limbal transplant to allow cells derived from transplanted limbal tissue (auto or allo) to re-populate the host corneal surface without 'contamination' from conjunctival epithelium.

2. Auto limbal transplantation. In patients where total stem cell deficiency affects only one eye, an auto limbal transplant procedure is the ideal option. It is important however, to be absolutely certain that the donor eye was not involved at the time of the initial injury. In unilateral manifestations of systemic diseases, harvesting tissue from the apparently normal eye is not recommended.

3. Allo limbal transplantation. When a living related donor, who is tissue matched to the recipient, is available, tissue is harvested from one donor eye and used on the recipient eye exactly as described above for auto limbal transplantation. In most instances, limbal tissue is obtained from cadaver donor eyes. In such an event, tissue matching is not usually practical. The whole limbus is harvested and sutured on to the recipient limbus after excision of any fibrovascular pannus. The threat of limbal graft rejection is considerable and prolonged systemic immunosuppression with cyclosporin A or tacrolimus is required postoperatively.

4. *Amniotic membrane grafts.* The amniotic membrane serves as a useful adjunct to stem cell grafting. Its mechanism of action is yet to be precisely defined but it serves two functions: (a) as a biological bandage affording protection and containing inflammation and (b) as a substrate that is favourable to epithelial growth and adhesion. One or both mechanisms may be invoked with stem cell grafting.

Further reading

Dua HS, Azuara-Blanco A. Allo-limbal transplantation in patients with limbal stem-cell deficiency. *British Journal of Ophthalmology* 1999; **83:** 414–19.

Dua HS, Azuara-Blanco A. Amniotic membrane transplantation. *British Journal of Ophthalmology* 1999; **83:** 748–52.

Dua HS, Azuara-Blanco A. Limbal stem cells of the corneal epithelium. *Surv Ophthalmol* 2000; **44:** 415–25.

Dua HS, Azuara-Blanco A. Autologous limbal transplantation in unilateral stem cell deficiency. *British Journal of Ophthalmology* 2000; **84:** 273–8.

Holland EJ, Schwartz GS. The evolution of epithelial transplantation for severe ocular surface disease and a proposed classification system. *Cornea* 1996; **15:** 549–56.

Rao SK. Limbal allografting from related live donors for corneal surface reconstruction. *Ophthalmology* 1999; **106:** 822–8.

Tseng SCG, Tsubota K. Important concepts for treating ocular surface and tear disorders. *American Journal of Ophthalmology* 1997; **124:** 825–35.

SUPERIOR OBLIQUE WEAKNESS

Robert H. Taylor

Weakness of the superior oblique muscle is the commonest cause of a vertical strabismus. It can be congenital or acquired. The exclusion of possible treatable intracranial lesions is of particular concern in acquired lesions.

Problem

Differentiating new from longstanding palsies is critical. Findings that indicate bilateral superior oblique weakness may be subtle, and may influence surgical planning.

Background

The fourth cranial nerve nucleus is situated in the lower midbrain. The fourth nerve decussates with its fellow in the anterior medullary velum and then exits the midbrain dorsally. It passes forward around the midbrain, between the superior cerebellar and posterior cerebral arteries, and pierces the cerebral layer of the dura of the lateral wall of the cavernous sinus, where it passes forward through the superior orbital fissure to supply the superior oblique muscle. The superior oblique muscle arises from the orbital apex and travels forward in the superiomedial aspect of the orbit. It has a long tendon, that passes through the trochlea complex. The attachment to the globe is wide, in the superior, posterior, lateral quadrant. The superior oblique causes downgaze, abduction and incyclotorsion.

Aetiology

Approximately one third of weaknesses of the superior oblique are congenital. The cause may remain idiopathic, or there may be absence or hypoplasia of the nerve nucleus, variation in tendon attachment or laxity of the tendon. When the tendon is lax the muscle belly has been shown to be smaller. Head trauma accounts for another third of cases. The unique exit pattern makes the nerve particularly vulnerable to head trauma. The site of damage following trauma is speculative, but may be the anterior medullary velum. Fourth nerve paresis following head trauma (which may be mild) may be unilateral or bilateral and, when bilateral, is often asymmetrical. Ischaemic lesions account for 20% of all superior oblique palsies. The site of ischaemia may be the brainstem affecting the nuclear or fascicular components, or the nerve itself. Giant cell arteritis can present with an isolated cranial nerve palsy. Intracranial neoplasms account for 5% of fourth nerve palsies. Other causes include haemorrhage and demyelination. Subarachnoid damage may be from tumour or meningitis. Cavernous sinus lesions include intracavernous aneurysms, meningiomas, pituitary adenomas and lymphomas. The fourth nerve may be involved in the orbital apex syndrome.

Differential diagnosis

Other causes of a vertical deviation include oculomotor palsy, thyroid eye disease, orbital fracture with entrapment, myasthenia gravis, orbital tumours, skew deviations and ipsilateral or asymmetric inferior oblique overaction. The ocular tilt reaction may be confused with a superior oblique weakness. This is a combination of an ipsilateral head tilt, an ipsilateral skew deviation, and extorsion. It is due to an imbalance of central otolithic projections from the vestibular nucleus to the intersitial nucleus of Cajal. If fixation is preferred in the infraducted eye, the contralateral eye is elevated and intorted, differentiating a superior oblique weakness, where the eye is elevated and extorted.

Clinical features

A decompensating congenital palsy may present with diplopia, aesthenopic symptoms or symptoms relating to the compensatory head posture. Decompensation may occur at any age. The characteristic head posture may have been noticed by the patient or others, but may be present and not remarked upon. A review of old photographs may be informative. Facial asymmetry may also be noted on careful inspection.

Acquired lesions usually present with diplopia except in young children. Diplopia is vertical and torsional and the diplopia is generally worse on down-gaze. The second image is lower and twisted.

A compensatory head tilt and turn to the contralateral side with chin depression may be present. Ipsilateral hypertropia (or hyperphoria breaking down to a tropia) is present, which is greater on contralateral version and ipsilateral head tilt (3 step test). If the deviation is small, dissociating the eyes using an alternating cover test may demonstrate the deviation. A 'V' pattern may be present. Torsion can be assessed by examining the fundus, and measured by using a single or double maddox rod or a synoptophore.

Longstanding lesions may become more concomitant and are associated with an increased vertical fusion range. This is best measured using a vertical prism bar. It does not rule out acquired lesions as an increased vertical fusion range can develop over several months.

There may be overaction of the contralateral inferior rectus (as a consequence of Hering's law) and secondary underaction of the contralateral superior rectus (as a consequence of Sherrington's law). Ipsilateral inferior oblique overaction may be marked. The ipsilateral superior rectus may become shortened. These secondary changes enhance any 'V' pattern.

The examiner should suspect bilateral palsies when there is a right hypertropia on left gaze and left hypertropia on right gaze, exclotorsion of over 20°, a large 'V' pattern or reversing height on contralateral tilt.

If an ipsilateral third nerve palsy is present, fourth nerve function is tested by assessing intorsion on attempted down-gaze which, if absent, confirms fourth nerve palsy. This may be best viewed at the slit-lamp. Nuclear or fascicular lesions of the fourth nerve may be associated with a contralateral Horner syndrome. A cavernous sinus lesion may affect some or all of the structures that pass through the sinus, namely the ophthalmic and maxillary division of the trigeminal nerve, the third, the fourth, the sixth and the sympathetic supply to the eye.

The orbital apex syndrome may affect all the nerves supplying the eye, with reduced vision from optic nerve involvement as well as total external and internal ophthalmoplegia. The inferior division of the oculomotor nerve may be spared.

Investigations

Cranial imaging is performed to exclude any intracranial pathology. Many clinicians would image all patients with acquired palsies. Those with ischaemic lesions require an appropriate work up. If the diagnosis is obscure and in the absence of an obvious cause, serial examination and imaging is suggested. Tumours may be detected years after initial negative cranial imaging.

Treatment

Treatment will depend on the presenting problem and the examination findings. Initially, the use of a vertically acting prism may be sufficient to relieve symptoms. It may be possible to manage the patient by incorporating the prism into their spectacle correction. Surgery may be required. Opinions will differ in individual cases regarding indications for surgery and surgical options. Ipsilateral inferior oblique weakening may suffice particularly when there is marked inferior oblique overaction. Other procedures include ipsilateral Harado Ito, superior oblique tuck (where tendon laxity is present) and contralateral inferior rectus recession. Clinically significant iatrogenic Brown's syndrome will occur in 30% of cases following superior oblique tuck. Surgical cure is less likely in trauma-induced lesions.

Further reading

Brazis PW. Palsies of the trochlear nerve: diagnosis and localization-recent concepts. *Mayo Clinic Proceedings* 1993; **68:** 501–9.

Keane JR. Fourth nerve palsy: historical review and study of 215 inpatients. *Neurology* 1993; **43**(12): 2439–43.

Knapp P. Classification and treatment of superior oblique palsy. *American Orthoptic Journal* 1974; **24:** 18–22.

Kraft SP, Scott WE. Masked bilateral superior oblique palsy: clinical features and diagnosis. *Journal of Pediatric Ophthalmology and Strabismus* 1986; **23**(6): 264–72.

Leigh RJ, Zee DS. Clinical features of ocular motor nerve palsies. In: *The Neurology of Eye Movements*, 3rd edn. New York, Oxford University Press, 1999; Section 9.8; 357–9.

Miller NR. Cerebrovascular disease. In: *Walsh and Hoyt's Clinical Neuro-Ophthalmology*, 4th edn., Vol. 4. Baltimore, MD: Waverly Press, 1991; 2371–89.

Richards BW, Jones FR, Younge BR. Causes and prognosis in 4278 cases of paralysis of the oculomotor, trochlear and abducens cranial nerves. *American Journal of Ophthalmology* 1992; **113:** 489–96.

Sato M. Magnetic resonance imaging and tendon anomaly associated with congenital superior oblique palsy. *American Journal of Ophthalmology* 1999; **127**(4): 379–87.

Scott WE, Kraft SP. Classification and surgical treatment of superior oblique palsies: I. Unilateral superior oblique palsies. *Transactions of the New Orleans Academy of Ophthalmology* 1986; **34:** 265–91.

Scott WE, Kraft SP. Classification and treatment of superior oblique palsies: II. Bilateral superior oblique palsies. *Trans New Orleans Acad Ophthalmol* 1986; **34:** 15–38.

Simons BD, Saunders TG, Siatkowski RM *et al.* Outcome of surgical management of superior oblique palsy: a study of 123 cases. *Binocular Vision and Strabismus* 1998; **13**(4): 273–82.

Related topics of interest

SYSTEMIC DRUGS USED IN GLAUCOMA

Shakti Thakur & Peter Shah

Problem

Whilst topical medication is the mainstay of glaucoma treatment, the use of systemic medication is often necessary to achieve rapid reduction of an acutely raised intraocular pressure or act adjunctively where topical medication is inadequate. It is important to be aware of the many side effects associated with their use, as some of these are potentially life-threatening.

Acetazolamide

Mechanism of action

This carbonic anhydrase inhibitor blocks the conversion of carbon dioxide to bicarbonate ions, which occurs in many tissues including the ciliary body.

Side effects

Side effects are common and lead to drug discontinuation in 40–50% of patients on long-term treatment. Acetazolamide causes a mild, usually self-limiting, metabolic disturbance with little risk of hypokalaemia, which does not necessitate intervention in healthy patients. An initial loss of potassium occurs which is usually insignificant and self-limiting. The metabolic acidosis is correlated with malaise, fatigue, depression, anorexia, weight loss and loss of libido. However, with coexisting renal impairment the drug can worsen pre-existing metabolic acidosis with serious, life-threatening consequences requiring immediate hospitalization. There are several case reports of this problem arising in the elderly, diabetics and other renal failure patients. The hypochloraemic acidosis induced by acetazolamide leads to late hypokalaemia.

Other specific side effects include altered taste, particularly of a metallic taste with carbonated beverages, gastritis, stomach burning and abdominal cramp due to local, gastrointestinal inhibition of carbonic anhydrase and diarrhoea due to decreased water reabsorption in the large intestine. Precipitation of renal calculi can occur and this may be more common in patients with a previous history of renal calculi. Reduced renal citrate excretion may be one mechanism of calculus formation. Lens-induced transient myopia may also occur.

Practical use

1. Acid–base balance/electrolytes. Do not use in marked renal impairment. Mild renal impairment may be present subclinically in the elderly and diabetics. Check urea and electrolytes in this group of patients before commencing treatment. If impaired, use low-dose acetazolamide, continue close monitoring of U&Es and watch serum bicarbonate. (Take advice from local chemical pathology lab since test may not be routinely available.) If serum bicarbonate concentration falls to 20 mmol (mEq)/l take advice of physicians as oral sodium bicarbonate may need to be given (with caution in cardiovascular disease) and/or stop acetazolamide.

Do not use in adrenal failure where sodium and potassium levels may already be depressed since with acute use of acetazolamide some potassium loss occurs.

In liver cirrhosis the increased risk of hepatic encephalopathy prohibits its use. In pulmonary obstruction or emphysema where the FEV1 is reduced to less than one litre the patient is unable to increase minute ventilation to compensate for the metabolic acidosis, resulting occasionally in respiratory acidosis and failure. Use low doses and monitor U&E and serum bicarbonate carefully.

In healthy patients on long-term treatment routine U&E measurements are only required if moderate symptoms of metabolic acidosis (the malaise complex) develop. Routine potassium measurements or supplements are not required unless potassium-depleting diuretics being used concomitantly require this.

2. Haematopoietic toxicity. These occur rarely (55 cases reported to the National Registry of Drug-Induced Ocular Side Effects, US, from 1972–1983, compared with an approximate one million prescriptions per year). However, since 32% of these resulted in death secondary to aplastic anaemia (idiosyncratic and not dose-related), thrombocytopenia or agranulocytosis, the following recommendations apply.

A full blood count, including reticulocyte count and white cell count with differentials, should be performed in all patients before initiating (long-term) CAI and 6 monthly thereafter. Monitoring is useful since recovery from haematologic toxicity has been seen after discontinuation of the drug unless allowed to progress to complete aplasia, which has a 50% mortality. Leucopenia occurs uncommonly (0.05–0.1%) of patients on treatment.

Note that the onset of adverse haematopoietic reactions most often occurred within 60–90 days after starting treatment, but six occurred within 14 days and rarely after 6 months.

Patients should be cautioned to report a persistent sore throat, fever, fatigue, pallor, easy bruising, epistaxis, purpura or jaundice at any time during treatment. A fall in the level of any single formed blood element requires immediate cessation of the drug.

Drug interactions

1. Aspirin. Concomitant use of aspirin may result in severe acidosis and central nervous disturbance. There are several case reports of severe metabolic acidosis, even coma, usually with a high dose of aspirin (3 g). The reaction may develop quickly or insidiously over days to weeks and has been well confirmed by animal studies. Although the mechanism is not fully established it is thought that the CAI-induced alteration of plasma pH promotes the non-ionized form of salicylate, which is lipid soluble and therefore penetrates the CNS more easily leading to salicylate toxicity. Alternatively, the salicylate inhibits plasma protein binding of acetazolamide impairing its renal excretion and causes acetazolamide toxicity which mimics salicitate toxicity. In either case the result is potentially serious and the patient should be well monitored if this is at all to be used. Naproxen has been used as a safer alternative to aspirin in one study and methazolamide suggested as a safer alternative to acetazolamide due to its minimal plasma-protein binding.

2. **Sulphonamide sensitivity.** Acetazolamide is a sulphonamide derivative and is contraindicated in patients with sulphonamide sensitivity.

3. **Drug metabolism.** Acetazolamide may potentiate the effects of folic acid antagonists, hypoglycaemics and oral anticoagulants. Doses of these drugs may therefore need to be reduced. Dose reduction may also be required for cardiac glycosides and hypertensive agents if blood pressure control is affected by the fluid shifts.

Advise physician/General Practitioner to monitor and adjust doses accordingly if patient is on long-term treatment.

Concomitant chronic phenytoin use may accelerate the development of osteomalacia.

Advise physician to monitor.

4. **Dosage.** The dose of acetazolamide required to achieve an optimum 4–10 micrograms/ml plasma level (to give the maximal IOP drop) is variable depending on individual metabolism and limitations due to side effects. Up to 1000 mg in divided doses may be given over 24 hours in a healthy individual by the oral route (effect within one hour, peaking at 2–4 hours) or intravenous route (effect within 5 minutes, peaking at 10–15 minutes). The slow-release preparation is effective at a lower dose i.e. 250 mg bd maximum which achieves a smooth plasma plateau and reduces the symptoms of mild metabolic acidosis (fatigue, malaise, etc.) linked with higher serum levels.

Finally, the intravenous route must be carefully employed since extravasation of the highly alkali solution (pH 9.1) of acetazolamide results in severe pain and tissue necrosis which may necessitate skin grafting. Subcutaneous sodium citrate 3.8% (1–2 ml) is generally recommended as an immediate measure, with massage and cold compresses to follow regularly for up to 24 hours and a plastic surgeon's advice.

Mannitol

Mechanism of action

Mannitol is an osmotic diuretic. It is administered most usefully by the intravenous route and distributes itself rapidly throughout all extracellular fluid compartments, remaining outside the blood–brain barrier and extraocular. Vitreous dehydration follows the shift of fluid along the osmotic gradient causing reduction of intraocular pressure in 30–60 minutes, lasting 4–8 hours. The osmotic diuresis is not accompanied by a loss of bicarbonate ions or alteration of plasma pH but potassium levels may rise acutely (variable). Virtually all the dose is excreted unchanged in the urine by glomerular filtration (80% within 3 hours, delayed in cardiac or renal failure up to 36 hours) after intravenous administration, undergoing no metabolism. This compares with nearly 20% absorption in the gastrointestinal tract when given orally, where some is metabolized and stored as liver glycogen and some metabolized by gut flora or lost in bile in renal failure.

Side effects

Intravenous administration has been associated with thirst, headache, fever, tachycardia, chest pain, urinary retention and blurred vision, which are related to the fluid shifts.

Drug interactions

Mannitol potentiates the ototoxic effects of aminoglycosides, may increase the renal excretion of lithium and enhance the effect of tubocurarine and other competitive or depolarizing neuromuscular blockers, which may be used in anaesthesia. The effect of oral anticoagulants may be reduced, as clotting factors may be concentrated secondary to dehydration. Acute changes in potassium concentration may affect digoxin toxicity and insulin action.

Practical use

Dose: 2 g/kg or 100 ml of a 20% solution given intravenously over 30 minutes is usual. Pulmonary oedema, congestive cardiac failure, inadequate urine flow (<30–50 ml/h), dehydration, acidosis and intracranial bleeding are absolute contraindications to its use.

Extravasation of the solution may cause thrombophlebitis and skin necrosis although the solution is not alkaline (pH 4.5–7.0).

Care with above drug interactions; monitor serum aminoglycosides, lithium, INR, digoxin, potassium as appropriate.

Glycerol

Mechanism of action

Reduction of intraocular pressure occurs secondary to osmotic vitreous dehydration. The pressure lowering and diuresis are less than with mannitol, but effective within 10 minutes, peaked at 30 minutes and lasting up to 4–5 hours. The glycerol is metabolized to glucose by the liver causing hyperglycaemia and glycosuria. It is therefore absolutely contraindicated in diabetics, as well as congestive cardiac failure, pulmonary oedema and inadequate urine flow.

Practical use

1–1.5 g/kg of a 50% solution (1 ml 50% solution = 0.62 g glycerol) is diluted in a flavoured drink e.g. orange juice, refrigerated to help mask the nasty taste and taken orally. It cannot be given intravenously as it causes severe vasoconstriction of the afferent glomerular arterioles with consequent haematuria.

Side effects

Headache and dehydration may occur in common with other osmotic diuretics. Nausea is not uncommon. Supportive measures i.e. rehydration and insulin to control the hyperglycaemia are only required if the patient becomes unwell, although the use of the drug should be avoided in those at risk of developing these complications.

Other uses

Glycerol may be applied topically to the anaesthetized cornea with the patient supine for 5–15 minutes. This dehydrates the cornea and restores transparency, facilitating examination.

Further reading

Barnes EA *et al.* Comment on, *Eye* 1996; **10:** 648–50.

Davis AR *et al.* Prevalence of chronic hypokalaemia amongst elderly patients on acetazolamide and diuretics. *Eye* 1995; **9:** 381–2.

Everritt D, Avorn J. Systemic effects of medications used to treat glaucoma. *Ann Intern Med* 1990; **112:** 120–5.

Fraunfelder FT *et al.* Hematologic reactions to carbonic anhydrase inhibitors. *American Journal of Ophthalmology* 1985; **100:** 79–81.

Ivan H. Stockley, Drug Interactions. In: *Aspirin or Salicylates & Carbonic Anhydrase Inhibitors,* 5th edn., Chapter 3, p. 44, 1999, Pharmaceutical Press.

Lichter PR. Reducing side effects of carbonic anhydrase inhibitors. *Ophthalmology* 1981; **88:** 266–9.

Maisey DN, Brown RD. Acetazolamide and symptomatic metabolic acidosis in mild renal failure. *British Medical Journal* 1987; **283:** 1527–8.

Wyeth Laboratories, Medical Information Dept, Data Sheet Compendium Diamox/ Literature Search.

THIRD (OCULOMOTOR) CRANIAL NERVE PALSY

Mike Burdon

The third cranial nerve has a complex nucleus, supplies all the extraocular muscles except for lateral rectus and superior oblique as well as the ciliary muscle and constrictor pupillae. It is less commonly affected than the fourth and sixth cranial nerves.

Problem

A third cranial nerve palsy is potentially a medical emergency. The correct management is firstly to rapidly determine the cause of the palsy and secondly to treat the diplopia.

Background

The third cranial nerve nuclear complex lies anterior to the periaqueductal grey matter of the midbrain. It extends from the posterior commissure superiorly to the fourth cranial nerve nucleus inferiorly. The complex contains a single midline subnucleus that innervates both levator palpebrae superioris muscles, and paired subnuclei that innervate the other muscles supplied by the third cranial nerves. Fibres from the superior rectus subnuclei decussate within the complex to join the contralateral third cranial nerve fascicle. The remaining subnuclei project ipsilaterally.

The third cranial nerve fascicle passes anteriorly through the medial longitudinal fasciculus, red nucleus, and the medial part of the cerebral peduncle. On leaving the midbrain, the nerve passes anterolaterally between the posterior cerebral and superior cerebellar arteries, lateral to the posterior communicating artery, and below the uncus of the temporal lobe. It then enters the lateral wall of cavernous sinus and divides into superior and inferior branches. Both branches enter the orbit through the annulus of Zinn. The superior branch innervates the superior rectus and levator palpebrae superioris muscles. The inferior branch innervates the medial and inferior recti, and the inferior oblique. The latter also provides parasympathetic drive to the ciliary muscle and constrictor pupillae via the ciliary ganglion.

Classification

Third cranial nerve palsies can be divided into those that are associated with other neurological deficits, and those that are isolated. The latter are further categorized into complete (total external and internal ophthalmoplegia), pupil sparing (complete external ophthalmoplegia but normal pupil reactions), and partial (incomplete external ophthalmoplegia with or without pupil involvement). Partial third nerve palsies include those with signs of aberrant regeneration.

Aetiology

Third cranial nerve palsy may occur as a result of disease anywhere along the course of the nerve. Other neurological signs may localize the site of the lesion. The majority of isolated third cranial nerve palsies are due to intracranial aneurysms (most commonly of the posterior communicating artery), microvascular infarction of the fascicle or peripheral nerve, parasellar tumours, or trauma. When third cranial nerve palsy is caused by an expanding intracranial aneurysm, there is a considerable risk of rapid progression to potentially fatal subarachnoid haemorrhage. This risk determines the urgency of investigation.

Differential diagnosis

A number of disorders may resemble a partial third cranial nerve palsy. Myasthenia gravis should be suspected if there is a history of variability in either the degree or direction of the diplopia, or if there is weakness or fatigue of other muscles, in particular the orbicularis oculi. An internuclear ophthalmoplegia may be mistaken for an isolated medial rectus palsy unless contralateral abducting nystagmus is specifically looked for. A careful history of exposure to medicines should be taken if the patient has an isolated fixed dilated pupil.

Clinical features

Patients with a complete third nerve palsy present with a marked ptosis, a fixed dilated pupil, and an eye that is displaced laterally and inferiorly because of the unopposed actions of the sixth and fourth cranial nerves. Paralysis may be incomplete and, on occasion, limited to a single extraocular muscle. Rarely, patients may present with an isolated dilated pupil.

Certain eye movement abnormalities are characteristic of a lesion within the third cranial nerve nuclear complex. They reflect the distribution of the various subnuclei (see above). Thus, patients with either a unilateral palsy associated with a contralateral superior rectus paresis and bilateral partial ptoses, or bilateral palsies with sparing of levator function, must have a nuclear lesion.

The eye movement abnormalities associated with a third cranial nerve palsy may be modified by aberrant regeneration of the nerve. The two most commonly observed patterns of aberrant regeneration are eyelid elevation on adduction or depression of the eye, and constriction of the pupil on adduction. Aberrant regeneration is associated with either compression or trauma to the third cranial nerve, and usually develop months after a known palsy. However, signs of aberrant regeneration are elicited at presentation, and indicate an underlying longstanding compressive lesion.

Once other causes for the observed eye movement and pupil abnormalities have been considered, a full neurological examination is required to determine whether the third cranial nerve palsy is isolated or associated with other neurological deficits. Particular attention should be paid to the visual fields, to the optic discs looking for papilloedema, to other cranial nerves, and to the contralateral limbs. Patients with other neurological deficits require immediate investigation beginning with neuroimaging.

Investigations

The urgency of investigation of an isolated third cranial nerve palsy is determined by whether it is complete, pupil sparing, partial, or associated with aberrant regeneration. This distinction is based on the observation that pupil fibres are located peripherally within the third cranial nerve, and are therefore less liable to micro-vascular disease, but more liable to compressive injury. Hence, a pupil sparing third nerve palsy is unlikely to be caused by an aneurysm. By contrast, an aneurysm may cause a complete or partial third cranial nerve palsy, with or without signs of aberrant regeneration.

Therefore, all patients, *except* those with pupil-sparing third cranial nerve palsies, must undergo an immediate magnetic resonance imaging (MRI) scan of the third cranial nerve pathway from brainstem to orbit, and magnetic resonance angiography (MRA) of the cerebral circulation. If the MRI and MRA are negative formal angiography should performed to exclude a small aneurysm or a carotid-cavernous fistula. If neuroimaging fails to establish a diagnosis, a lumbar puncture should be performed to look for inflammatory, infective, or neoplastic disease.

Patients with a pupil-sparing third cranial nerve palsy should be reviewed every 2 days for a week to make sure that they do not develop pupil involvement. As mentioned above, such palsies are likely to be due to ischaemia, and patients should be screened for vasculopathic risk factors (blood pressure, full blood count, glucose, lipid profile) and giant cell arteritis. Neuroimaging should be performed on patients with presumed microvascular third cranial nerve palsies if there is no evidence of recovery by 12 weeks.

Treatment

Treatment is initially directed at the underlying cause. Microvascular palsies usually recover spontaneously within 4 months. Surgery to intracranial tumours and aneurysms may lead to partial or complete recovery over a period of 6 months to a year. Traumatic third cranial nerve palsies may recover over a similar period of time. Repeated prism cover tests, Hess charts and fields of binocular single vision should be used to monitor improvements in ocular motility. An eye patch or occlusive contact lens may be required to provide symptomatic relief from diplopia (if there is no associated ptosis).

The definitive treatment of a third cranial nerve palsy is determined by the degree of recovery. If there is no recovery surgical options are limited. Combined horizontal muscle and ptosis surgery may return the eye to primary position and improve cosmesis. Such procedures do not eliminate (and may worsen) diplopia. When partial recovery has occurred muscle surgery may result in a useful field of binocular single vision.

Further reading

Payne JW, Adamkiewicz J. Unilateral internal ophthalmoplegia with intracranial aneurysm. *American Journal of Ophthalmology* 1969; **68**: 349–52.

Rucker WC. The cause of paralysis of the third, fourth, and sixth cranial nerves. *American Journal of Ophthalmology* 1966; **61**: 1293–8.

Rush JA, Younge BR. Paralysis of cranial nerves III, IV, and VI. Course and prognosis in 1000 cases. *Archives of Ophthalmology* 1981; **99**: 76–9.

Schumacher-Feero LA, Yoo KW, Solari FM, Biglan AW. Results following treatment of third cranial nerve palsy in children. *Transactions of the American Ophthalmology Society* 1998; **96:** 455–72.

Young TL, Conahan BM, Summers CG, Egbert JE. Anterior transposition of the superior oblique tendon in the treatment of oculomotor nerve palsy and its influence on postoperative hypertropia. *Journal of Pediatric Ophthalmology and Strabismus* 2000; **37:** 149–55.

Related topics of interest

Diplopia work-up (p. 105); Sixth (abducens) cranial nerve palsy (p. 289); Superior oblique weakness (p. 298).

THYROID DISORDERS: MEDICAL ASPECTS

Paul Dodson & Amanda Butcher

Thyroid disorders are common. Hyperthyroidism affects approximately 2% of women and 0.2% of men. Hypothyroidism affects 1.5% of women and 0.1% of men. The rationale for treatment is the relief of symptoms in hyper- and hypothyroidism and to reduce the risk of the sequelae of a suppressed thyroid-stimulating hormone (TSH) i.e. atrial fibrillation and osteoporosis, risks that remain, even in the absence of symptoms and signs of hyperthyroidism.

Problem

It is not the thyroid status of the patient that causes ocular complications but the, as yet poorly understood, autoimmune process underlying the thyroid disorder. Thyroid eye disease (TED), acropachy and pretibial myxoedema occur almost exclusively in those patients with an autoimmune aetiology for their thyroid dysfunction.

Background

1. *Causes of primary hyperthyroidism include:*
- overproduction of thyroid hormone (e.g. Graves' disease, toxic multinodular goitre, toxic thyroid adenoma.) Graves' disease is the overproduction of thyroid hormones (T4 or T3 or both) mediated by autoantibodies against the thyroid-stimulating hormone (TSH) receptor. It is the condition most likely to present with thyroid eye disease and classically presents with goitre, hyperthyroidism and exophthalmos;
- inflammation-induced leakage of thyroid hormone (thyroiditis, post-radiotherapy to the neck for Hodgkin's disease).

2. *Causes of secondary hyperthyroidism include:*
- ingestion of excess thyroid hormone;
- extra thyroidal hormonal stimulation/production [rare] (e.g. TSH-producing pituitary tumour, HCG-producing tumours);
- selective pituitary resistance to thyroid hormone;
- ingestion of excess iodine (Jod–Basedow phenomenon).

3. *Causes of primary hypothyroidism include:*
- loss of thyroid tissue from previous treatment of hyperthyroidism, e.g. surgery, radioactive iodine;
- autoimmune destruction of thyroid tissue (e.g. Hashimoto's thyroiditis), Hashimoto's disease is an autoimmune thyroiditis and the commonest cause of hypothyroidism. It can present with hyperthyroidism initially but eventually leads to destruction of the gland leaving a woody goitre and a hypothyroid patient. In keeping with its autoimmune aetiology TED can be present in up to 3% of patients with this condition;
- congenital.

4. Causes of secondary hypothyroidism include:

- inadequate TSH production resulting from pituitary disease (e.g. tumour, sarcoidosis);
- drugs (e.g. amiodarone, lithium);
- iodine deficiency.

Baseline investigations should include a serum-free thyroxine level (Free T4) and a thyroid-stimulating hormone level (TSH).

Interpretation of results:

	Hyperthyroidism	Hypothyroidism
FT4	High or normal	Low
TSH	Suppressed	High

Note: In the presence of a suppressed TSH and normal Free T4 a free triiodothyronine (Free T3) should be requested. A raised Free T3 indicates hyperthyroidism due to 'T3 toxicosis'. A raised or normal TSH in the presence of a raised Free T4 is suggestive of the very rare TSH-secreting pituitary adenoma.

Graves' disease and Hashimoto's thyroiditis are autoimmune diseases although the precise immunopathology is still not clear. Some patients with Graves' disease have thymic hyperplasia, lymphadenopathy or splenomegaly as well as concurrent autoimmune conditions such as pernicious anaemia, myasthenia gravis, polymyalgia rheumatica, vitiligo and rheumatoid arthritis. Graves' disease and Hashimoto's have histological abnormalities in common with a lymphocytic infiltration of the thyroid gland. Many autoantibodies have been detected associated with these diseases.

In clinical practice there are three antibodies detectable that can help with the diagnosis of autoimmune thyroid disease and suspected euthyroid TED.

1. TSH receptor antibodies (TRAbs). These are present in almost all patients with Graves' disease at some point in their illness. They can be present in 40–95% of patients with TED even in the absence of other signs of thyroid autoimmune disease. This is one of the most useful antibody tests in patients suspected of having euthyroid TED.

2. Antithyroid peroxidase antibodies (anti-TPO) previously known as anti-microsomal antibodies. These are present in up to 90% of Hashimoto's disease and 80% of Graves' disease.

3. Antithyroglobulin antibodies. These are present in 55% of Hashimoto's and 25% of Graves' patients. They are also present in 10% of elderly, healthy women. Unlike TRAbs, anti-TPO and antithyroglobulin antibodies rarely disappear during the course of the disease.

Thyroid swelling or goitre can occur in euthyroid, hyperthyroid or hypothyroid patients, depending on the aetiology of the thyroid dysfunction. Simple euthyroid goitre is usually due to iodine deficiency leading to a reduction of thyroid hormone production leading to increase in TSH from the pituitary and growth of the gland. Other types of goitre include multinodular, colloid, single nodular, cystic and carcinoma. The presence of a goitre (both or one lobe) or a thyroid nodule will necessitate investigation. Methods available include ultrasound, isotope scanning and fine needle aspiration, employed usually to exclude thyroid carcinoma. However, thyroid carcinoma in the presence of hyperthyroidism is very rare. Isotope scanning may be useful to identify hot or cold nodules.

Clinical features

	Hyperthyroidism	Hypothyroidism
General	Weight loss Heat intolerance Malaise Hair loss Thyroid acropachy (a) Onycholysis Gynaecomastia +/– Goitre	Weight gain Cold intolerance Tiredness/malaise Hair dry and thin Loss of eyebrows Deep voice Serous effusions e.g. pleural, pericardial, ascites, joint +/– Goitre
Gynaecological	Amenorrhoea Raised sex hormone binding globulin	Menorrhagia Infertility
Gastrointestinal	Diarrhoea	Constipation
Muscle	Proximal myopathy Periodic paralysis	Muscular chest pain Muscle cramps Raised creatine kinase
Cardiovascular	Dyspnoea Atrial fibrillation Angina High output cardiac failure	Bradycardia Hypercholesterolaemia Ischaemic heart disease
Bone	Osteoporosis Hypercalcaemia	Arthralgia
Neurological	Poor concentration Tremor	Deafness Slow mentation Carpal tunnel syndrome Slow relaxing reflexes Cerebellar signs
Eyes	Thyroid eye disease (a)	Thyroid eye disease rare
Blood	Leucopenia	Macrocytic anaemia
Skin	Urticaria Pretibial myxoedema (a)	Skin dry and coarse

(a) denotes sign associated with autoimmune aetiology.
Hyperthyroidism may be occult in the elderly and present in the apathetic form.

Treatment

1. Hyperthyroidism

- **A finite course of carbimazole (CMZ).** Thionamide drugs e.g. CMZ work by blocking the production of thyroid hormone and are given in a reducing course to control hyperthyroidism, with a starting dose of 20–60 mg depending on the severity of the hyperthyroidism. The dosage reduction is titrated according to FT4 levels and needs to be continued for up to 18 months to obtain maximum remission rate off therapy. Factors associated with relapse are male sex, large goitre, severe disease, large maintenance of thionamide therapy and slow response to antithyroid drugs. The side effects of the thionamaide drugs include rash, arthralgia and rarely agranulocytosis. Patients should be advised to stop the treatment and have a full blood count should they develop a sore throat. Patients who are pregnant or breast-feeding should have propylthiouracil (PTU) due to its reduced teratogenic effects and excretion in breast milk.

- **Radioactive iodine (RAI).** This is a definitive treatment and involves the administration of a single radioactive dose of iodine by an accredited physician and nuclear medicine department. After the dose is given the patient undertakes to restrict bodily contact with others, particularly children for a dose-related period of time. The usual dose is 400–500 megaBq. Non-response after 4–6 months can be treated with a repeat dose but more than two doses are rarely required. Apart from the risk of post-treatment hypothyroidism there are no apparent side effects and no excess risk of secondary malignancy. Currently RAI is not recommended for patients with active TED as there are reports suggesting that the TED may deteriorate. There is controversy whether this effect can be mitigated by the use of oral steroids for 1 month prior to and following the RAI dose. Other contraindications include retrosternal goitre, uncontrolled thyro-toxicosis and risk of pregnancy.

- **Surgery.** This is a definitive treatment usually reserved for large goitres causing symptoms of neck compression or thyroid cancer. This is an option for treatment in of patients with controlled hypertension and TED, as there is no evidence of deterioration of TED when compared to medical therapy. It should be carried out in a surgical unit highly experienced in the procedure. Potential complications include hypocalcaemia, recurrent laryngeal nerve paralysis and paralysis of the external branch of the superior laryngeal nerve.

- **Beta blockers.** These are an adjunct to treatment only. They are used to ameliorate symptoms such as palpitations and tremor. Non-cardioselective agents are preferable (e.g. propanolol).

After definitive treatments and during treatment with thionomide drugs patients may become hypothyroid, the risk of hypothyroidism increasing with time post-treatment. It is important to monitor TFTs and clinical effects post-treatment to minimize the severity and length of time that a patient is hypothyroid, hence frequent follow-up is recommended. There have been suggestions that profound hypothyroidism post-treatment itself can provoke or worsen TED.

Thyroid storm or thyroid crisis can be precipitated in a hyperthyroid patient by induction of anaesthesia, surgery, systemic illness and radioiodine therapy. It is manifest by fever, confusion, tachycardia, hypotension, vomiting and diarrhoea. This is a medical emergency requiring rapid iv infusion of fluids, steroids and large doses of PTU, used in this situation as it prevents peripheral conversion of T4 to T3. High dose beta-blockade is also required to control heart rate. Thyroid storm is prevented by ensuring that hyperthyroidism is rendered at least partially controlled prior to surgery or RAI by an adequate course of thionamides. The use of beta-blockade or oral potassium iodide (to block release of thyroid hormones) alone is not adequate.

2.   Hypothyroidism.   A deficiency of thyroid hormones is corrected by replacing them with an analogue thyroxine. The patients are monitored with TFTs until rendered biochemically and clinically euthyroid. Subsequently, monitoring is required until a full replacement dose of thyroxine is required i.e. 150–200 micrograms daily.

Myxoedema coma is a rare profound hypothyroidism and usually presents in the elderly with hypothermia, bradycardia and confusion/coma. The treatment includes general resuscitation measures and T3 administration with steroid cover.

Further reading

Bartalena L, Marcocci C, Bogazzi F *et al.* Use of corticosteroids to prevent progression of Graves' ophthalmopathy after radioiodine treatment for hyperthyroidism. *New England Journal of Medicine* **321:** 1349–52.

Gittoes N, Franklin J. Hyperthyroidism current treatment guidelines. *Drugs* 1998; **55:** 543–53.

Thyroid Eye Disease D. Butterworth and Heinemann, 1997.

Related topic of interest

Thyroid eye disease (p. 315).

THYROID EYE DISEASE

Robert H. Taylor

Thyroid eye disease (TED) is characterized by swelling of the extraocular muscles and orbital fat. Graves' disease is associated with thyroid eye disease in 25–50% of cases. However, TED is also seen with clinically and biochemically hypothyroid and euthyroid patients. An auto-immune condition is present in almost all patients with TED. The condition is usually bilateral but may be clinically unilateral. It is the most common cause of a unilateral and bilateral proptosis.

Problem

The aetiology remains poorly understood and treatment is therefore difficult to rationalize. There is no widely accepted definition of what constitutes a diagnosis. Many names are in use. Potential blindness can occur from optic nerve compression and corneal exposure can lead to perforation. Minimal proptosis does not exclude optic nerve compression. Immunomodulation in the active inflammatory phases has limited effect and is associated with significant treatment side effects.

Background

The swelling of the orbital muscles and fat is immunologically mediated. The immune reaction is directed at proteins expressed by the orbital fat that are transcripts of the thyroid-stimulating hormone receptor (TSH receptor). Muscles undergo lymphocytic infiltration and become oedematous, secondary to the hydrophobic properties of the glycosaminoglycans and collagen produced by fibroblasts. This 'wet phase' is followed by or co-exists with a fibrotic reaction particularly in the inferior and medial rectus muscles. This is followed by a static phase where there is no active inflammation, just the fibrotic sequelae.

Diagnosis

Despite the abundance of clinical signs there is no widely accepted definition of what constitutes thyroid eye disease. Bartley and Gorman suggested eyelid retraction plus one of thyroid abnormality, proptosis, optic nerve dysfunction or extraocular movement disorder. In the absence of eyelid retraction, thyroid dysfunction needs to be present in association with proptosis, optic nerve dysfunction or extraocular muscle involvement after excluding other causes.

Clinical features

Ocular symptoms include gritty red eyes, photophobia and swollen lids. General history and examination explores for systemic thyroid dysfunction. Risk factors for TED include smoking and female sex. However when males are affected the disease tends to be more severe. There is an association with myasthenia gravis. Reduced vision may occur, with colour desaturation (particularly in the tritan axis). Diplopia (commonly worse on waking or when fatigued) is a feature in the later stages.

Diagnosis (after Bartley and Gorman)

One

Eyelid retraction *plus*
> Thyroid dysfunction or abnormal regulation *or*
> Proptosis *or*
> Optic neuropathy *or*
> Motility disturbance
> Or **two**

In the absence of eyelid retraction and after excluding other causes

Thyroid dysfunction or abnormal regulation *plus*
> Proptosis *or*
> Optic neuropathy *or*
> Motility disturbance

Other ocular features include: proptosis (21–23 mm: mild; over 28 mm: marked), swelling or pigmentation of the lids, lid lag and retraction, prolapse of orbital fat, conjunctival oedema, superior limbic keratitis, corneal exposure, episcleral injection over the rectus muscles, limitation of movement particularly of up-gaze and abduction, a rise in intraocular pressure (often worse on elevation), choroidal folds and macular oedema. Pain, tenderness, conjunctival injection and oedema may be used as indicators of active inflammation.

Optic nerve compression in particular must be excluded. This may be severe in patients with minimal proptosis due to a tight orbital septum. Monitor visual acuity, colour vision, visual field changes, pupil function for an afferent defect and fundal examination, including the disc for swelling or engorged veins.

Investigations

Biochemical investigations include thyroid-stimulating hormone (TSH) levels and free T4. Free T3 assay is indicated if the TSH is low and T4 normal. Antibody assays include anti-TSH receptor antibody, anti-thyroid peroxidase antibody (anti-TPO), and anti-thyroglobulin antibodies.

Imaging studies are very useful and although some authors recommend MRI and in particular the STIR sequence, computer tomography gives useful information and is much cheaper. In the STIR sequence of the T2-weighted MRI, oedematous tissues return a prominent signal. A significant proportion of patients with Graves' disease (71% in one series) will have swelling of the extraocular muscles demonstrated on MRI without clinical orbitopathy. The swelling characteristically affects the belly of the muscles (as opposed to myositis when the tendon is also swollen) and the muscle margin is usually distinct. A bilateral picture often emerges on imaging even if the clinical picture is unilateral.

Treatment

It is important to involve a physician to manage the systemic disorder. There is controversy about methods of control of hyperthyroidism when associated with active TED. Medical control of the thyroid disorder is important and is beneficial for TED.

Radioactive iodine may exacerbate TED. However, recent publications retract a little from this view; suggesting avoidance of post-ablation hypothyroidism is prudent, but the treatment *per se* may be associated with an increase, decrease or no change in activity of TED. The use of thyroid ablation (with radioactive iodine or surgery) has been suggested as a treatment for TED, claiming that this will promote stability, a reduction in cross-reacting antigens and a fall in lymphocytic activity. The authors point out that such a strategy (with radioactive iodine) is covered with oral steroids for 3 months. It has yet to gain widespread acceptance.

Ocular treatment is divided into treatment of the expanding orbital tissues, supportive therapy for the ocular surface and rehabilitation of the motility and lid appearance once the inflammatory disease is quiescent.

The expansion may respond to the cessation of smoking, although there is only anecdotal evidence to support this. The head of the bed should be raised and some effect may be gained by using diuretics.

Ocular surface problems require supportive treatment, with tear replacements and ointments at night. Superior limbic keratitis is treated with topical steroids. Treatment of raised intraocular pressure may be required.

Vision-threatening signs (ocular surface exposure and optic nerve compression) need to be addressed immediately. Medical decompression consists of oral or intravenous steroids. Plasma exchange may be a useful adjunct. Azathioprine or cyclosporin may be used to enable a reduction in the dose of steroid. Conflicting results have been published regarding the use of high-dose immunoglobulin. At present this is not used in routine clinical practice.

In fulminant cases, surgical decompression should not be delayed for more than 24–48 hours if there is no improvement with medical treatment. The type of surgery is debated, and consultation with an orbital surgeon is appropriate. Medial wall decompression alone may be sufficient, but it may be necessary to decompress the floor, lateral wall or even the roof. Emphasis is on decompressing the posterior orbit, as optic nerve compression is often maximal at the orbital apex. General anaesthesia may be hazardous in a thyrotoxic patient and discussion with the anaesthetist is advised.

Early irradiation to the orbit during the wet phase may be considered to control the immune process. Fractionated treatment totalling 2000 rad is given over 10 days. The extraocular muscles are targeted via a lateral approach to minimize irradiation of the lens and cornea.

Diplopia is monitored with serial examinations involving the prism cover test in pertinent directions of gaze and duction deficits. Hess charts and fields of binocular single vision add a pictorial representation. Fresnel prisms or botulinum toxin injection can be used initially to relieve diplopia. Botulinum toxin given to vertically acting muscles may reverse the vertical diplopia, and so be poorly tolerated. Botulinum toxin can also be injected into Müller's muscle for mild cases of upper lid retraction. Muscle surgery can be performed if the patient is euthyroid and the motility parameters are stable for at least 6 months. Levator muscle surgery for upper lid retraction can be considered once all surgery for proptosis and strabismus is complete. Surgery can be performed on Müller's muscle or the aponeurosis. A spacer can be used if the levator is fibrosed. For lower lid retraction, the use of a spacer is essential. A lateral tarsorrhaphy may antagonize optic nerve compression and is rarely used. Blepharoplasty can be used to remove prolapsed orbital fat.

Complications of surgical decompression include postoperative diplopia (usually an esotropia with an A pattern) and lacrimal drainage problems. Long-term steroid use is complicated by osteoporosis, hypertension, weight gain, diabetes mellitus and peptic ulceration. Complications of radiation include skin changes, conjunctival hyperaemia, cataract and radiation retinopathy. Treatment leading to hypo-thyroidism may make thyroid eye disease worse.

Conclusion

Treatment is far from satisfactory. The eye disease runs a course of relapse and remission, even after metabolic stability. Vision is lost through optic nerve compression, corneal exposure, chronic choroidal folds or macular oedema and iatrogenic injury.

Further reading

Bartalena L, Marcocci C, Bogazzi F et al. Relation between therapy for hyperthyroidism and the course of Graves' ophthalmopathy. New England Journal of Medicine 1998; 338(2): 733–78.

Bartley GB, Fatourechi V, Dakrmas EF et al. The chronology of Graves' ophthalmopathy in an incidence cohort. American Journal of Ophthalmology 1996; 121: 426–34.

Bartley GB, Gorman CA. Diagnostic criteria for Graves' ophthalmopathy. American Journal of Ophthalmology 1995; 119(6): 792–5.

Burch HB, Wartofsky L. Graves' ophthalmopathy: current concepts regarding pathogenesis and management. Endocrine Reviews 1993; 14: 747–93.

Fells P, Kousoulides L, Pappa A, Munro P, Lawson J. Extraocular muscle problems in thyroid eye disease. Eye 1994; 8: 497–505.

DeGroot LJ. Radioiodine and the immune system. Thyroid 1997; 7(2): 259–64.

Marcocci C, Bartalena L, Tanda ML et al. Graves' ophthalmopathy and 131I therapy. Quarterly Journal of Nuclear Medicine 1999; 43(4): 307–12.

Munro D. Thyroid eye disease. British Medical Journal 1993; 306: 805–6.

Tallstedt L, Lundell G, Tørring O et al. Occurrence of ophthalmopathy after treatment for Graves' hyperthyroidism. The Thyroid Study Group. New England Journal of Medicine 1992; 326(26): 1733–8.

Weetman AP, Harrison BJ. Ablative or non-ablative therapy for Graves' hyperthyroidism in patients with ophthalmopathy. Journal of Endocrinology 1998; 21(7): 472–5.

Villadolid MC, Yokoyama N, Izumi M et al. Untreated Graves' disease patients without clinical ophthalmopathy demonstrate a high frequency of extraocular muscle (EOM) enlargement by magnetic resonance. Journal of Clinical Endocrinology and Metabolism 1995; 80(9): 2830–3.

Related topics of interest

Diplopia work-up (p. 105); Myasthenia gravis (p. 168); Thyroid disorders: medical aspects (p. 310).

TOXICOLOGY: DRUGS FOR NON-OCULAR DISEASES

Gavin Walters & Robert H. Taylor

Systemic administration of certain drugs may produce a variety of side effects in the eye and visual system.

Problem

Adverse effects often occur in the first 2 weeks of therapy, although there may be a long latent period between drug administration and toxic effects. These changes occasionally persist or even progress after withdrawal of the drug. The ophthalmologist should be aware of such potential toxic effects and take a thorough past and current drug history.

Clinical features

The drugs mentioned are those which have potentially important toxic effects on the visual system. The list is not comprehensive but includes mainly drugs of importance in ocular toxicology, which are used in current clinical practice.

1. Antimalarials. *Chloroquine* and *hydroxychloroquine* were originally used for their antimalarial properties. Currently they are mainly used for their anti-inflammatory effects in the treatment of rheumatoid arthritis, discoid lupus and systemic lupus erythematosus. The major side effect of these drugs is retinal toxicity. The mechanism of the toxicity of hydroxychloroquine is in doubt. Currently it appears that retinal damage is caused by a direct toxic effect on the retinal cells rather than toxicity mediated by binding to the retinal pigment epithelium (RPE) alone. This has usually occurred at total doses in excess of those currently recommended. Hydroxychloroquine appears to have a higher margin of safety compared with chloroquine. Chloroquine should only be used where hydroxychloroquine has failed as there are insufficient data to recommend a safe maximum dose.

It is recommended that the maximum daily dose of hydroxychloroquine should not exceed 6.5 mg/kg lean body weight daily. Characteristic early ophthalmic findings include loss of the foveal reflex (reversible) with irregular macular pigmentation (premaculopathy stage). Later there is a 'bull's eye' maculopathy (irreversible) which is associated with reduced visual acuity and central field disturbance. A paracentral scotoma, 4–7° from fixation to a red target may be the earliest objective finding. Corneal verticillata, lens deposits and abnormalities of ocular motility and accommodation can also occur. Visual problems may be reversible if the drug is stopped in the premaculopathy stage. Further deterioration in visual acuity can occur after discontinuing the drug in advanced stages.

The Royal College of Ophthalmologists recommend that rheumatologists measure a patient's near visual acuity and, if normal, treatment with hydroxychloroquine can commence. The patient should be monitored yearly by the prescribing physician, enquiring about visual symptoms and rechecking near acuity. If the patient develops blurred vision or a change in measured acuity the treatment should be stopped and the patient referred to an ophthalmologist. The ophthalmologist should assess distance and near acuity, colour vision and visual field along with corneal and retinal examination. In patients requiring long-term treatment (> 5 years) an individual arrangement should be made with the ophthalmologist.

Quinine, another antimalarial, is currently used mainly in the treatment of nocturnal cramps. Taken in large quantities, as in suicide attempts, quinine is highly toxic and can lead to severe visual loss. Initially there may be profound visual loss with dilated pupils. The fundus appearance is often normal or there may be mild venous dilatation. Over time there is disc pallor and arteriolar narrowing, occasionally with bone spicule pigmentation. The natural course is for improvement, although there are often residual visual field defects. The pathological insult is likely to be a direct toxic effect on the retinal cells especially photoreceptors and ganglion cells. The value of treatment, including vasodilators, stellate ganglion block and iv ACTH, is unclear.

2. Antimycobacterial drugs.   *Ethambutol* causes an optic neuropathy. Patients can present with a loss of visual acuity, colour vision defects (especially red) and field defects (typically centrocaecal, occasionally bitemporal). Toxicity is more common where excessive dosage is used or where renal impairment occurs. The incidence in patients receiving 15–25 mg/kg is estimated at 1–6%. Patients should be advised to discontinue therapy immediately if they develop visual symptoms. Visual function usually, but not always, returns after discontinuation of the drug. Visual acuity should be tested before starting ethambutol.

Rifabutin is indicated for prophylaxis against *Mycobacterium avium* infections in AIDS patients with a low CD4 count as well as the treatment of pulmonary TB. It has been associated with an acute non-granulomatous iritis which usually resolves on drug withdrawal. *Isoniazid* has been implicated in cases of optic neuropathy. Both *rifampicin* and *rifabutin* can discolour soft contact lenses red-orange.

Clofazimine used in the treatment of dapsone-resistant leprosy and *Mycobacterium avium* infections in AIDS patients has been reported to be associated with a bull's eye maculopathy with relatively normal vision.

3. Antibiotics.   Optic neuropathy has been described in cystic fibrosis patients taking *chloramphenicol* systemically for long periods. *Nalidixic acid* and *tetracyclines* have been associated with idiopathic intracranial hypertension (pseudotumour cerebri). *Aminoglycosides* impair neuromuscular transmission and can exacerbate myasthenia gravis as well as producing a transient myasthenia syndrome in normal patients. *Sulphonamides* (and many other drugs) can precipitate Stevens–Johnson syndrome. *Metronidazole* may cause transient visual loss, hallucinations, photophobia and ocular motility disturbances, including oculogyric crises. Optic neuritis has also been reported. Tetracycline stains teeth in children less than 12 years old.

4. Anticonvulsants.   *Vigabatrin* is indicated in epilepsy not controlled by other drugs and in infantile spasms. It is thought to be retinotoxic. Up to 1/3 of patients receiving vigabatrin develop visual field defects which are irreversible. There is a concentric constriction of the fields of both eyes, more marked nasally than temporally. Centrally (within 30 degrees of fixation) there is frequently an annular nasal defect, although central visual acuity is not impaired. All patients old enough to do so should have perimetry (ideally static) performed before commencing vigabatrin. Pre-existing visual field defects are a contraindication to treatment. Patients on treatment should be screened 6 monthly and should be instructed to report any visual symptoms. If field constriction is noted consideration should be given to the gradual discontinuation of vigabatrin. Alternatives to field testing include ERG and field-specific VEPs although these have not been validated in detecting vigabatrin-associated field defects.

Phenytoin can cause nystagmus (gaze-evoked, periodic-alternating, down-beat and opsoclonus) as well as ophthalmoplegia. Phenytoin has also been implicated in Stevens–Johnson syndrome. *Carbamazepine* can cause diplopia at peak plasma concentrations and can precipitate an oculogyric crisis.

5. Tamoxifen is a non-steroidal oestrogen receptor antagonist used in the treatment of breast cancer. Ocular toxicity, occurring in up to 12% of cases, includes corneal verticillata, optic neuritis and retinopathy. Previously it was thought that such toxicity only occurred at high doses but toxicity is now known to occur at doses as low as 20 mg/day. Total accumulative dose appears important in the development of toxicity. The retinopathy is characterized by numerous tiny white refractile retinal lesions in the macula and paramacula area often associated with cystoid macular oedema. The retinopathy may be reversible in some cases on discontinuing tamoxifen. The keratopathy is visually insignificant and reversible on stopping treatment. The retinal lesions appear to be confined to the nerve fibre layer and inner plexiform layers.

6. Antipsychotics. *Chlorpromazine* can cause pigmentary granular deposits in the palpebral portion of the cornea and conjunctiva and beneath the anterior capsule of the lens. Retinal toxicity has also been reported with a salt and pepper granularity of the RPE but vision usually remains good.

Thioridazine can cause a pigmentary retinopathy at doses of greater than 800 mg/day. It is characterized by visual loss, occurring a few weeks after commencing therapy, with pigment deposits between the equator and the posterior pole. Nyctalopia occurs later. The retinopathy is usually reversible on stopping the thioridazine.

7. Anti-arrythmics. *Amiodarone* causes reversible corneal verticillata in most patients but they rarely cause symptoms. It has also been reported rarely to cause an optic neuropathy.

Cardiac glycosides, such as digoxin can cause visual anomalies including blurring, xanthopsia ('yellow vision') and other colour vision aberrations possibly due to cone dysfunction. Changes are reversible on stopping the drug.

8. Isotretinoin is used in the treatment of severe acne. Ocular side effects include dry eye, conjunctivitis, contact lens intolerance, corneal opacities, nyctalopia, optic neuritis and idiopathic intracranial hypertension.

9. Corticosteroids are used to control inflammation in many wide ranging conditions. Corticosteroids can cause posterior subcapsular cataract. Factors, which may be involved in the formation of cataract include the inhibition of the lens sodium-potassium-ATPase mechanism and changes in specific amino groups of the lens crystallins. The relationship between dose, duration of therapy and the development of cataract in unclear. There appears to be some genetic susceptibility and disease-specific influences. Corticosteroids can also produce raised intraocular pressure by reducing aqueous outflow, although the mechanism is unclear. Withdrawal of systemic corticosteroids is associated with idiopathic intracranial hypertension.

10. Sildenafil (Viagra) is a phosphodiesterase-5(PDE5) inhibitor used in the treatment of male erectile dysfunction. The drug also has an inhibitory effect on PDE6 which controls the levels of c-GMP in the retina. Some patients report a bluish haze to their vision or increased light sensitivity although long-term retinal damage has not been reported. Sildenafil is relatively contraindicated in patients with a pre-existing retinal dystrophy.

11. Non-steroidal anti-inflammatory drugs. *Indomethacin* can cause a vortex keratopathy (verticillata). *Ibuprofen* has been implicated in causing optic neuropathy.

12. Sex hormones. Both the oral contraceptive and hormone replacement therapy may increase the risk of thromboembolic phenomena in the eye.

13. Oxygen. Exposure to high concentrations of oxygen for long periods can lead to visual problems. Retinal arteriolar constriction and visual field defects can occur but are usually transient. The situation is very different in the pre-term infant where uncontrolled high oxygen partial pressure is known to be an aetiological factor in retinopathy of prematurity.

14. Antimuscarinics. Any drugs with antimuscarinic properties have the potential to cause dry eye, accommodation problems and precipitate acute angle closure glaucoma in susceptible eyes. These include phenothiazines, the inhaler ipratropium bromide, anti-parkisonism drugs, such as benzhexol, tricyclic antidepressants and premedications, such as hyoscine and atropine.

15. β-Blockers. Conjunctival shrinkage has been associated with systemic *practolol* usage. β-Blockers have been reported to produce dry eye.

16. D-Penicillamine is used in the treatment of severe rheumatoid arthritis, Wilson's disease and cystinuria. It can produce a myasthenia-like syndrome with ocular signs and generalized muscle involvement associated with the formation of antiacetylcholine receptor antibodies. **Gold**, also used in the treatment of rheumatoid arthritis, causes ocular chrysiasis when gold crystals are deposited in the cornea, conjunctiva and lens.

17. Desferrioxamine is an iron-chelating agent used mainly to prevent iron overload in patients requiring repeated blood transfusion. High-dose intravenous desferrioxamine has been associated with a toxic retinopathy with abrupt onset of reduced visual acuity and colour vision. The fundus is either normal or shows fine mottling of the RPE. Rarely, a more florid pseudo-retinitis pigmentosa may develop. The vision improves after cessation but does not return to normal.

18. *Methanol* toxicity occurs usually after ingestion of contaminated illicit spirit alcohol. Toxicity appears to be in the ganglion cell layer of the retina and the optic nerve. Retinal oedema as well as optic disc swelling can be visible. Symptoms occur 18–48 hours after ingestion and consist of reduced visual acuity, central scotomas and eventually optic atrophy. If the patient survives any visual recovery will occur in the first 4–6 days. Most patients remain blind.

19. *'Talc' retinopathy.* Intravenous drug abusers sometimes inject crushed tablets containing talc and cornstarch. Talc may also be an unknown additive to other powdered white illicit drugs. The talc lodges in the lung capillaries eventually leading to shunt vessels, allowing the particles to pass to the retina. Bilateral fine glistening opacities associated with small vessels of the inner retina are visible. Peripheral retinal ischaemia can occur leading to proliferative retinopathy.

20. *Proton pump inhibitors.* *Omepreole* has been reported as causing an anterior ischaemic optic neuropathy. *Pantoprazole* and *lansoprazole* may have similar associations. Vasoconstriction secondary to inhibition of the potassium ion/proton pump has been suggested as a possible mechanism.

21. *Antivirals.* Cidofovir is a DNA polymerase chain reaction inhibitor indicated for CMV retinitis. Reports exist of it causing reduced intraocular pressure.

Further reading

General reading

Grant WM, Schuman JS. *Toxicology of the Eye*, 4th edn. Springfield, Il: Charles C Thomas, 1993.

More specific reading for some of the drugs mentioned above

Hydroxychloroquine: Ocular toxicity and hydroxychloroquine: Guidelines for screening. The Royal College of Ophthalmologists, 1998.

Quinine: Brinton GS, Norton EWD, Zhan JE *et al.* Ocular quinine toxicity. *American Journal of Ophthalmology* 1980; **90**(3): 403–10.

Ethambutol: Salmon JF, Carmichael TR, Welsh NH. Use of contrast sensitivity measurement in the detection of subclinical ethambutol toxic optic neuropathy. *British Journal of Ophthalmology* 1987; **71**(3): 192–6.

Vigabatrin: Kalviainen R, Nousiainen I, Mantyjarvi M *et al.* Vigabatrin, a gabaergic antiepileptic drug, causes concentric visual field defects. *Neurology* 1999; **53**(5): 922–6.

Tamoxifen: Noureddin BN, Seoud M, Bashshur Z *et al.* Ocular toxicity in low-dose tamoxifen a prospective study. *Eye* 1999; **13**: 729–33.

Chlorpromazine: Isaac NE, Walker AM, Jick H *et al.* Exposure to phenothiazine drugs and the risk of cataract. *Archives of Ophthalmology* 1991; **109**(2): 256–60.

Thioridazine: Cameron ME, Lawrence JM, Olrich JG. Thioridazine (Melleril) retinopathy. *British Journal of Ophthalmology* 1972; **56**(2): 131–4.

Sildenafil: Marmor MF, Kessler R. Sildenafil (Viagra) and Ophthalmology. *Surv Ophthalmol* 1999; **44**(2): 153–62.

Practolol: Rahi AH, Chapman CM, Garner A *et al.* Pathology of practolol induced ocular toxicity. *British Journal Ophthalmology* 1976; **60**(5): 312–23.

D-Penicillamine: Katz LJ, Lesser RL, Merikangas JR, Silverman JP. Ocular myasthenia gravis after D-penicillamine administration. *British Journal Ophthalmol* 1989; **73**(12): 1015–18.

Desferrioxamine: Lakhanpal V, Schocket SS, Rouben J. Deferoxamine (Desferal)-induced toxic retinal pigmentary degeneration and presumed optic neuropathy. *Ophthalmology* 1984; **91**(5): 443–51.

Talc: Tse DT, Ober RR. Talc retinopathy. *American Journal of Ophthalmology* 1980; **90**(5): 624–40.

Omeprezole: Schonhofer PS, Werner B. Ocular damage with proton pump inhibitors. *British Medical Journal* 1997; **314**: 1805

Related topic of interest

Corneal opacity (p. 75).

TOXICOLOGY: DRUGS FOR OCULAR DISEASE

Gavin Walters & Robert H. Taylor

Drugs, mainly in the form of topical medications, are commonly given for ocular conditions. Before prescribing the ophthalmologist should be aware of a patient's medical history and care must be taken especially in the elderly, the young, the pregnant and patients with any systemic disease.

Problem

All topically applied drugs have the potential for local side effects, often affecting the ocular surface. Significant systemic absorption of eye drops can occur, via the nasal mucosa, avoiding first-pass metabolism, having the potential to produce systemic toxicity. Although relatively uncommon, systemic side effects can be life threatening.

Background

The ophthalmologist should have a good working knowledge of all potential side effects and drug interactions trying to avoid them where possible. Infants and children have a greater susceptibility to toxicity and care should be taken when prescribing in these groups. Most topical eye medications have not been implicated in fetal abnormalities. Care should always be exercised in prescribing in pregnancy and drugs should only be used as necessary, limiting systemic absorption with punctal occlusion.

Clinical features

The more common side effects and interactions are mentioned here and the lists are by no means exhaustive.

1. β-blocker drops infrequently have local side effects. Allergic blepharoconjunctivitis can occur sometimes due to preservatives. Conjunctival hyperaemia, super-ficial punctate keratitis, dry eye and corneal anaesthesia have been reported.

Although generally well tolerated significant systemic side effects can occur. Cardiovascular (β_1-antagonist) effects include bradycardia, heart block, congestive cardiac failure, hypotension, Raynaud phenomenon and worsening of peripheral vascular disease. Respiratory (β_2-antagonist) side effects include bronchospasm (predominantly a problem in patients with pre-existing lung disease and in the elderly), respiratory failure and reduced exercise tolerance. Respiratory problems may be less in cardioselective β-blockers (e.g. *betaxolol*), although they should still be avoided in asthma. CNS side effects include fatigue, depression, anxiety, hallucinations, confusion and myasthenia gravis can be exacerbated. Decreased libido and impotence can occur. β-blockers can mask symptoms of hypoglycaemia in insulin-dependent diabetics.

β-blockers are contraindicated in patients with asthma or obstructive airways disease, heart failure, bradycardia, heart block and peripheral vascular disease. β-blockers should not be prescribed in patients already taking the calcium channel-blocker verapamil.

2. *Adrenergic agonists.*

- *Adrenaline*, a non-selective α- and β-agonist, results in more than 50% of patients becoming intolerant because of local reactions. Initially, after instillation, the conjunctiva blanches followed by rebound hyperaemia. Allergic reactions can lead to follicular conjunctivitis. Adrenaline is oxidized to adrenochrome which causes black conjunctival deposits in up to 20% of cases. Adrenaline can also exacerbate anterior uveitis and cause cystoid macular oedema in up to 20% of aphakic patients. Systemic side effects include tachycardia, hypertension and arrhythmias. *Dipivefrine*, a pro-drug of adrenaline, has similar side effects. Both drugs induce mydriasis and can cause angle-closure glaucoma.
- *Apraclonidine*, a relatively selective α_2-agonist, can cause mydriasis, lid retraction and conjunctival blanching. Allergic blepharoconjunctivitis is common in up to 48% of patients after chronic use, although less common in children. Systemic effects include headache, dry mouth and a potential to exacerbate ischaemic heart disease.
- *Brimonidine*, a highly selective α_2-agonist, most commonly results in allergic blepharoconjunctivitis occurring in 9.6% of patients. Dry mouth, fatigue/drowsiness, headache and rarely depression have been reported. Drowsiness can occur in children. Acute hypotension, bradychardia and apnoea can occur in infants. The use of brimonidine is contraindicated in the first year of life. Both *apraclonidine* and *brimonidine* should be avoided in patients taking tricyclic antidepressants or monoamine-oxidase inhibitors.
- *Phenylephrine*, an α_1-agonist, can result in local allergy. Systemic side effects include arrhythmias, hypertension and coronary artery spasm. The 2.5% solution should be used in infants.

3. *Prostaglandins.*

- *Latanoprost* is a prostaglandin $F_{2\alpha}$-agonist. No significant systemic side effects have been reported although caution is advised in severe brittle asthma. Latanoprost produces an increase in iris pigmentation, especially in mixed coloured irides, in 8–15% of eyes within 3–12 months. This is thought to be due to an increase in melanin production rather than due to proliferation of melanocytes. Darkening, thickening and lengthening of the lashes has been reported. There is a risk of cystoid macular oedema. Cystoid macula oedema has been reported in aphakes.

4. *Carbonic anhydrase inhibitors.*

- *Acetazolamide* is administered both orally and parenterally but is not active topically. Acetazolamide is a sulphonamide and as such sulphur-allergic patients can rarely have reactions and rashes as well as blood dyscrasias such as idiosyncratic aplastic anaemia. The most common symptom complex associated with acetazolamide is that of fatigue, anorexia, weight loss, malaise, depression and loss of libido. Patients also frequently experience nausea, diarrhoea, paraesthesias of the extremities and headache. Acetazolamide causes diuresis. Chronic ingestion leads to a 10-fold increase in renal calculi (due to a metabolic acidosis). In therapeutic doses acetazolamide causes a metabolic and respiratory acidosis which can be a major problem in chronic pulmonary disease and in renal and hepatic failure. Long-term use can lead to hypokalaemia and hyponatraemia. It is recommended that monitoring of electrolytes and blood counts be undertaken in long-term use. Local ocular effects include a transient myopia.

- *Dorzolamide* is a topical carbonic anhydrase inhibitor. There is the potential for sulphonamide-related idiosyncratic blood dyscrasias. Other systemic reactions are greatly reduced compared with acetazolamide but include headache, dizziness, parasthesia and nausea. Superficial punctate keratitis occurs in up to 15% of cases and local allergy is a problem in up to 10% of cases.

5.   Osmotic diuretics.
- *Mannitol* is given intravenously. Many patients develop headache and back pain combined with a diuresis during treatment. Frail elderly patients and those with cardiac and renal failure can develop circulatory overload which can lead to heart failure and pulmonary oedema. Mannitol clears slowly in renal failure. Subdural haematomas and anaphylactic reactions can occur.
- *Glycerol* is administered orally and being very sweet can produce nausea and vomiting. It is metabolized by the liver and so is safer in renal failure.

6.   Parasympathomimetics.   Local side effects are common with pilocarpine. The most common include miosis with reduced acuity and darkening of vision, myopia (due to ciliary muscle contraction with forward lens displacement), and brow and temporal headache. Retinal detachments have been reported with miotic therapy. Allergic reactions, iris cysts, posterior synechiae and possibly cataract formation are other local effects. Angle-closure glaucoma can be exacerbated due to increased lens curvature. Systemic side effects are rare with pilocarpine but high doses can lead to sweating, nausea, vomiting, diarrhoea, intestinal colic, bradycardia and bronchospasm.

- *Ecothiopate iodide* drops are only available in the UK on a named patient basis. The muscle relaxant suxamethonium must not be used if patients are taking topical ecothiopate iodide.

7.   Parasympatholytic agents.
- *Atropine, homatropine, cyclopentolate* and, to a lesser extent, *tropicamide* all have the potential for systemic side effects especially in infants and children. Symptoms of toxicity include dry skin and mouth, flushing, hyperthermia (due to the inability to sweat), tachycardia (due to vagal inhibition), and irritability or delerium with hallucinations. Parents should be warned of these side effects when administering these drugs at home. The risks can be reduced by using ointment rather than drops as well using 0.5% atropine rather than 1%. In infants 0.5% cyclopentolate should be used rather than 1%. All parasympatholytics can cause an increase in aqueous outflow resistance causing a rise in intraocular

pressure in susceptible individuals. Mydriasis can induce pupillary block causing angle-closure glaucoma.

8. **_Topical and parenteral corticosteroids_** can cause elevated intraocular pressure (IOP) in up to 30% of normal individuals. Patients with open-angle glaucoma, diabetes and high myopia have an increased IOP sensitivity to corticosteroids. The IOP appears to be elevated because of increased outflow resistance, although the exact mechanism is unknown. _Fluorometholone_ may have less of an effect on IOP. Topical corticosteroids can induce posterior subcapsular cataract but are less of a problem than systemic corticosteroids. As anti-inflammatory drugs and immune modulators corticosteroids can mask the signs of infection as well as increasing suseptibility to infection. Corticosteroids should not be used in the undiagnosed red eye. Topical corticosteroids can inhibit corneal healing and have been associated with corneal and scleral melts. Periocular corticosteroid injections can have an effect on the hypothalamic/pituitary/adrenal axis.

9. **_Local anaesthetics._** Topical local anaesthetics can disrupt the corneal epithelium. Periocular local anaesthetics can have significant systemic absorption leading to toxicity. The main effects are on the central nervous and cardiovascular systems. Initially nausea, perioral numbness and tingling occur. Later there is a fall in blood pressure, muscle twitching leading to seizures, respiratory depression and circulatory collapse. Direct injection into the subdural space can induce immediate respiratory arrest. It is recommended that someone experienced in resuscitation, ideally an anaesthetist, is available during periocular local anaesthetic procedures. Diplopia can result from effects on the extraocular muscles. A possible mechanism is a direct intramuscular injection.

10. **_Antibiotics._** Topical antibiotics may cause localized allergy and corneal epithelial toxicity. _Chloramphenicol_ topically has been implicated in cases of aplastic anaemia although a causal effect has not been established. Chloramphenicol should be avoided in patients with a history, or family history, of bone marrow failure.

11. **_Fluorescein._** Fluorescein is well tolerated topically. Intravenous fluorescein most commonly leads to nausea (about 5%). Severe systemic reactions, such as laryngeal oedema, anaphylaxis, bronchospasm and circulatory collapse, are rare. The risk of death from a fluorescein injection is less than 1 in 100 000.

12. **_Preservatives_** such as benzalkonium chloride, are often a constituent of topical eye medications. They can be a source of localized allergy as well as causing corneal epithelial toxicity.

Further reading

General reading

Grant WM, Schuman JS. _Toxicology of the Eye_, 4th edn. Springfield, Il: Charles C Thomas, 1993.
Mauger TF, Elson CL, editors. _Ocular Pharmacology_, 6th edn. St Louis: Mosby, 1994.

More specific reading for some of the drugs mentioned above

β-blockers: Diggory P, Cassels-Brown A, Vail A, Hillman JS. Randomised, controlled trial of spirometric changes in elderly people receiving timolol or betaxolol as initial treatment for glaucoma. *British Journal of Ophthalmology* 1998; **82**(2): 146–9.

Apraclonidine: Araujo SV, Bond JB, Wilson RP *et al.* Long term effect of apraclonidine. *British Journal Ophthalmology* 1995; **79**(12): 1098–101.

Brimonidine: Cantor LB, Burke J. Drug evaluation: brimonidine. *Expert opinion in investigative drugs* 1997; **6**: 1063–83.

Walters G, Taylor RH. Severe systemic toxicity caused by brimonidine drops in an infant with presumed juvenile xanthogranuloma. *Eye* 1999; **13**(6): 797–8.

Latanoprost: Alm A, Stjernschantz J, Scandanavian Latanoprost Study Group. Effects on intraocular pressure and side effects of 0.005% latanoprost applied once daily, evening or morning. A comparison with Timolol. *Ophthalmology* 1995; **102**(12): 1743–52.

Dorzolamide: Strahlman E, Tipping R, Vogel R *et al.* A double-masked, randomised 1-year study comparing dorzolamide (Trusopt), timolol and betaxolol. *Archives of Ophthalmology* 1995; **113**: 1009–16.

Chloramphenicol: Walker S, Diaper CJ, Bowman R *et al.* Lack of evidence for systemic toxicity following topical chloramphenicol use. *Eye* 1998; **12**(5): 875–9.

Related topic of interest

Toxicology: drugs for non-ocular diseases (p. 319).

TOXOPLASMOSIS

Philip I. Murray

Toxoplasmosis results from infection by the obligate intracellular parasite, *Toxoplasma gondii*. Ocular disease is the commonest disabling consequence of toxoplasma infection and is a major and preventable cause of severe visual handicap.

Problem

Misunderstanding arises with regards to route of transmission, use of serological investigations in diagnosis, indications for treatment, choice of treatment options, and the value of screening pregnant women.

Background

Young cats are the definitive hosts and excrete oocytes in their faeces for 14 days after having become infected. Thereafter a healthy cat will not normally be a source of infection again. The cat is the only known host in which the reproductive cycle of *Toxoplasma gondii* takes place. It is not the infected cats that are the primary source of infection for humans, but the result of eating raw/partly cooked meat from other infected animals acting as intermediate hosts. Infection also occurs from the ingestion of unwashed fruit or vegetables through contamination of soil. In earth, cats' faeces may remain infective for up to 18 months. Similarly, the handling of used cat litter may be a source of infection. There may also be a risk of catching toxoplasmosis from handling sheep at lambing time.

Human infection occurs by either the congenital or acquired route. Congenital infection arises when a pregnant woman becomes infected. In 40% of these women toxoplasma crosses the placenta to infect the fetus. The severity of infection is greatest in the first trimester, but the frequency of transmission to the fetus is higher in the third trimester. Although a number of babies per year may be born infected with toxoplasmosis, only a small number of these will exhibit clinical symptoms directly after birth. A surveillance study based on all UK births in 1989/90 detected only 14 severely affected congenitally infected offspring. Once maternal immunity has developed, subsequent fetuses will be protected against congenital infection. Likewise, a woman with congenital toxoplasmosis cannot transmit the infection to her children.

Acquired disease is usually asymptomatic or may take the form of a non-specific glandular fever-like illness. It is believed that 30–50% of the adult population has serological evidence of previous toxoplasma infection. Immunocompromised patients, such as those with the acquired immunodeficiency syndrome (AIDS) are at risk of developing acquired toxoplasmosis as well as reactivation of pre-existing ocular lesions.

Congenital infection is by far the commonest route of transmission, but necrotizing toxoplasmic retinochoroiditis has been reported to occur in 1–21% of acquired systemic infection. Although it is still believed that the vast majority of ocular infections are due to recurrences of congenital disease, a number of recent studies have questioned this, particularly as recurrences of acquired disease are visually indistinguishable from recurrent congenital infection.

Clinical features

The disease is bilateral in 40% of cases, and in immunocompetent individuals is almost never active simultaneously in both eyes. Patients usually present complaining of floaters and, if the disc or macula is affected, reduced visual acuity. Often, this is a reactivation of a previous lesion occurring at the edge of an old scar (satellite formation). Active retinitis usually appears as an oval or circular white, fluffy area with overlying vitreous activity. As it heals, it becomes more circumscribed with evidence of pigment clumping. Inactive lesions take the form of atrophic scars with hyperpigmentation along the borders. Retinal vasculitis (periphlebitis) may be seen, sometimes in all four retinal quadrants. Rarely, multifocal grey-white lesions at the level of deep retina and retinal pigment epithelium have been described with little or no overlying vitreous inflammation (punctate outer retinal toxoplasmosis). Toxoplasmic retinochoroiditis in AIDS may be bilateral in the form of multifocal lesions and may co-infect the retina with other organisms, such as cytomegalovirus. A subgroup of older patients with large lesions has been described.

Permanent loss of visual acuity may occur as a result of the retinitis directly involving the disc, macula or papillo-macular bundle. Macular oedema may be associated with lesions adjacent to the macula. Congenital lesions have a predilection for the macula and not uncommonly do so bilaterally resulting in severe permanent visual compromise. Other complications include vascular occlusions, sub-retinal neovascular membrane (SRNVM) formation and retinal detachment.

Active ocular toxoplasmosis is a clinical diagnosis. The finding of typical scars in the affected or contralateral eye will help in diagnosis. There are numerous serological tests available, the commonest being the dye test. Due to the high prevalence of positive sera in the general population a positive dye test or the detection of IgG antibodies is of little use. A negative dye test (performed on undiluted serum) makes the diagnosis improbable. The finding of IgM antibodies would imply acquired infection particularly IgM ISAGA. Using the polymerase chain reaction to look for toxoplasma gene products in intraocular fluid may be helpful but is not yet completely reliable. Intraocular antibody production may also be of use.

Treatment

Ocular toxoplasmosis is a self-limiting disease. Small peripheral retinal lesions usually require no treatment. Associated anterior uveitis can be treated with topical steroid and mydriatic. The indications for systemic treatment are: (1) lesions affecting the disc, macula or papillo-macular bundle, (2) marked vitritis, (3) lesions threatening a major vessel and (4) all lesions in immunocompromised individuals.

If systemic treatment is required, a variety of regimes have been shown to be effective and should be given for at least 4 weeks: (1) pyrimethamine/sulphadiazine/prednisolone plus folinic acid supplements, (2) clindamycin/sulphadiazine/prednisolone or (3) cotrimoxazole/prednisolone. One should be aware of the potential side-effects of these therapies. Corticosteroids should not be used on their own as they may lead to fulminant disease. Similarly, periocular injections of corticosteroids are contraindicated. Unfortunately, these treatments are unable to eradicate the encysted form of toxoplasma (bradyzoites) in the retina thus failing to prevent recurrences. A relatively new drug, atovaqone, which acts by selective inhibition of mitochondria electron transport chain in protozoa has been shown to have significant *in vivo* and *in vitro* activity against the encysted stage of toxoplasma infection. Recent clinical studies have found it to be effective but recurrences still occurred. In those women who seroconvert during pregnancy, spiramycin is the drug of choice. Although only 60% effective it reduces the risk of transmission across the placenta. It can be used throughout the pregnancy. In immunocompromised patients, long-term maintenance therapy is required and corticosteroids are not given. Laser photocoagulation is occasionally used, particularly in patients in who systemic therapy may be contraindicated, such as during pregnancy; and in patients with a SNRVM. Vitrectomy may be required for persistent, visually disabling floaters, for those that detach, or combined with removal of SNRVM.

As most cases of ocular disease are a result of congenital infection, measures should be directed at preventing maternal infection during pregnancy. Education on eating only washed fruit and vegetables, avoiding unpasteurized goat's milk, cooking meat thoroughly and wearing rubber gloves when handling used cat litter needs to be widely available to pregnant women. In several European countries, repeated serological screening during the antenatal period allows the detection of active infection during pregnancy thereby allowing treatment to be initiated. A recent study has shown the estimated lifetime risk of symptomatic ocular toxoplasmosis by age 60 years in British-born individuals to be 18/100 000 This relatively low risk indicates limited potential benefits of prenatal or postnatal screening in the UK. However those born in West Africa have a 20-fold higher lifetime risk.

Further reading

Bosch-Driessen EH, Rothova A. Recurrent ocular disease in postnatally acquired toxoplasmosis. *American Journal of Ophthalmology* 1999; **128**: 421–5.

Gilbert RE, Dunn DT, Lightman S *et al*. Incidence of symptomatic toxoplasma eye disease: aetiology and public health implications. *Epidemiol Infect* (**Q125**) 1999; **123**: 283–9.

Holland GN. Perspective. Reconsidering the pathogenesis of ocular toxoplasmosis. *American Journal of Ophthalmology* 1999; **128**: 502–5.

Holland GN, Muccioli C, Silveira C, Weisz JM, Belfort Jnr R, O'Connor GR. Intraocular inflammatory reactions without focal necrotizing retinochoroiditis in patients with acquired systemic toxoplasmosis. *American Journal of Ophthalmology* 1999; **128**: 413–20.

Rothova A. Ocular involvement in toxoplasmosis. *British Journal of Ophthalmology* 1993; **77**: 371–7.

Rothova A, Meenken C, Buitenhuis HJ *et al*. Therapy for ocular toxoplasmosis. *American Journal of Ophthalmology* 1993; **115**: 517–23.

UVEAL MELANOMA

Ian Rennie

Uveal melanomas are the commonest primary intraocular malignancy in adults with an incidence of approximately 6–7 cases per million population per year in Western countries. Ciliary body and choroidal (posterior uveal) melanomas have a peak instance in late middle age (mid 50s) whereas iris melanomas occur most frequently one decade earlier. Melanoma can also, rarely, occur in childhood.

Problem

Posterior uveal melanoma poses a significant threat to life with approximately 50% of patients dying from their disease.

Background

Uveal melanoma is predominantly a disease of Caucasians and is extremely uncommon in non-white races. It occurs more frequently in patients with blond hair and blue eyes in contrast to brown-haired, dark-eyed individuals. Choroidal naevi are extremely common, occurring in 2–6% of the normal population. The role of pre-existing naevi in the development of uveal melanomas is uncertain. It is probable that some melanomas do arise from pre-existing naevi. Patients with ocular and ocular-dermal melanocytosis have an increased risk of developing uveal melanomas.

The role of sunlight and UV light in the development of uveal melanomas remains controversial. The fact that melanoma tends to occur in lightly pigmented individuals and that iris melanomas have a predilection for the lower half of the iris suggests a possible aetiological role. However, the dramatic rise in the instance of cutaneous melanomas which has been attributed to increase exposure to sunlight in fair-skinned individuals has not been seen in uveal melanomas where the instance appears to have remained relatively constant. Furthermore, the natural crystalline lens is an effective UV light filter, which protects the posterior uveal tract from excessive UV light exposure. This property of the lens increases with age. It is theoretically possible that excessive exposure to sunlight in early childhood may contribute to the development of uveal tumours in later life.

Uveal melanomas metastasize via the blood stream and have a strong predilection to develop metastases in the liver. Most patients develop metastases within 5 years of diagnosis. Occasionally, the advent of metastatic disease may be delayed for many years. In general, tumours arising from the ciliary body have a less favourable prognosis than those that arise in the choroid. Prognostic factors include tumour size and histological cell type. In contrast, iris melanomas rarely metastasize, this event occurring in only 3% of cases. Recent studies have shown that evaluation of tumour vascular patterns and cytogenetic analysis are additional indices of prognosis. In particular, tumours which are found to have lost one copy of chromosome 3 and/or have additional copies of all or part of chromosome 8 have a particularly unfavourable prognosis.

Clinical features

Improved screening techniques by optometrists, particularly in the use of indirect ophthalmoscopy or 90 dioptre lens through the dilated pupil has led to the increase in finding of small, asymptomatic melanomas.

Symptomatic tumours present in a variety of ways, dependent on their size and location. Choroidal tumours involving the posterior pole usually present with either a loss or distortion of central vision. Peripheral choroidal tumours may present with photopsias and/or a shadow in the vision: particularly if they are associated with a retinal detachment. Ciliary body tumours may attain a relatively large size before detection, particularly presenting with visual loss either due to lenticular astigmatism associated with dislocation of the lens, or as a result of extensive retinal detachment. Iris lesions usually manifest as a change in the appearance of the iris or secondary glaucoma. This latter presentation is particularly common in diffuse melanomas of the iris where the diagnosis may be missed or delayed because of their unusual appearance.

Typically, posterior melanomas appear as a raised pigmented mass often with an associated retinal detachment. The degree of pigmentation is extremely variable and completely amelanotic tumours are not uncommon. Abnormalities of the overlying retinal pigment epithelium are common: the presence of significant amounts of orange pigment (lipofuscin) on the surface may act as a useful indice of malignancy. Herniation of the tumour through Bruch's membrane typically produces a 'collar stud' appearance.

To the experienced observer a typical large, elevated, pigmented, posterior uveal melanoma does not present a diagnostic challenge. However, small atypical lesions, particularly those which are amelanotic, may present considerable diagnostic difficulty. The list of conditions that may simulate a choroidal melanoma is extremely lengthy and includes: large atypical naevi, choroidal metastases, choroidal haemangioma and eccentric disciforms.

Investigations

B-scan and standardized A-scan ultrasonography are useful ancillary diagnostic tools. Typically, melanomas are seen as an elevated solid mass with relatively low internal reflectivity. Other features, such as choroidal excavation and orbital shadowing may be seen but their absence does not exclude a melanoma. Fluorescein and indocyanine angiography may also be useful to differentiate pseudomelanomas from melanomas, and may be of particular value in differentiating them from vascular tumours such as choroidal haemangiomas. CT and MRI imaging are of little value in differentiating melanomas from other intraocular lesions. However, they may be of some value in demonstrating extraocular extension of the primary tumour.

Fine needle aspiration biopsy of the primary tumour may be helpful in certain circumstances. This technique may be of particular value when the patient presents with an amelanotic tumour in the eye and a history of previous malignant disease, which raises the possibility of ocular metastasis. However, ocular complications may occur, the most common being vitreous haemorrhage. Therefore, biopsy should be restricted to specialized centres where the necessary expertise is available, not only to perform the biopsy but also to interpret the results.

Treatment

In recent years, a number of techniques have been developed aimed at destroying the primary tumour without the need to remove the eye. No single technique is ideal for all tumours and a careful assessment must be made of both the tumour and the patient, prior to initiating treatment. A number of parameters must be taken into account before developing a treatment plan. These include: size, location and degree of pigmentation of the primary tumour, state of the fellow eye, age, physical status of the patient and patient preference. Although opinions vary between experts as to the relative merits of certain treatments, there is uniform agreement that the aims of treatment in order of descending importance are: eradication of the primary tumour, retention of the globe and preservation of useful vision.

1. Radiotherapy. The use of radioactive isotope plaques (brachytherapy) are a well established and effective way of treating small and medium-sized posterior segment uveal melanomas. The plaques are placed on the sclera overlying the base of the tumour. Accurate localization of the tumour and placement of the plaque so that it completely covers the borders of the tumour is essential. The plaque is removed when a calculated dose of radiation has been delivered. Commonly used radioactive isotopes include ruthenium 106 which emits beta radiation and is suitable for tumours less than 6 mm thick or iodine 125 which emits gamma irradiation and can be used for thicker tumours.

Uveal melanomas may also be treated by external beam irradiation. Localizing rings are placed on the sclera around the tumour base to facilitate accurate location of the charged particle beam. Opinions vary as to the usefulness of this technique with some experts preferring brachytherapy as a routine treatment and using external beam irradiation for larger tumours which cannot be adequately treated with a plaque.

In recent years, a number of centres have successfully treated uveal melanomas using either a gamma knife or LINAC (Linear Accelerator) unit. This treatment is generally reserved for tumours that are either too large or unfavourably located for simple brachytherapy.

Complications of irradiation include radiation retinopathy and optic neuropathy. Severe retinopathy including retinal or optic disc neovascularization leading to rubeosis and secondary glaucoma can occur particularly if the tumour is large, retinal detachment is extensive and/or the optic nerve is included in the treatment field.

2. Transpupillary diode thermotherapy. This is a relatively new treatment modality where the aim of the treatment is to raise the core temperature of the tumour by approximately 8–20°C. The diode laser is used with a wavelength of 810 nanometres, covering the tumour with overlapping 3 mm spots each of 1 minute duration. The power of the laser is adjusted to produce a faint whitening of the tumour surface at the end of each spot application. Indocyanine green has been used to augment the treatment and may be of particular value in amelanotic lesions. The treatment is most suitable for posteriorly placed lesions that are less than 3.5 mm in elevation. Several treatment sessions may be required to eradicate the tumour. Complications include tumour regrowth, vascular occlusions and wrinkling of the internal limiting membrane. The latter may cause visual loss or distortion if the lesion is close to the fovea.

3. *Argon laser photocoagulation.* Laser has been used for small tumours with a thickness of less than 3 mm. Late tumour recurrence has proved to be a common problem with this form of therapy. It has now been superseded by transpupillary diode thermotherapy.

4. *Local resection.* Trans-scleral resection of uveal tumours may be of value in selected cases in particular iris and ciliary body tumours, which extend for less than three clock hours. Anterior choroidal tumours with a maximum base diameter of less than 14 mm can also be resected. Local resection of choroidal tumours usually requires profound hypotensive anaesthesia which limits the use of this technique to those individuals with a healthy cardiovascular system.

Operative complications include severe intraocular haemorrhage and retinal detachment. Local tumour recurrence has proved to be a relatively common complication causing some ocular oncologists to advocate the use of low-dose plaque brachytherapy in combination with surgical resection.

5. *Enucleation.* Enucleation is still the treatment of choice for large tumours, tumours that cannot be treated easily by other modalities, or where the visual prognosis for the eye is already extremely poor. Enucleation is also recommended for patients not wishing to undergo other forms of therapy. Exenteration is rarely used in the treatment of uveal melanoma. It is reserved in general for neglected cases where there is extensive intrascleral spread into the orbit and ocular adnexa.

Further reading

Rennie IG. Uveal Melanoma: The Past, The Present and the Future. *Eye* 1997; **II:** 255–64.

Shields JS, Shields CL. *Intraocular Tumours: A Text and Atlas.* WB Saunders Company, 1992.

Sisley K, Rennie IG, Parson MA *et al.* Abnormalities of chromosomes 3 and 8, in posterior uveal melanoma, correlates with prognosis. *Genes, Chromosomes and Cancer* 1997; **18:** 1–7.

UVEITIS: WHO AND WHAT TO INVESTIGATE

Philip I. Murray

Uveitis, a term used to describe inflammation of the uveal tract (iris, ciliary body, chorid) alone, actually comprises a large group of diverse diseases affecting not only the uvea but also the retina, optic nerve and vitreous. The International Uveitis Study Group classification separates uveitis by anatomical localization of the disease, according to the major visible signs: anterior, posterior, pan and intermediate. The course of the disease can be described as acute, chronic (greater than 3 months duration) or recurrent. In the majority of cases of endogenous uveitis, the aetiology is unknown. Some cases are a manifestation of a systemic disease, such as sarcoidosis or Behçet's disease, whilst others are only associated with various conditions, such as the HLA-B27 related group of diseases. Although one can attach a label to a number of uveitis syndromes, such as Fuchs' heterochromic cyclitis or Vogt–Koyanagi–Harada, the actual cause underlying these diseases is unknown. Despite this, classifying uveitis patients into different subgroups is important, even if an aetiology is never found, as evidence exists on how best to manage these distinct uveitis entities and their likely prognosis.

Problem

One of the most pressing questions that arises in the mind of every ophthalmologist who sees a new case of uveitis is 'what is the cause of this disease?'. Because this problem is inextricably linked to other salient issues, such as the natural course of the disease and the most appropriate therapy, pathogenesis is of prime importance. Thus, performing various investigations may be of value in determining the cause of the intraocular inflammation particularly as it may form part of a systemic disease process. Yet, it is the choice and appropriateness of the investigations that are problematic.

Background

Little is known about the pathogenesis of uveitis, but disturbances of immune mechanisms have long been suspected of playing a central role with immunological abnormalities found in many patients. In cases of endogenous uveitis in which no link with an infectious agent can be identified, autoimmunity has been invoked as the cause, mainly on the basis of immunopathological findings from eyes removed as a result of serious sight-threatening complications. In most uveitis patients routine investigations, serological and radiological are unhelpful. There are no serological markers of disease activity as can be found in patients with systemic vasculitis. Also, any abnormalities found in peripheral blood are unlikely to reflect what is going on inside the eye. Nevertheless, in view of the puzzling nature of uveitis and the common association with systemic disease, many patients are frequently overinvestigated by being subjected to a vast battery of unnecessary tests. Yet, it is important not to miss a readily treatable (e.g. infective) cause.

The management of uveitis should be a systematic approach tailored to each patient's particular type of uveitis. It is essential that a detailed history is taken and direct questioning should include asking about back/joint problems, skin disease, respiratory disease, neurological disease, gastrointestinal disease, mouth and genital ulcers and sexually transmitted disease. When seeing a patient with chronic or recurrent disease it is important to pay attention to previous findings in the notes for any clues to diagnosis, such as an absence of posterior synechiae in a white and painless eye as seen in patients with Fuchs' heterochromic cyclitis; or unilateral uveitis often associated with raised intraocular pressure recurring within a few months of stopping topical steroids as seen in patients with herpes simplex or varicella zoster virus uveitis. A careful ocular examination should be performed. Details, such as iris nodules (e.g. tuberculosis, sarcoidosis, Fuchs' heterochromic cyclitis), iris atrophy (e.g. herpetic uveitis) may all be a pointer to a specific diagnosis. It is often the history and examination findings that are far more informative than any laboratory investigations, particularly in Behçet's disease where the diagnosis is made according to criteria based on symptoms and signs. An accurate history and examination can prevent the patient undergoing unnecessary investigations.

Clinical features

Unfortunately, no large studies exist which demonstrate the value of investigating patients with uveitis. A number of specific uveitis entities can often be diagnosed solely on clinical examination. These include Fuchs' heterochromic cyclitis and a recurrence of presumed congenital ocular toxoplasmosis. Investigations may not be needed.

Debate exists as to whether patients with the commonest type of uveitis, acute anterior uveitis (AAU), should be investigated. It is well recognized that approximately 50% of patients with AAU are HLA-B27 positive. A number of these patients will give a history of an associated HLA-B27 disease. In the others, HLA typing is unnecessary because it will be unlikely that the result will help in the future management of the patient. Also, HLA-B27-associated AAU often presents with a number of clinical clues that help in diagnosis: it is usually recurrent, unilateral but alternating, often severe anterior chamber inflammation with extensive posterior synechiae, fibrin and even hypopyon.

Even if investigations are undertaken, the likelihood of a 'definitive' aetiology being found for the uveitis is remote. A 'definitive' aetiology of herpes simplex or varicella zoster virus uveitis can only be made in a few patients, usually by detecting herpesviral DNA in intraocular fluid using the polymerase chain reaction, but a 'presumed' aetiology identified on clinical grounds can be made in larger numbers. Although laboratory investigations can diagnose sarcoidosis, the precise cause of sarcoidosis is unknown. In children, systemic disease is more commonly identified, in particular ANA-positive juvenile arthritis. Laboratory investigations are often more fruitful in paediatric uveitis.

It is important to understand the reasons for ordering any investigation:

- will it identify an underlying systemic disease process or association?
- will it provide a 'definitive' aetiology?
- will it confirm or reject a diagnosis?
- will it help in the management of the patient?

Interpretation of results is also very important, particularly with regards to false negatives and false positives. The latter are not uncommon particularly with regards to syphilis serology, rheumatic fever and the Mantoux test.

Ordering large numbers of tests in the hope that one may turn out to be positive should be actively discouraged. If one does enough investigations on any patient there is the chance that something will turn up abnormal but it may have no relevance to the uveitis.

Attention should be paid to the sensitivity and specificity of each test. In the clinical setting, one should perform the minimum number of investigations that will give the maximum information regarding the management of the patient. There are a number of tests that would be common to all uveitis patients, and additional tests that might be relevant to a particular type of uveitis. If investigating the patient was considered appropriate then a number of baseline tests could be undertaken as they may pick up an underlying disease that could be treated.

General investigations

These include:

- full blood count;
- plasma viscosity/ESR;
- syphilis serology;
- urinalysis (e.g. protein for TINU; glucose for diabetes);
- chest X-ray (TB, sarcoidosis);
- ANA (in children).

Any other tests that need to be ordered should depend on the clinical findings and the ophthalmologist's index of suspicion for a particular diagnosis.

Specific investigations

These tests may include:

- angiotensin-converting enzyme (sarcoidosis);
- toxoplasma dye test/IgG antibodies (if negative in undiluted serum to exclude congenital toxoplamosis), IgM antibodies for acquired disease;
- toxocara ELISA;
- HLA-A29 or HLA-B27;
- anti-neutrophil cytoplasmic antibody (Wegener's);
- Mantoux test (TB, sarcoidosis);
- fundus fluorescein angiography;
- electrophysiology;
- CT scan of chest (sarcoidosis);
- CT scan of orbits/B-scan ultrasound;
- MRI head scan (demyelination, sarcoidosis, lymphoma);
- Gallium scan (sarcoidosis);
- Lumbar puncture (demyelination, lymphoma);
- conjunctival biopsy (sarcoidosis) NB 'blind' biopsies should be discouraged);
- polymerase chain reaction of intraocular fluid (usually for infective causes, e.g. herpesviruses, *P. acnes*);

- vitreous biopsy (lymphoma, candida, *P. acnes*);
- choroidal biopsy (lymphoma);
- lyme serology.

In some patients with recurrent or chronic uveitis, repeating investigations 3–5 years later may increase the yield of positive results. Those patients in whom an underlying systemic disease is suspected should be referred to the appropriate specialist as they may require more detailed/invasive investigations.

Conclusion

Uveitis is a puzzling, potentially sight-threatening disease. Do not expect to find a 'definitive' aetiology in the vast majority of patients. A detailed history and thorough clinical examination remains essential in establishing a diagnosis of underlying systemic disease in these patients. Except in children baseline screening investigations should be avoided, as they do not contribute to finding a cause or help in management, and are often expensive. Tests should be ordered only if there is a strong suspicion of systemic disease and tailored to the clinical findings. Performing an ACE and CXR may assist in the diagnosis of sarcoidosis, particularly in those patients with clinical signs compatible with this disease.

Further reading

Barile GR, Flynn TE. Syphilis exposure in patients with uveitis. *Ophthalmology* 1997; **104:** 1605–9.

Marr JE, Stavrou P, Moradi P, Murray PI. Should we investigate patients with uveitis? *Invest Ophthalmol Vis Sci* 1998; **39:** S608.

Murray P. Serum autoantibodies and uveitis. *British Journal of Ophthalmology* 1986; **70:** 266–8.

Rosenbaum JT, Wernick R. The utility of routine screening of patients with uveitis for systemic lupus erythematosus or tuberculosis. A Bayesian analysis. *Archives of Ophthalmology* 1990; **108:** 1291–3.

Stavrou P, Linton S, Young DW, Murray PI. Clinical diagnosis of ocular sarcoidosis. *Eye* 1997; **11:** 365–70.

VISION IMPAIRMENT IN CHILDREN AND THEIR EDUCATION

John Christmas & Robert H. Taylor

The role of the ophthalmologist is primarily in providing diagnosis, treatment, prognosis and information to parents, teachers and other members of the team of allied professionals. This team may include orthoptists, low vision optometrists, teachers, speech therapists, occupational therapists, psychologists, paediatricians and general practitioners. A basic understanding of the problems that a visually impaired child may encounter at home and at school is advised. An understanding of who to communicate with in the community is also essential.

Problem

The community set up in different parts of the country and in different countries will vary. Access to the system can be a challenge for parents if professional guidance is not available.

Background

Until the 1980s in the United Kingdom, children with a visual impairment were as a rule taught in segregated provision, either in a school for the blind or in a school for the partially sighted. This would often mean living away from home in a residential school, with financial implications for the Local Education Authority (LEA). Those with a visual impairment not placed in these schools had to make the most of mainstream schooling without qualified support. Since then, there has been a 'Climate of Change' in the approach to Special Educational Needs (SEN). Following the 1981 Education Act, LEAs took on responsibility for the teaching of children with all kinds of disabilities in mainstream settings. This included those with a visual impairment. Qualified teachers of the visually impaired (VI) were employed.

1. Location of provision. Most primary school-aged pupils who have visual impairment without learning difficulties are provided for in their local schools. There is a slight tendency for some to move to a special school for the visually impaired at secondary level but still the majority is based locally. Children with additional learning difficulties will often be provided for regionally at a special school with the VI Service visiting to advise, as they would do in a mainstream setting.

Over the last 15 to 20 years, the proportion of children with additional handicaps has increased to about 50% of visually impaired children. The general philosophy of inclusion, which saw VI children as well as those with other impairments, being taught in their local mainstream school is being extended to those with more complex needs. There are examples of schools throughout the world where multiply handicapped children are now finding placements, either full- or part-time in a mainstream setting. The expertise of the special school staff is being 'exported' to these schools and the special schools themselves are being looked upon more as a resource base or a location for short-term teaching placement rather than as a place for segregated learning. Both the receiving school and the multiply handicapped child will benefit from this experience. The included child is supported by experienced and specialist staff in this mainstream placement.

Clinical features

To provide the appropriate support the input of health professionals is needed at an early stage. This would include pre-school groups and reception classes that are able to alert VI teachers to the child and develop a dialogue between health, education and, very importantly, the family. The visual diagnosis and prognosis will assist in planning for appropriate schooling at a later date. Within the concept of 'visual impairment' is a continuum of sensory abilities. The ophthalmologist can provide important information to the VI teacher, such as likely progression or associated neurological deficit. Continuing links between health and education services will allow for the more effective monitoring of provision and progress during the school years. The ophthalmologist should be familiar with the various forms, which must be completed to help the child gain access to the low vision system.

Provision may need to be changed as the pupil moves through the school system and demands increase. The school may not be able to support the child from within its own resources and the LEA or other higher funding organization may need to intervene. A 'Statement of Special Educational Needs' or equivalent may need to be completed.

Braille users traditionally have full-time support from a Learning Support Assistant. It is often more difficult to assess the level of such support for a partially sighted child since their needs vary, not just their visual acuity, but also attitude, independence and stage of schooling.

1. Assessment of vision. VI teachers carry out their own 'Functional Vision Testing' in the school situation to advise on matters such as placement in the classroom; the need for braille or the print size required; safety issues; or alternative provision, for example, in physical education. Multiply handicapped visually impaired (MHVI) children are often difficult to assess.

In some ways the actual diagnosis is of limited importance to the provision of appropriate education. It does not appear to matter whether the malfunction is in the eye, the optic nerve or the brain or what the clinically appraised visual acuity might be. What matters is the level of functioning in the school situation. A visual acuity worked out under clinical conditions is often of little relevance in a school where lighting varies and where visual demands are made from a variety of distances. The visual performance of MHVI children may vary considerably depending on a variety of factors. However, the clinically assessed visual acuity can be valuable as a benchmark against which other tests made by the teacher might be judged. Direct input and information from health colleagues is of vital importance to low vision children. Schools benefit enormously from copies of reports from health colleagues about the children in their schools. Often, these reports reach schools only via the VI Service.

2. Spectacles and low vision aids. The need to wear spectacles, or otherwise, as assessed by the low vision ophthalmologist/optometrist is useful knowledge for VI teachers, schools and the family. Near vision spectacles are increasingly used for brain-damaged children where poor accommodation has been demonstrated. The VI teacher needs to know which set of spectacles to use, what to do if spectacles are refused and how to obtain a spare pair of spectacles.

3. Equipment. Low-tech equipment, such as sloping reading/writing boards are often very popular since they aid access. Similarly, good contrast rulers, lined paper and items such as large display calculators may be as useful. For others, a laptop computer with modified display or speech, or a closed circuit television (CCTV) may be indicated. Monoculars are particularly useful for distance vision such as looking at a blackboard. Unfortunately, in children anything that makes a child stand out may not be used as it is a source of teasing. Neurologically normal children rarely use near aids, preferring to hold the text very close and accommodate. Types of stand magnifiers which rest on the page are possible exceptions.

4. Reading materials. What really matters in the school situation is how the child functions. Advising on type of reading material such as Braille or other methods is not easy. A braillist in mainstream school may be more successfully provided for than some partially sighted large- print readers. Braille books are often more easy to obtain than large-print ones, especially in the top primary and early secondary years.

Reading materials for the partially sighted have to be gauged as to what size print, spacing or font style is required. As a rough guide if the near vision is less than N10, large print may be useful. Similarly, layout of the printed page needs to be varied. This may be a trial and error exercise.

Conclusion

Many questions remain unanswered. For example, who requires mobility training or other life skills: just the braille user or the partially sighted child as well? Who knows best – school or home? What programme of work is thus best suited to the child? One that emphasizes listening skills or touch or one that takes into account that the child might just be seeing something and we need to keep visual stimulation going?

Visual impairment in school is a fascinating and challenging situation. Provision for the child is complex and benefits from a joint approach between education and health working with the concerned families. Combined clinics mean fewer professionals for the families to see. An exchange of reports and information is similarly beneficial. These closer professional working relationships are for the good of the child who is, after all, central to the work that we all do.

Further reading

Chapman EK, Stone JM. *The Visually Impaired Child in Your Classroom*. Cassell Educational Limited, London, UK, 1988.

Mason, HL. *Spotlight on Special Educational Needs: Visual Impairment*. Nasen Enterprises Ltd, 1995.

VISUAL-EVOKED POTENTIAL TESTING IN CHILDREN

Carole M. Panton & Carol A. Westall

The visual-evoked potential (VEP) is a gross electrical response (voltage change) elicited from the visual cortex in response to a changing visual stimulus. These voltage changes vary with time and can be plotted as waveforms. The VEP reflects the central 6–10 degrees of the visual field and is dominated by cone activity.

Problem

Successful VEP recording requires co-operation and attention from the subject. Changes in attention can adversely effect the VEP, particularly when used for acuity assessment. The time taken to record VEPs may be too long to maintain a young child's attention for binocular and then monocular testing. VEPs recorded from children with developmental delay or seizures may reflect abnormalities of the EEG rather than abnormalities of visual acuity. Poor accommodation or nystagmus rather than pathology of the visual pathways may result in poor-quality VEPs. There can be large variations in acuity obtained by VEPs compared with behavioural testing techniques.

Background

The VEP reflects the activity of the visual pathway from the retina to the striate cortex. Abnormalities occurring anywhere in the visual pathway may give abnormal VEPs (e.g. optic nerve disease such as glioma or optic nerve hypoplasia may result in increased latency of the VEP). Retinal disease affecting primarily cone function may also result in abnormal VEPs.

The amplitude of VEP response (1–20 uv) is small compared with the amplitude of the background electroencephalogram (60–100 uv). Signal averaging is required to allow the VEP waveform to emerge from the background EEG activity. An on-line artefact reject capacity is required to exclude unwanted noise from head or eye movements.

For clinical paediatric testing, direct observation of waveforms allows response reliability to be assessed. This is achieved most easily by use of transient stimulus presentation: two or less repetitions per second. The typical transient waveform is complex with negative troughs and positive peaks. Latency is the time measured in milliseconds from the stimulus onset to the peak of the component of interest. Amplitude is the size, measured in microvolts, of a component. Usual amplitude measurement is from a preceding negative trough to the peak of the component of interest. Variability in amplitude is large between subjects but latency is a more reliable measure of VEPs, particularly in children. Differences in amplitude and latency between the eyes are assessed and results compared with normal age-matched control data. Equal vision is associated with responses of similar amplitudes and latencies. In cases of horizontal nystagmus a more accurate acuity assessment can be obtained by using horizontal stripes or pattern onset-offset.

The VEP develops rapidly during the first few months of life, reaching adult levels between 4 and 6 months. The latency of components of the VEP to an alternating stimulus decreases with age. Age-matched data from visually normal children are required for correct interpretation of VEPs.

Testing methods

The attention and cooperation of the child is essential and the presence of two testers is usually required. During electrode placement and testing, speed is essential, as children will lose attention quickly. The child should be tested in a room with minimal distraction from the computer equipment and operator; a separate testing booth is often preferable. The person monitoring a baby (sitting on a parent's lap) is hidden from view so that the visual stimulus is the most compelling thing for the baby to look at. While one observer watches the child at all times during testing to monitor fixation, the other tester operates the computer equipment. A remote control switch is required to ensure that data are collected only when the child is fixating the stimulus. There is degradation of the VEP signal during any period of inattention, so keeping the child involved and amused is of the utmost importance. A young child's interest in the stimulus can be enhanced by talking to the child, jingling keys in front of the screen, having pop-up cartoons on the screen and by singing. Older children are instructed to fixate and focus on the stimulus or cartoons. Simple counting games relating to the stimulus can be used to enhance concentration.

A repetitive flashing light is used to record the flash VEP. A photostimulator most easily delivers the flash (e.g. a Grass photostimulator held 40 cm from the subject). The stimulus for a pattern VEP is usually a checkerboard or stripes. A pattern repeatedly appearing and disappearing, while the mean screen luminance remains constant, provides the stimulus for a pattern onset-offset VEP. A pattern with stripes or checks alternating in contrast provides the stimulus for pattern alternation. For a paediatric population pattern onset-offset is helpful in stabilizing fixation.

Electrode placement for recording VEPs follows the commonly used 10–20 system. Three active electrodes are placed over the occipital cortex. The central electrode OZ is placed on the midline approximately 2 cm above the inion. Active electrodes are placed to the left and right respectively of OZ. A distance of 5% of the head circumference separates them from OZ. Clip electrodes attached to each ear can be used for reference and ground. Before electrode placement the scalp is cleaned and abraded slightly with prepping gel. Gold disc electrodes filled with conductive electrode paste are attached with tape at the desired active electrode positions and secured with a headband such as Coban (3M).

Paediatric protocol

Refraction should be known before VEP assessment and any necessary optical correction worn. Electrode impedance is checked before recording begins and should be under 5 kilohms. The initial stimulus depends on apparent visual behaviour. A medium check size such as 60 minutes of arc is usually chosen. Repeatability should be confirmed for each check size presented (latency of component of interest within 5 milliseconds of preceding trial). Repeatable responses are followed by a decrease in check size. Check size is increased with non-repeatability.

In new cases, binocular recording is attempted first to ensure that a response can be obtained. Monocular recordings, if the child's co-operation allows, are then attempted after one eye has been occluded with a self-adhesive patch. In cases of obvious monocular deficit, monocular testing begins immediately. At least 40 repetitions should be recorded for each stimulus presentation. In cases of monocular severe visual impairment (no response to pattern) a flash stimulus is indicated. To prevent light leakage the better eye is patched with two adhesive patches and a black opaque patch.

Clinical applications

1.   *Visual acuity.* VEPs can also be used to assess visual acuity in a child who is preverbal, developmentally delayed or who has multiple handicaps. An estimate of acuity is obtained by recording VEPs to a series of decreasing check sizes until there are no responses discernible from the background noise. Refractive error should be corrected before acuity assessment. In the presence of optic nerve disorders, acuity results are measured lower with VEPs than with forced choice preferential looking (FCPL). Conversely, in patients with neurological disorders resulting in severe cognitive delays, acuity levels are better using VEPs than FCPL. VEPs are very sensitive to detecting interocular differences and provide an effective way of detecting amblyopia and monitoring occlusion treatment.

2.   *Albinism.* Most children with ocular cutaneous and ocular albinism demonstrate an abnormal decussation of nerve fibres at the optic chiasm. In normal subjects the VEP recorded between the ipsilateral and contralateral cortices are fairly symmetrical with monocular stimulation (50–60% decussation). In albinism (80% decussation) flash VEP asymmetry exists, the pattern of asymmetry reversing between right and left eye testing.

3.   *Cerebral visual impairment.* The VEP is useful to determine the presence of cerebral visual impairment. This should be suspected in a child with poor vision in the presence of a normal eye examination including pupil reflexes and a normal ERG. In cases with no previous neurologic abnormalities (i.e. post-surgery, trauma, hypoxia or infectious disease) VEP responses to flash or pattern can be important prognostic indicators for visual recovery. Poor VEP responses generally predict a poor visual outcome. Care is needed to exclude confounding factors such as poor accommodation and EEG abnormality.

4.   *Delayed visual maturation.* Alternatively, a young baby may present for examination because of failure to fixate or follow due to delayed visual maturation. Examination reveals normal pupillary responses, no structural defect, no nystagmus and a normal-appearing fundus. VEPs can be used to monitor visual development and will show a progressive improvement in latency and amplitude, which is not normally seen in children with cerebral visual impairment.

5.   *Ocular motor apraxia.* Young babies with ocular motor apraxia who are unable to initiate saccades may appear to have a visual impairment. Compensatory head thrusts develop by 6 months of age. Before the development of the head thrusts, the diagnosis can be supported by the presence of normal age appropriate pattern VEP responses.

6. *Functional visual loss.* Lastly, a child may complain of reduced acuity in the absence of any pathology. Normal functioning of the afferent visual pathway can be demonstrated by obtaining VEPs with normal latencies and amplitude to small patterns thus confirming the presence of a normal visual system.

Conclusion

VEPs can provide diagnostic information and assess visual function in a quick, objective and noninvasive manner. Care must be taken that any observed abnormality in the VEP is genuine and not a reflection of poor attention or other testing difficulties.

Further reading

Harding GFA, Odom VJ, Spileers W, Spekreijse H (on behalf of the International Society of Clinical Electrophysiology and Vision). Standard for visual evoked potential. *Vision Research* 1996; **36:** 3567–72.

McCulloch D, Skarf B. Development of the human visual system: monocular and binocular pattern VEP latency. *Investigative Ophthalmology and Visual Science* 1994; **32:** 2372–81.

Sokol S. Visual evoked potential: theory, techniques and clinical applications. *Survey of Ophthalmology* 1976; **21:** 18–44.

Westall CA. Electrophysiological testing. In: Leat SJ, Shute RH, Westall CA (eds). *Assessing Children's Vision: A Handbook.* Oxford, Butterworth-Heinemann, 1999; 311–343.

VISUAL FIELD TESTING

S. Ramanathan, Robert H. Taylor & Peter Shah

Traquair described the visual field as 'an island of vision in a sea of darkness'. This island is subject to differing patterns of erosion by time and various diseases. The aim of visual field testing is to map the topography of this island to aid diagnosis and monitor change. The two areas of ophthalmology in which visual field testing is most essential are glaucoma and neuro-ophthalmology. A thorough understanding of the principles involved in visual field testing will enable clinicians to gain maximum information from their use. Sitting as a test subject at each of the machines described below is strongly recommended, as it gives a unique insight into the difficulties of performing the test and the sources of error.

Problem

The three problems commonly faced with visual field testing are: selection of the most appropriate form of test, dealing with variability in results due to subjective responses, and considering learning curves and other sources of artefact which complicate interpretation of data.

Background

- *Fixation* is the part of the field corresponding to the fovea. The central field lies within 30° of fixation.
- The *arcuate area* (Bjerrum area) is the part of the field arching from the blind spot above and below fixation to end at the horizontal raphe.
- A *stimulus* is a light or target presented to the patient.
- An *isopter* is a threshold line joining points of equal sensitivity on a visual field chart.
- *Visual threshold* is a statistical concept defined as the stimulus value at which the stimulus is seen by the patient 50% of the time. This is measured in decibels (dB), a logarithmic scale.
- *Short-term fluctuation* is the variability in repeated measurements during the same session. *Long-term fluctuation* is the change between different testing sessions.
- *Generalized depression* is a reduction in the sensitivity of the whole visual field. It causes a constriction of the peripheral field and enlargement of scotomas.
- A *scotoma* is an area of the visual field surrounded by an area with greater sensitivity than itself. An *absolute scotoma* is a field defect present despite using the maximal stimulus. A *relative scotoma* is a field defect seen using a weak stimulus but disappearing as the stimulus gets stronger. A *positive scotoma* is characteristic of macular disease and vitreous opacities where the patient notices that an area of the visual field (often central) is missing. A *negative scotoma* is more characteristic of neurological disease, patients are often unaware of these scotomas until they are demonstrated. Patients often notice that objects may appear suddenly in their visual field as they emerge from an area of scotoma.
- *Perimetry* is field testing carried out on a hemispherical surface such as the Goldmann and Humphrey machines. The stimulus is at a constant distance from the

eye. *Campimetry* is field testing where the stimulus moves on a flat surface such as with the Tangent or Bjerrum screen. Campimetry is limited to the central 30° due to the diminishing size of the target as it moves further from fixation.

- In *kinetic perimetry* the stimulus is moved from non-seeing to seeing areas in order to find locations in the field just sensitive to preselected test objects.
- In *static perimetry* the stimulus is stationary but changes its intensity to find the sensitivity of the eye at preselected locations in the visual field.
- *Confrontational field testing* using finger counting is quick, simple and effective in detecting neurological field defects. A hat pin will enable more subtle defects to be mapped. A red hat pin increases the sensitivity for early neurological defects.

Kinetic perimetry

The commonest form of kinetic perimetry in use is the *Goldman perimeter* which can be used in static as well as kinetic modes. It consists of a hemispherical bowl with a central chin rest on which the patient is comfortably positioned. A lens holder allows the patient's near refractive correction to be held without touching the lashes. Fixation is monitored by a telescope incorporating a fixation target. The stimulus is projected onto the inside of the bowl and is moved towards the centre at approximately 2°/sec. The patient is asked to press a button on first seeing the light stimulus and this point is plotted by the perimetrist.

The stimulus can be varied in two ways: (1) by altering the stimulus size, which is indicated by Roman numerals: 0, I is 0.25 mm², II, III is 4 mm², IV and V is 64 mm²; (2) by altering the stimulus intensity by a series of primary filters indicated by Arabic numerals: 1, 2, 3 and 4. Filter 1 reduces the light intensity to 3.15% transmission, filter 2 allows 10% transmission, filter 3 allows 31.5% and filter 4 equals 100% transmission. There is a second set of auxiliary filters which can be used to reduce the light intensity still further: designated a (40% transmission), b (50%), c (60%), d (80%) and e (100% transmission). The auxiliary filters are not used in routine clinical practice and as the 'e' filter does not reduce light intensity it is the one most commonly used. The maximal stimulus is therefore V-4e and the minimal stimulus is 0-1a. In practice the suggested initial stimuli used are **I-4e** and **I-2e**. It is important to check that the stimulus values are kept the same for repeat tests since this affects the size of the field. In performing field for the the driving test, a **III-4e** target is used.

One of the limitations of Goldmann perimetry is that the speed of target movement will affect the size of field. The technique requires a skilled operator to get consistent fields which may otherwise vary with different operators. Though kinetic perimetry has the advantage of rapid comprehensive coverage of the whole visual field with the production of recognizable isopters, static testing is much more accurate at measuring the depth, slope and extent of the defect.

Static perimetry

Manual static perimetry is very time consuming. Computerization of visual field testing has brought static perimetry to the fore, examples being the Humphrey and Octopus field analysers. The more precision that is required the more data that must be collected and the longer the test. There are various strategies available which vary in duration and data collected.

Threshold-related (suprathreshold) tests, such as the Armaly and Humphrey 120 point are quick to perform and are most often used for screening purposes. They work by calculating the threshold either according to age and/or by testing a few pre-defined points. This is used to extrapolate a hill of vision. Then a suprathreshold stimulus (4–6 dB brighter) is presented at predetermined points and recorded as being seen or not seen. These will detect most moderate to severe defects. Unfortunately, they do not document the exact degree to which the field is lost in any particular area and may miss subtle variation in the contour of the scotoma. Hence they have little value in the follow-up of patients with established field loss who should proceed to having a full threshold test. Screening tests have limitations in the detection of early glaucomatous visual field loss.

Threshold tests, in general, take more time, collect more data and are more useful in the follow up of patients with field loss. They work by establishing the threshold for every point tested, thus mapping the actual contour of the hill of vision. Some tests using this principal are the Octopus 32 and Humphrey 24-2 and 30-2. Because of the time constraints due to patient fatigue, testing is limited to the central 24° or 30° of field. Using a bracketing strategy the computer initially increases the stimulus by large steps (4 dB) till the threshold is crossed and the patient is able to see the stimulus. Then it re-crosses the threshold in smaller steps (2 db) to check and refine the threshold measurement. The computer also re-tests points to assess the patient's variability, monitor fixation and calculate false-positive and false-negative rate to give a profile of patient reliability with testing. Though the gold standard for monitoring it can be difficult to learn and thus is not suitable for all patients. The learning curve effect is usually seen in the first few tests and one should interpret initial tests with caution.

The raw data allow statistical analysis to aid clinical judgement. Mean deviation can be calculated by comparing the patient's measurement with age-matched controls. One of the most useful statistical analysis is the pattern standard deviation which highlights focal depressions in the field, which can be masked by the generalized depression in sensitivity that occurs with media opacity, such as cataract.

The challenge has been to devise ways to improve data collection without increasing the test duration. One of the more recent test algorithms to be developed is the *SITA (Swedish interactive threshold algorithm) standard and fast* which take 50% less time to perform. These rely on repeatedly recalculating all the test points during the entire test as patient responses are registered. This allows the likely threshold values to be established more rapidly (i.e. the field machine spends less time working up to the threshold). This allows testing to be carried out more efficiently with fewer stimulus exposures without decreasing the quality of test results.

Short-wavelength automated perimetry (SWAP) also known as blue/yellow perimetry has been suggested to be more sensitive to early glaucomatous damage than 'white on white' standard perimetry. SWAP has been proposed to selectively test for parvocellular retinal ganglion cell loss, although some authorities have questioned the validity of the absolute distinction between the parvocellular and magnocellular systems. SWAP is not routinely used in most clinical settings due to increased total testing time, difficulty of test set-up, higher short-term fluctuation and because data are affected by lens opacity (many elderly patients have both nuclear sclerosis and glaucoma).

Clinical features

The key points to appreciate when using visual field tests to assist in the diagnosis and management of disease states are:

1. In order to get good data one needs to have skilled perimetrists with adequate time to test patients.
2. Each of the two 'gold standards' of visual field testing (Goldmann and Humphrey automated perimetry) will be useful in different clinical situations.

   For example, Goldmann visual field testing is commonly used in neuro-ophthalmic practice and in those patients with glaucoma or retinal dystrophies who cannot produce reliable fields with automated perimetry. In advanced glaucoma Humphrey field analysis may not be useful, whereas a Goldmann field with a peripheral isopter may help management. In some clinical situations (e.g in normal tension glaucoma), it may be advantageous to perform both Humphrey and Goldmann perimetry. Children can usually do reliable Goldmann perimetry at a younger age than Humphrey perimetry.
3. The results of any test must be assessed in the context of the patient and their disease and not studied in isolation.
4. One must be alert to the potential pitfalls inherent in using any clinical test. A thorough understanding of the principles involved in visual field testing will enable clinicians to gain maximum information from their use. Sitting as a test subject at each of the machines described above is strongly recommended, as it gives a unique insight into the difficulties of performing the test and the sources of error.

Summary

Age causes a loss of sensitivity of 0.8 dB per decade concentrated more in the upper field due to neural loss. Changes in refractive status can cause dramatic changes in the field (e.g. over-correction by 1 dioptre will cause a reduction in sensitivity of 3.6 dB). Edge artefact from the trial frame lens is a common cause of dense peripheral field depression. Media opacity, ptotic lids, prominent brows and co-existing retinal disease, such as macular degeneration can all influence the field. It is important to look for these and to compensate for them to avoid misdiagnoses. With serial fields it is important to understand the settings and to make sure the refractive status, background luminance, stimulus size, intensity and exposure times are standardized in order to get data that can be used to assess disease progression. The difficulty of using serial visual fields to detect change and disease progression in glaucoma is an area of active research. Recent sophisticated statistical packages based on linear regression models (e.g. 'Progressor' developed by the Institute of Ophthalmology and Moorfields Eye Hospital) are available to aid in the detection of pointwise change and progression, but are not yet in mainstream clinical practice.

Further reading

American Academy of Ophthalmology Section 10. *Glaucoma* (1994–1995) 46–65.

Bajandas FJ, Kline LB. *Neuro-Ophthalmology Review Manual*, 3rd edn. Thorofare, NJ: Slack, 1988; 1–43.

Bengtsson B, Heijl A. SITA Fast, a new rapid perimetric threshold test. Description of methods and evaluation in patients with manifest and suspect glaucoma. *Acta Ophth Scand* 1998: **76:** 431–7.

Ritch R, Shields NB, Krupin T. *The Glaucomas.* St Louis: CV Mosby Company, 1996.

Related topics of interest

VITRECTOMY

Andy B. Callear

Three-port pars plana vitrectomy, developed during the 1970s, is now universally accepted as an invaluable tool by retinal surgeons. Recent refinements, particularly the development of narrow gauge instruments, have given vitrectomy a place in a wide range of clinical situations.

Problem

Vitrectomy may be a treatment option in a diverse range of conditions. Many of these conditions are complex and surgical outcomes are by no means certain. In some cases, most notably retinal detachment it may not be the only therapeutic option. The patient often plays a large part in the postoperative management. Careful planning and counselling are therefore vital before surgery is undertaken.

Background

An understanding of the benefits of vitrectomy can be gained from examining the mechanical advantages:

- visual axis opacity can be removed from the posterior segment of the eye;
- traction bands within the vitreous cavity can be divided;
- samples of vitreous gel can be obtained;
- volume can be removed from the posterior segment of the eye to facilitate the injection of vitreous substitutes;
- access is provided to the retinal surface and subretinal space for fine manipulations;
- intraocular pressure can be controlled peroperatively with hydrostatic pressure;
- simultaneous cataract surgery can be performed without opening the anterior segment of the eye.

The number of indications is steadily growing. The following disorders account for the bulk of a vitreoretinal surgeon's workload but the list is by no means complete:

- rhegmatogenous retinal detachment (see below);
- traction retinal detachment;
- macular hole (see separate topic);
- non-clearing vitreous haemorrhage;
- retained lens fragments following complicated phakoemulsification cataract surgery;
- epiretinal membrane;
- trauma (penetrating or intraocular foreign body);
- rare conditions such as amyloid, lymphoma, aqueous misdirection, uveal effusion;
- severe ectopia lentis and complete lens dislocation.

Technique

In all vitrectomy procedures a standard approach is adopted:

- pharmacologic dilation of the pupil;
- the conjunctiva is removed at the limbus and three scleral entry sites are fashioned over the pars plana;
- an infusion is plugged into one of the three sclerostomies and connected to a reservoir of saline the height of which can be varied;
- an aspirating vitreous cutter and a light source are manipulated by the surgeon through the other two sclerostomies;
- core vitrectomy is performed;
- instrumentation varies depending on the condition involved. Scissors, forceps and laser may be employed. Air, oil or heavy liquid may be used as tools.;
- substances may be left in the posterior segment to facilitate surgery. They may have a pharmacological role (e.g. antibiotics) or be temporary vitreous substitutes such as gases and silicone oil;
- careful examination of the retina posterior to the entry sites is performed to exclude iatrogenic retinal tears;
- conjunctival closure may be accompanied by antibiotic and steroid injection into the subconjunctival space.

Complications

Complications can be minimized by careful surgical technique:

- Cataract may rarely be caused by lens touch intraoperatively. More commonly it takes the form of accelerated development of nuclear sclerosis following surgery.
- Retinal detachment may occur either due to entry site tears or retinal trauma caused by instrumentation.
- Postoperative haemorrhage usually clears spontaneously but occasionally warrants reoperation.
- Glaucoma may occur by just about any mechanism. Specific entities include ghost cell glaucoma, rubeotic glaucoma and angle-closure glaucoma secondary to choroidal effusion.
- Endophthalmitis is rare.
- Others include corneal decompensation and visual field loss.

Clinical features

There follows a brief description of three of the conditions that can be managed with vitrectomy. These three conditions are topical as there is still debate over some of the details of patient management.

1. Diabetic retinopathy. Vitrectomy is indicated in proliferative diabetic retinopathy if traction retinal detachment threatens the macula or is complicated by rhegmatogenous retinal detachment. Recently the 'Diabetic Vitrectomy Study' has shown clear benefit from early vitrectomy for non-clearing vitreous haemorrhage. This treatment effect is greater in type I diabetics. Vitrectomy may also lead to resolution of intractable macular oedema, especially if the posterior hyaloid face is still attached preoperatively.

Core vitrectomy is followed by separation of the posterior hyaloid face from the retina using sharp dissection. Meticulous attention to haemostasis with endo-diathermy protects against recurrent haemorrhage in the postoperative period. Sufficient laser is performed intraoperatively to control the neovascular process. Whenever possible lens-sparing surgery is performed to reduce the risk of rubeosis iridis.

Identification of pre-existing or iatrogenic retinal holes is essential. Treatment of retinal holes with laser or cryotherapy should be supplemented by scleral buckling and gas or oil injection. This reduces the risk of postoperative retinal detachment, a complication that can be devastating.

2.   *Rhegmatogenous retinal detachment.*   This occurs with an incidence of 1 in 10 000 and is more common in highly myopic eyes. Retinal tears usually form at the time of posterior vitreous detachment, allowing fluid to pass into the subretinal space.

Vitrectomy enables the treatment of retinal detachment in circumstances where conventional surgery may be difficult or inappropriate for example:

- giant retinal tear;
- very posterior tears;
- multiple tears situated on different meridia;
- myopic macular hole;
- proliferative vitreoretinopathy;
- thin sclera.

Some surgeons routinely perform vitrectomy in all aphakic and pseudophakic eyes with retinal detachment. The high magnification afforded enables the characteristi-cally tiny retinal tears to be identified more readily. Subretinal fluid may be drained internally during vitrectomy using a flute needle held directly over the retinal tear whilst air enters the eye under pressure. Alternatively, adjuncts such as heavy liquid or oil may be used to flatten the retina.

3.   *Sub-foveal choroidal neovascularization.*   May be secondary to age-related macular degeneration (ARMD) or, less commonly, other conditions which tend to affect younger adults. The latter group include idiopathic neovascular membranes and those secondary to inflammation, myopia or angioid streaks. These patients can benefit from vitrectomy and direct removal of the membrane via a small retinotomy. The pressure in the eye is maintained artificially high following removal of the membrane for 2 minutes to prevent subretinal haemorrhage. Recurrence of the membrane is not uncommon but may be amenable to repeat surgery. Neovascular membranes secondary to ARMD are associated with a very diseased retinal pigment epithelium (RPE). Hence removal of the membrane is almost invariably accompan-ied by loss of RPE. The results of surgery are often poor in spite of attempts to graft RPE.

Two other approaches to ARMD-related choroidal neovascularization are gaining popularity:

- Relocation of the macula by creation of a retinal fold. The retina is artificially detached at vitrectomy and a gas bubble inserted into the posterior segment of the eye. As the retina reattaches in the postoperative period the patient is slowly turned to create a retinal fold. This has the effect of relocating the macula away from the diseased RPE. Scleral plication or resection can be used to shorten the eye wall thus maximizing the distance the macula moves. The diseased RPE is then treated with laser as if it were an extrafoveal membrane.

- Relocation of the macula by retinal rotation. The retina is artificially detached and a 360-degree retinectomy performed. The retina is then rotated about the optic nerve such that the macular retina moves away from the diseased RPE. The retina is reattached with gas and laser applied to the edge of the retinectomy. Four-muscle squint surgery can be performed later to correct the cyclotorsion created.

Further reading

Benson MT, Callear AB, Tsaloumas M, Chinna J, Beatty S. Surgical excision of subfoveal neovascular membranes. *Eye* 1998; **12:** 768–74.

Eifrig DE, Lochart DL, Berglund RD, Knobloch WH. Pars Plana Vitrectomy. *Ophthalmic Surgery* 1978; **9:** 76–88.

Ratner CM, Michels RG, Aver C, Rice TA. Pars plana vitrectomy for complicated retinal detachment. *Ophthalmology* 1983; **90:** 1323–7.

Scott JD. *Surgery for retinal and vitreous diseases,* 1st edn., London: Butterworth-Heinemann, 1998.

Smiddy WE, Flynn HW Jr. Vitrectomy in the management of diabetic retinopathy. *Survey of Ophthalmology* 1999; **43:** 491–507.

Related topics of interest

WEGENER'S GRANULOMATOSIS: MEDICAL ASPECTS

Clara Day & Caroline O.S. Savage

Wegener's granulomatosis (WG) is an autoimmune disease with multisystem involvement, which was first described by Friedriech Wegener in 1936.

Problem

Aetiology is still uncertain. There is no single defining pathognomonic feature and the spectrum of organ involvement can be wide. Glomerulonephritis is common but not invariable. Diagnosis may be difficult and requires a high incidence of clinical suspicion as there is often a considerable delay from onset of symptoms to diagnosis and commencement of treatment. There is often a normochromic, normocytic anaemia with a leucocytosis. Non-specific markers of inflammation like C-reactive protein (CRP) and (ESR) are usually raised but these are also raised in many other disorders.

Complications can arise as the result of the powerful immunosuppressive treatment, they include opportunistic infection, which can be severe and life threatening, and neoplasms. It is important that Wegener's granulomatosis is diagnosed as early as possible in order that appropriate treatment can be initiated, and permanent organ damage limited.

Background

A recent estimate of incidence was 8.5 per million in a population in eastern England and incidence appears to be rising although this may be due to increased diagnosis. Sufferers are usually Caucasian and there appears to be an equal sex distribution. In some series presentation appears to be seasonal with most patients reporting onset of symptoms in autumn and winter. Pathologically, Wegener's granulomatosis is defined by the Chapel–Hill criteria as being granulomatous inflammation of the respiratory tract with widespread necrotizing vasculitis affecting small and medium vessels.

Although there is some evidence of a genetic predisposition to Wegener's granulomatosis, no consistent HLA association has been found. Recent reports suggest a link with α-1-antitrypsin polymorphisms with an increased frequency of the null 'z' allele amongst patients with vasculitis. Interestingly, α-1-antitrypsin is the natural inhibitor of proteinase 3, a neutrophil serine proteinase and the cANCA antigen. Some investigators have suggested an infectious cause for the disease and the seasonal presentation could concur with this theory. There is some evidence that nasal carriage of staphylococcal species may have a role in disease relapse. Anti-staphylococcal treatment is being trialled currently.

Clinical features

WG tends to present in the fifth decade but can occur at any age. It is rare in childhood and often has an atypical presentation. Patients often present with non-specific flu-like symptoms, myalgia, fever and weight loss before developing respiratory tract symptoms. The disease may progress to involve the kidneys or remain in its limited respiratory form. Long-term damage from disease activity itself includes blindness from retinal vasculitis, deafness from cochlear nerve damage, subglottic stenosis requiring tracheostomy from major airway involvement, pulmonary fibrosis secondary to pulmonary vasculitis and dialysis-dependent renal failure.

- Upper respiratory tract involvement is common occurring in up to 90% of patients.
- Nasal involvement with mucosal inflammation and ulceration can give rise to several symptoms including epistaxis, rhinorhoea, nasal discomfort and crusting. The classic saddle nose deformity is caused by destruction of cartilage.
- Sinus involvement leads to chronic sinusitis and facial pain, which can be mistaken for toothache.
- Ear involvement gives rise to a serous otitis media or a conductive hearing loss secondary to Eustachian tube blockage. Sensorineural hearing loss may also occur with cochlear nerve vasculitis.
- Laryngeal, tracheal and large airway inflammation can produce hoarseness or subglottic stenosis.
- Pulmonary involvement is less common at presentation (40–70%) but occurs in an estimated 85% at some point in the illness. Common features include cough, haemoptysis, pleuritic pain and dyspnoea. A particularly severe manifestation is alveolar haemorrhage caused by small vessel vasculitis.
- Renal disease, occurring in 76% in one meta-analysis, can present as microscopic haematuria, mild proteinuria and/or red cell casts with a normal renal function, impaired renal function that progresses over weeks to months, or rapidly progressive acute renal failure requiring dialysis.

Chest radiographs show pulmonary infiltrates, which may cavitate and hence it may be necessary to exclude tuberculosis or neoplasms. Other systems can also be affected:

- Musculoskeletal; vasculitis can give myalgia and arthralgia although true arthritis is uncommon.
- Ocular involvement; conjunctivitis, episcleritis, scleritis, corneal ulceration, marginal infiltrates, uveitis, retinal vasculitis, optic neuropathy, orbital mass, orbital cellulitis and nasolacrimal duct obstruction have all been described. Despite advances in therapy, significant ocular morbidity can occur (blindness, enucleation, exenteration).
- Nervous system; cerebral vasculitis presents in many ways ranging from behavioural changes to coma depending on the vessels involved. Cerebral granulomatous disease may also occur and pituitary involvement has been reported. Peripheral nerve vasculitis may give rise to an asymmetrical mononeuritis multiplex.
- Skin; splinter haemorrhages, nailbed infarcts, palpable purpura and isolated necrotic lesions can all be caused by a leucocytoclastic vasculitis. Granulomatous inflammation can give rise to isolated skin nodules.

Diagnosis

In the early 1980s antineutrophil cytoplasmic antibodies (ANCA) were detected in the serum of patients with Wegener's granulomatosis and have been of considerable help in aiding diagnosis and monitoring disease. ANCA directed against proteinase 3, when detected by indirect immunofluorescence and ELISA are over 90% sensitive and specific for active Wegener's granulomatosis. There is, however, a small subset of patients who have ANCA directed against myeloperoxidase and a further small group who remain persistently ANCA negative. ANCA levels tend to fall with treatment and rise prior to relapse and are therefore helpful in monitoring disease activity in addition to aiding diagnosis.

Tissue biopsy is necessary for a firm diagnosis. Nasal biopsy is often unhelpful and shows only non-specific inflammation in about 50% of cases. Open lung biopsy produces results far superior to those obtained by the transbronchial route and shows granulomatous inflammation or small vessel vasculitis. Renal biopsy, in the presence of an active urinary sediment or renal impairment, shows a focal, segmental, necrotizing glomerulonephritis, which can extend to diffuse involvement with crescents in severe disease. This glomerulonephritis is pauci-immune. Focal sclerosis may also be present if scarring of previously active disease has already occurred.

Treatment and prognosis

Prognosis improved somewhat with the introduction of corticosteroid treatment but the major breakthrough came in the 1970s with the use of oral cyclophosphamide. Standard treatment consists of high-dose oral corticosteroids with cyclophosphamide to induce remission. After a variable time, the doses are reduced and eventually stopped giving a 5-year survival of 70–80%. Until recently the maintenance phase was for at least 1 year after achievement of remission and therefore drug side effects were considerable. These include haemorrhagic cystitis (up to 40% in some series), bladder cancer, gonadal toxicity, other neoplasms and opportunistic infection. Recent research has focused on less toxic drugs for remission induction and maintenance therapy, which is necessary in a disease where 50% of patients have been shown to relapse on long-term follow-up. Various treatments to induce remission have been tested including pulsed intravenous cyclophosphamide (giving a lower total dose than with oral treatment), methotrexate, intravenous immunoglobulin, anti-tumour necrosis factor (TNF) therapy, anti-thymocyte globulin and monoclonal antibodies directed against T-cells, azathioprine, mycophenolate mofetil, co-trimoxazole have been investigated as maintenance therapies. Initial small-scale trials have been promising, but results from multicentred, randomized, controlled trials are awaited.

Poor prognostic features include dialysis dependency at presentation or alveolar haemorrhage. In these cases adjunctive therapy including high-dose intravenous corticosteroids or plasma exchange/immunoabsorption have been shown to be helpful. These treatments are also currently being subjected to large-scale trials. Older patients also tend to be in a poor prognostic category but this can be helped somewhat with specific tailoring of immunosuppressive regimes.

Further reading

Cockwell P, Savage COS. Pathogenesis of Wegener's granulomatosis. In: *Inflammatory Disease of Blood Vessels.* GS Hoffman, CM Weyand (ed.). Marcel Dekker, Inc., New York, 1999.

Hewins P, Cohen Tervaert JW, Savage COS, Kallenberg CGM. Is Wegener's granulomatosis an autoimmune disease? *Current Opinion in Rheumatism* 1999; **912:** 3–10.

Jennette JC, Falk RJ. Small vessel vasculitis. *New England Journal of Medicine* 1997: **337:** 1512–23.

Kallenberg CGM, Brouwer E, Weening JJ, Cohen Tervaert JW. Anti-neutrophil cytoplasmic antibodies: Current diagnostic and pathophysiological potential. *Kidney International* 1994; **46:** 1–15.

Savage COS, Harper L, Adu D. Primary systemic vasculitis. *Lancet* 1997; **349:** 553–8.

INDEX

Polyarteritis nodosa, 76, 209, 217, 235
Polycarbonate, 251
Polyhexamethylene biguanide (PHMB), 3
Polymyalgia rheumatica, 311
Polymyositis pernicious anaemia, 169
Porencephalic cyst, 213
Porphyria cutanea tarda, 56, 57
Port wine stain (PWS), 83
Posterior
  capsular opacification, 35
  embryotoxon, 177
  polymorphous dystrophy, 76
  uveitis, 235
Post-infectious optic neuritis, 214
Postocclusion surge, 227
Povidone iodine 5%, 240
Power pulse, 227
Practolol, 57
Prader – Willi, 9
Preseptal cellulitis, 84
Pretibial myxoedema, 87, 310
Primary biliary cirrhosis, 86
Primary proliferative endotheliopathy, 146
Prism adaption trial, 116
Progressive oculomotor apraxia, 232
Progressive outer retinal necrosis, 128, 235
Proliferative diabetic retinopathy, 102
Proliferative vitreoretinopathy, 273
Propionibacterium acnes, 241
Proptosis, 28, 84, 181, 223, 315, 316
Protanomaly, 61
Protanopia, 61
Protease inhibitors, 129
Protein kinase C inhibitors, 103
Proximal, 113
Pseudo-hole, 154
Pseudohypoparathyroidism, 49
Pseudomembranous conjunctivitis, 56
Pseudomonas aeruginosa, 157
Pseudoxanthoma elasticum, 88, 249
Pterygium, 77
Ptosis, 134, 168
Pubic lice, 42
Punctate inner choroiditis, 235
Pupil block, 172
Pursuit movement, 143
Purtscher retinopathy, 22, 285
Pyridostigmine, 170

Quinine, 320

Quinolones, 239

Radial keratotomy, 253
Radial perineuritis, 2
Radioactive iodine, 313, 317
Radiotherapy, 335
Raeder's syndrome, 162
Raised intracranial pressure, 289
Raynaud phenomenon, 187
Rebleeding, 24
Refib, 220
Refraction, 47
Refractive surgery, 253
Refsum disease, 183, 184, 265
Reis – Bücklers dystrophy, 75
Reiter syndrome, 148
Rejection, 73
Relative afferent pupil defect (RAPD), 260
Renal calculi, 301
Renal cell carcinomas, 232
Rete, 295
Retinal
  astrocytic hamartoma, 230
  correspondence, 46
  detachment, 5, 25, 39, 51, 88, 154, 173, 265, 271,
    283
  dysplasia, 69
  dystrophies, 256
  fat embolization, 22
  haemorrhages, 285
  neovascularization, 259
  periphlebitis, 278
  pigment epithelitis, 235
  telangiectasia, 79
  vasculitis, 79, 86, 235
  vein occlusion, 79
Retinitis pigmentosa, 66, 79, 81, 110, 182, 210, 249,
  265
Retinitis punctata albescens, 182, 183, 266
Retinitis, 235
Retinoblastoma, 47, 206
Retinochoroidal coloboma, 69
Retinoic acid, 14
Retinopathy of prematurity, 48, 69, 284
Retinoschisis, 183, 273
Rhabdomyosarcoma, 180
Rhegmatogenous retinal detachment, 154, 353
Rhese view, 23
Rheumatoid arthritis, 75, 169, 281
Rieger's anomaly, 178